Update of Dental Local Anesthesia

Guest Editors

PAUL A. MOORE, DMD, PhD, MPH
ELLIOT V. HERSH, DMD, MS, PhD
SEAN G. BOYNES, DMD, MS

DENTAL CLINICS OF NORTH AMERICA

www.dental.theclinics.com

October 2010 • Volume 54 • Number 4

SAUNDERS an imprint of ELSEVIER, Inc.

W.B. SAUNDERS COMPANY
A Division of Elsevier Inc.

1600 John F. Kennedy Boulevard ● Suite 1800 ● Philadelphia, Pennsylvania 19103-2899

http://www.dental.theclinics.com

DENTAL CLINICS OF NORTH AMERICA Volume 54, Number 4
October 2010 ISSN 0011-8532, ISBN-978-1-4377-2441-7

Editor: John Vassallo; j.vassallo@elsevier.com
Developmental Editor: Donald Mumford

Dental Clinics of North America (ISSN 0011-8532) is published quarterly by Elsevier Inc., 360 Park Avenue South, New York, NY 10010-1710. Months of issue are January, April, July, and October. Business and Editorial Offices: 1600 John F. Kennedy Boulevard, Suite 1800, Philadelphia, PA 19103-2899. Periodicals postage paid at New York, NY and additional mailing offices. Subscription prices are $240.00 per year (domestic individuals), $420.00 per year (domestic institutions), $113.00 per year (domestic students/residents), $287.00 per year (Canadian individuals), $529.00 per year (Canadian institutions), $347.00 per year (international individuals), $529.00 per year (international institutions), and $170.00 per year (international and Canadian students/residents). International air speed delivery is included in all *Clinics* subscription prices. All prices are subject to change without notice. **POSTMASTER:** Send address changes to *Dental Clinics of North America*, Elsevier Health Sciences Division, Subscription Customer Service, 3251 Riverport Lane, Maryland Heights, MO 63043. **Customer Service (orders, claims, online, change of address): Elsevier Health Sciences Division, Subscription Customer Service, 3251 Riverport Lane, Maryland Heights, MO 63043. Tel: 1-800-654-2452 (U.S. and Canada). Fax: 314-447-8029. E-mail: journalscustomerservice-usa@elsevier.com (for print support); journalsonlinesupport-usa@elsevier.com (for online support).**

Reprints. For copies of 100 or more, of articles in this publication, please contact the Commercial Reprints Department, Elsevier Inc., 360 Park Avenue South, New York, NY 10010-1710. Tel.: 212-633-3812; Fax: 212-462-1935; E-mail: reprints@elsevier.com.

The *Dental Clinics of North America* is covered in *MEDLINE/PubMed (Index Medicus), Current Contents/Clinical Medicine, ISI/BIOMED* and *Clinahl*.

Printed in the United States of America.

Contributors

GUEST EDITORS

PAUL A. MOORE, DMD, PhD, MPH
Professor of Pharmacology and Dental Public Health; Chair, Department of Dental Anesthesiology, University of Pittsburgh School of Dental Medicine; Adjunct Professor of Pharmacology, University of Pittsburgh School of Pharmacy; Adjunct Professor of Epidemiology, University of Pittsburgh Graduate School of Public Health, Pittsburgh, Pennsylvania

ELLIOT V. HERSH, DMD, MS, PhD
Professor of Pharmacology, Department of Oral Surgery and Pharmacology, University of Pennsylvania School of Dental Medicine; Chair, Institutional Review Board #3, Office of Regulatory Affairs, University of Pennsylvania, Philadelphia, Pennsylvania

SEAN G. BOYNES, DMD, MS
Director, Anesthesia Research, Department of Dental Anesthesiology, University of Pittsburgh School of Dental Medicine, Pittsburgh, Pennsylvania

AUTHORS

MOHAMMAD ABDULWAHAB, DMD, MPH
Clinical Assistant Professor, Department of Anesthesiology, University of Pittsburgh School of Dental Medicine, Pittsburgh, Pennsylvania

SEAN G. BOYNES, DMD, MS
Director, Anesthesia Research, Department of Dental Anesthesiology, University of Pittsburgh School of Dental Medicine, Pittsburgh, Pennsylvania

DAVID CARSTEN, DDS
Resident, Dental Anesthesiology Residency, Lutheran Medical Center, Brooklyn, New York

TAYLOR M. CLARK, DDS
Chief Resident, Dental Anesthesiology Residency Program, School of Dentistry, University of California, Los Angeles, Los Angeles, California

MICHAEL A. CUDDY, DMD
Assistant Professor, Department of Anesthesiology, University of Pittsburgh School of Dental Medicine, Pittsburgh, Pennsylvania

RAYMOND A. DIONNE, DDS, PhD
Scientific Director, National Institute of Nursing Research, National Institutes of Health, Rockville, Maryland

ZYDNIA ECHEVERRIA, DMD
Resident, Department of Anesthesiology, University of Pittsburgh Graduate Dental Anesthesiology Program, University of Pittsburgh, School of Dental Medicine, Pittsburgh, Pennsylvania

EDGAR P. FAYANS, DDS
Director, Dental Anesthesiology Residency, Lutheran Medical Center, Brooklyn, New York

STEVEN GANZBERG, DMD, MS
Professor of Clinical Anesthesiology, Section of Anesthesiology, College of Dentistry, College of Medicine and Public Health; Dental/Maxillofacial Anesthesiology Residency Program Director, The Ohio State University, Columbus, Ohio

HELEN GIANNAKOPOULOS, DDS, MD
Assistant Professor of Oral and Maxillofacial Surgery, Department of Oral Surgery and Pharmacology, University of Pennsylvania School of Dental Medicine, Philadelphia, Pennsylvania

JOSEPH A. GIOVANNITTI Jr, DMD
Associate Professor, Department of Anesthesiology, University of Pittsburgh School of Dental Medicine, Pittsburgh, Pennsylvania

SHARON M. GORDON, DDS, MPH, PhD
Associate Professor, Department of Oral-Maxillofacial Surgery, Baltimore College of Dental Surgery, Dental School, University of Maryland, Baltimore, Maryland

DANIEL A. HAAS, DDS, PhD
Associate Dean, Clinical Sciences; Professor and Head of Dental Anesthesia, Chapman Chair in Clinical Sciences, Faculty of Dentistry; Professor, Department of Pharmacology, Faculty of Medicine, University of Toronto; Active Staff, Sunnybrook Health Sciences Centre, Ontario, Canada

ELLIOT V. HERSH, DMD, MS, PhD
Professor of Pharmacology, Department of Oral Surgery and Pharmacology, University of Pennsylvania School of Dental Medicine; Chair, Institutional Review Board #3, Office of Regulatory Affairs, University of Pennsylvania, Philadelphia, Pennsylvania

HANNA KIM, DDS
Resident, Dental Anesthesiology Residency, Lutheran Medical Center, Brooklyn, New York

KYLE J. KRAMER, DDS
Chief Resident, Section of Anesthesiology, College of Dentistry, College of Medicine and Public Health; Dental/Maxillofacial Anesthesiology Residency Program, The Ohio State University, Columbus, Ohio

ROCHELLE G. LINDEMEYER, DMD
Assistant Professor of Pediatric Dentistry, Director of the Pediatric Dental Graduate Program, Department of Preventive and Restorative Sciences, University of Pennsylvania School of Dental Medicine, Philadelphia, Pennsylvania

QUEN LY, DDS, DMD
Resident, Dental Anesthesiology Residency, Lutheran Medical Center, Brooklyn, New York

STANLEY F. MALAMED, DDS
Dentist Anesthesiologist, Professor of Anesthesia & Medicine, The Herman Ostrow School of Dentistry of USC, Los Angeles, California

JOHN G. MEECHAN, BDS, PhD, FDSRCS, FDSRCPS
Senior Lecturer in Oral Surgery, School of Dental Sciences, Newcastle University, Newcastle Upon Tyne, United Kingdom

ANASTASIA V. MISCHENKO, DDS, MS
Clinical Faculty, Department of Endodontics, Prosthodontics, and Operative Dentistry, Baltimore College of Dental Surgery, Dental School, University of Maryland, Baltimore, Maryland

PAUL A. MOORE, DMD, PhD, MPH
Professor of Pharmacology and Dental Public Health; Chair, Department of Dental Anesthesiology, University of Pittsburgh School of Dental Medicine; Adjunct Professor of Pharmacology, University of Pittsburgh School of Pharmacy; Adjunct Professor of Epidemiology, University of Pittsburgh Graduate School of Public Health, Pittsburgh, Pennsylvania

KELLIE PAXTON, DMD, MS
Private Endodontic Practice, Executive Endodontics of Weston, Weston, Florida

ROBERT M. PESKIN, DDS
Clinical Associate Professor, Department of Hospital Dentistry and Dental Anesthesiology, School of Dental Medicine, Stony Brook University, Stony Brook, New York

SUSAN POORSATTAR, DDS
Resident, Pediatric Dentistry, San Francisco, California

KENNETH REED, DMD
Dentist Anesthesiologist, Clinical Assistant Professor of Anesthesia & Medicine, The Herman Ostrow School of Dentistry of USC, Los Angeles, California

CHESTER J. SOKOLOWSKI, DDS
Postdoctoral Fellow in Anesthesiology, Department of Anesthesiology, University of Pittsburgh School of Dental Medicine, Pittsburgh, Pennsylvania

STEVEN J. SPECA, DMD
Post-Doctoral Fellow, Department of Anesthesiology, University of Pittsburgh School of Dental Medicine, Pittsburgh, Pennsylvania

HUNTER R. STUART, DDS, MS
Chief Resident, Dental Anesthesiology Residency, Lutheran Medical Center, Brooklyn, New York

DAVID E. THOME, DDS
Private Pediatric Dental Practice, Westside Orthodontics and Pediatric Dentistry, Miramar, Florida

LARRY TRAPP, DDS, MS
Associate Professor, Department of Dental Anesthesiology, Loma Linda University School of Dentistry, Loma Linda, California

JOHN WILL, DDS
Loma Linda University School of Dentistry, Loma Linda, California; Private Practice of Dental Anesthesiology, Leoma, Tennessee

JOHN A. YAGIELA, DDS, PhD
Director, Dental Anesthesiology Residency Program; Professor and Chair, Division of Diagnostic and Surgical Sciences, School of Dentistry, University of California, Los Angeles, Los Angeles, California

JAYME ZOVKO, RDH, BS
Faculty Research Associate, Department of Anesthesiology, University of Pittsburgh School of Dental Medicine, Pittsburgh, Pennsylvania

Contents

The development of safe and effective local anesthetic agents has possibly been the most important advancement in dental science to occur in the last century. The agents currently available in dentistry are extremely safe and fulfill most of the characteristics of an ideal local anesthetic. These local anesthetic agents can be administered with minimal tissue irritation and with little likelihood of inducing allergic reactions. A variety of agents are available that provide rapid onset and adequate duration of surgical anesthesia. This introductory article provides a brief update of the clinical pharmacology of local anesthetic agents and formulations used in dentistry at present.

Local anesthetics are commonly used in both dentistry and medicine. These drugs are also used in some office-based medical practices. Except for minor procedures, most physicians who require complicated nerve blocks rely on anesthesiologists to administer the local anesthesia. Both ester and amide local anesthetics are routinely used in medical practice. This article reviews the types and uses of local anesthesia in anesthesiology.

Although the use of long-acting local anesthetics has become a useful therapeutic approach for managing peri- and postoperative pain, recent evidence reveals unexpected outcomes. This article reviews the clinical use of long-acting local anesthetics, presents current clinical research findings, and makes recommendations for their use.

Infiltration is preferred to regional block techniques in the maxilla as the former offers a number of advantages. This paper considers the evidence for the efficacy of infiltration anesthesia in the mandible in the adult dentition, both as a primary and as a supplemental method.

Phentolamine mesylate, at dosages from 0.4 to 0.8 mg in adults and adolescents and at dosages from 0.2 to 0.4 mg in children aged 4 to 11 years, has been proven to be safe and effective for the reversal of soft tissue anesthesia (lip and tongue numbness) and the associated functional deficits resulting from a local dental anesthetic injection containing a vasoconstrictor. Its ability to block a-adrenergic receptors on blood vessels induces vasodilation and enhances the redistribution of the local anesthetic away from the injection site. The low dosages administered for dental local anesthetic reversal in all likelihood accounts for the lack of significant cardiovascular effects that are associated with the medical use of the drug for hypertensive conditions associated with catecholamine excess.

In 2000, the US Food and Drug Administration (FDA) approved the use of 4% articaine with epinephrine 1:100,000, and with epinephrine 1:200,000 in 2006. Articaine has been commonly compared with its predecessor, lidocaine hydrochloride. Since its introduction in 1948, lidocaine has maintained a status as the most widely used local dental anesthetic in most countries. Proven efficacy with low allergenicity and toxicity over long-term clinical use and research have confirmed the value and safety of this drug. Thus, it became the gold standard to which all new local anesthetics are compared. Despite the gold standard status of lidocaine, numerous reports and editorials have supported and recognized the use of articaine.

True allergic reactions to local anesthetics are rare adverse reactions. At the most, they represent less than 1% of all adverse local anesthetic reactions. When true allergic reactions have been confirmed, the reactions are most commonly the type I anaphylactic and type IV delayed hypersensitivity responses. The type I immediate hypersensitivity reactions are the most severe and may be life-threatening. In the event a potential allergic reaction occurs in a dental office, the dentist needs to properly evaluate the events leading up to the reaction and provide a differential diagnosis. A referral should be given to any patient when an allergic reaction cannot be ruled out as an intravascular injection, toxic overdose, psychogenic reaction, or an idiosyncratic event.

Dentistry has two medications in its pain management armamentarium that may cause the potentially life-threatening disorder methemoglobinemia. The first medications are the topical local anesthetics benzocaine and prilocaine. The second medication is the injectable local anesthetic prilocaine. Acquired methemoglobinemia remains a source of morbidity and mortality in dental and medical patients despite the fact that it is better understood now than it was even a decade ago. It is in the interest of all dental patients that their treating dentists review this disorder. The safety of dental patients mandates professional awareness.

The most widely used method for controlling pain during dental procedures is the intraoral administration of local anesthetics in close proximity to a specific nerve or fiber to obtund nerve conduction. The most commonly anesthetized nerves in dentistry are branches or nerve trunks associated with the maxillary and mandibular divisions of the trigeminal nerve (cranial nerve V). However, other nerves may be inadvertently affected by intraoral local anesthesia injections, resulting in anesthetic complications of structures far from the oral cavity. Practitioners should be aware of potential ocular complications following intraoral injections in dentistry. These complications include oculomotor paralysis and vision loss. The knowledge of these conditions and their potential cause should alert the dentist to the importance of appropriate injection techniques and an understanding of management protocol.

A clinically significant interaction between epinephrine or levonordefrin with nonselective beta-adrenergic blocking agents, although apparently rare in the dental setting, is potentially serious and can lead to significant hypertension with a concomitant reflex bradycardia. Based on the results of epinephrine infusion studies, the severity of the interaction seems dose related; small epinephrine doses cause less of a pressor response than larger doses. The interaction can be seen after intraoral submucosal injections but is generally of a smaller magnitude, at least with only 1 or 2 cartridges of lidocaine plus 1:100,000 epinephrine. However as demonstrated by 1 case report, some individuals are hypersensitive to this interaction. Inadvertent intravascular injections of local anesthetic plus vasoconstrictor and the use of high doses of vasoconstrictor are likely to result in a more pronounced response. Patients with significant cardiovascular disease may be especially vulnerable to the most serious sequelae resulting from the pressor reactions of the drug combination.

The use of systemically absorbed drugs in the gravid and in the lactating patient is of concern to the dentist. This article reviews concerns for the health and safety of the mother, developing fetus, and neonate involving local anesthetics. The available literature on the use of local anesthetics for dentistry in the pregnant and postpartum patient is also reviewed. In addition, the physiology of the pregnant and postpartum woman is discussed because this is essential to understanding potential interplay with local anesthesia and the stress of a dental appointment.

Paul A. Moore and Daniel A. Haas

Alterations to normal oral sensory function can occur following restorative and surgical dental procedures. Paresthesia is defined as an abnormal sensation, such as burning, pricking, tickling, or tingling. Paresthesias are one of the more general groupings of nerve disorders known as neuropathies. This article reviews the extent of this oral complication as it relates to dental and surgical procedures, with specific emphasis on paresthesias associated with local anesthesia administration. This review establishes a working definition for paresthesia as it relates to surgical trauma and local anesthesia administration, describes the potential causes for paresthesia in dentistry, assesses the incidence of paresthesias associated with surgery and local anesthesia administration, addresses the strengths and weaknesses in research findings, and presents recommendations for the use of local anesthetics in clinical practice.

Chester J. Sokolowski, Joseph A. Giovannitti Jr, and Sean G. Boynes

Needle phobia has profound health, dental, societal, and legal implications, and severe psychological, social, and physiologic consequences. There is genetic evidence for the physiologic response to needle puncture, and a significant familial psychological component, showing evidence of inheritance. Needle phobia is also a learned behavior. The dental practitioner must recognize patients with needle phobia before the administration of local anesthetics to identify patients who are potentially reactive and to prevent untoward sequelae. Needle phobia is highly associated with avoidance behavior, and the dentist must exhibit compassion and respect. To avoid bradycardia, hypotension, unconsciousness, convulsions, and possibly asystole, oral premedication with benzodiazepines or other antianxiety agents must be considered for patients who are needle phobic. Management of needle phobiaeinduced syncope includes perioperative monitoring, oxygen administration, positioning, atropine, and vasopressors.

Stanley F. Malamed, Kenneth Reed, and Susan Poorsattar

Since the introduction of nonreusable, stainless steel dental local anesthetic needles, needle breakage has become an extremely rare complication of dental local anesthetic injections. But although rare, dental needle breakage can, and does, occur. Review of the literature and personal experience brings into focus several commonalities which, when avoided, can minimize the risk of needle breakage with the fragment being retained from occurring.

Computer-controlled local anesthetic delivery (C-CLAD) devices and systems for intraosseous (IO) injection are important additions to the dental anesthesia armamentarium. C-CLAD using slow infusion rates can significantly reduce the discomfort of local anesthetic infusion, especially in palatal tissues, and facilitate palatal approaches to pulpal nerve block that find special use in cosmetic dentistry, periodontal therapy, and pediatric dentistry. Anesthesia of single teeth can be obtained using either C-CLAD intraligamentary injections or IO injections. Supplementary IO anesthesia is particularly suited for providing effective pain control of teeth diagnosed with irreversible pulpitis.

Within the last 30 years, the role of dental hygienists has expanded to include the administration of local anesthesia. Several studies have been performed to assess practice characteristics and effectiveness of these changes in state licensure regulations. Findings indicate an acceptance of this expansion in dental hygiene practice; however, the delegation of this pain control procedures remains controversial. To address this controversy, the authors have reviewed of current literature to assess the practice of local anesthesia administration by dental hygienists.

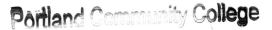

THE CLINICS ARE NOW AVAILABLE ONLINE!

Access your subscription at:
www.theclinics.com

Preface

Update of Dental Local Anesthesia

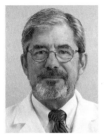
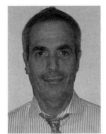
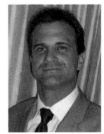

Paul A. Moore, DMD, PhD, MPH   Elliot V. Hersh, DMD, MS, PhD   Sean G. Boynes, DMD, MS

Guest Editors

Possibly the most important skill required of all dental practitioners is the ability to provide safe and effective local anesthesia. The agents and anesthetic delivery equipment available today provide the practitioner an array of options to effectively manage the pain associated with dental procedures. We have come a long way from the time when the numbing properties of cocaine were first recognized; to its topical application for ophthalmologic surgery; to the introduction of needles and syringes to permit nerve block anesthesia; to the synthesis of procaine and ester anesthetics; and to the development of the amide anesthetics used today.

This issue of *Dental Clinics of North America* focuses on the most recent developments in dental local anesthesia. As an introduction, a brief description of the pharmacology and toxicology of therapeutic agents currently available in dentistry is presented, followed by an update of agents used in medicine. Recent research findings associated with the use of the long-acting local anesthetic bupivacaine are then provided. A review of the efficacy and potential indications for mandibular infiltration anesthesia to supplement nerve blocks follows. The clinical research findings for the novel application of phentolamine to reverse soft tissue anesthesia are provided as well as the results of a meta-analyses assessing the efficacy of articaine formulations. Advances in armamentarium used for dental anesthesia are updated as well.

The current knowledge regarding rare complications is also critically reviewed. Topics specifically addressed include allergic reactions, unusual ocular complications, methemoglobinemia, paresthesias, drug interactions with beta-antagonists, and needle breakage. Recommendations for safe use of local anesthetics for pregnant and lactating patients are then provided. The basis for patient fears of needles, a significant cause of psychogenic reactions, is additionally reviewed. Finally, regulations established for the administration of local anesthesia by dental hygienists are described and the safety record supporting this widening scope of practice is presented.

Dent Clin N Am 54 (2010) xiii–xiv
doi:10.1016/j.cden.2010.07.001
0011-8532/10/$ – see front matter © 2010 Elsevier Inc. All rights reserved.

As the editors of this issue, we are grateful for the support of the authors, and their willingness to prepare the articles. They represent the leaders in the field of pharmacology and local anesthesia in dentistry. Several are authors of popular textbooks. A few have established productive research careers. Many are program directors for graduate programs in dental anesthesiology. All are teachers, dedicated to the safe and effective use of local anesthesia by general dentists, dental specialists, and dental hygienists.

Many of the articles in this issue have been authored or coauthored by students enrolled in graduate programs and anesthesiology residencies. These CODA-approved programs are educating the future leaders in dental anesthesia. It will be through their vision of the future and their innovative efforts that safer and more effective methods for pain control will be developed. In 10 or 20 years, we hope that their discoveries will be described in a follow-up "Update of Dental Local Anesthesia" issue of *Dental Clinics of North America*. One could imagine articles entitled "Effective Alternatives to Nerve Block Anesthesia;" "Pulpal Anesthesia Using Novel Topical Anesthetics;" "Latex and Antioxidant-Free Local Anesthetic Cartridges;" or "Local Anesthetic Agents Selective for Nociception."

We look forward to reading them.

Paul A. Moore, DMD, PhD, MPH
Department of Dental Anesthesiology
University of Pittsburgh
School of Dental Medicine
623 Salk
3501 Terrace Street
Pittsburgh, PA 15261, USA

Elliot V. Hersh, DMD, MS, PhD
Department of Oral Surgery and Pharmacology
University of Pennsylvania
School of Dental Medicine
240 South 40th Street
Philadelphia, PA 19104-6030, USA

Sean G. Boynes, DMD, MS
Department of Dental Anesthesiology
University of Pittsburgh
School of Dental Medicine
622A Salk
3501 Terrace Street
Pittsburgh, PA 15261, USA

E-mail addresses:
pam7@pitt.edu (P.A. Moore)
evhersh@pobox.upenn.edu (E.V. Hersh)
sgb10@gmx.com (S.G. Boynes)

Local Anesthetics: Pharmacology and Toxicity

Paul A. Moore, DMD, PhD, MPH[a,b,c,*], Elliot V. Hersh, DMD, MS, PhD[d,e]

KEYWORDS

• Local anesthetics • Pharmacology • Toxicity reaction • MRD

The development of safe and effective local anesthetic agents has been possibly the most important advancement in dental science to occur in the last century. The agents currently available in dentistry are extremely safe and fulfill most of the characteristics of an ideal local anesthetic (**Box 1**). These local anesthetic agents can be administered with minimal tissue irritation and with little likelihood of inducing allergic reactions. A variety of agents are available that provide rapid onset and adequate duration of surgical anesthesia. The agents provide anesthesia that is completely reversible, and systemic toxicity is rarely reported. An ideal local anesthetic agent, one that would induce regional analgesia by selectively inhibiting pain pathways without interrupting transmission of other sensory modalities, has not yet been discovered.

This issue of *Dental Clinics of North America* updates the advancements in local anesthesia therapeutics currently available in dentistry and provides an insight into a wide range of concerns related to the agents used for local anesthesia. This introductory article provides a brief update of the clinical pharmacology of local anesthetic agents and formulations used in dentistry at present. Following this update, a review of the dosing strategies needed to prevent local anesthetic toxicity reactions is presented.

CLINICAL PHARMACOLOGY OF LOCAL ANESTHETICS

For the last 20 years, amides are predominantly used in dentistry as local anesthetic agents. Lidocaine and mepivacaine, 2 of the most commonly used amide local

[a] Department of Dental Anesthesiology, University of Pittsburgh School of Dental Medicine, Pittsburgh, PA 15261, USA
[b] University of Pittsburgh School of Pharmacy, Pittsburgh, PA 15261, USA
[c] University of Pittsburgh Graduate School of Public Health, Pittsburgh, PA 15261, USA
[d] Department of Oral Surgery and Pharmacology, University of Pennsylvania School of Dental Medicine, 240 South 40th Street, Philadelphia, PA 19104-6030, USA
[e] Office of Regulatory Affairs, University of Pennsylvania, 240 South 40th Street, Philadelphia, PA 19104-6030, USA
* Corresponding author. Department of Dental Anesthesiology, University of Pittsburgh School of Dental Medicine, Pittsburgh, PA 15261.
E-mail address: pam7@pitt.edu

Dent Clin N Am 54 (2010) 587–599
doi:10.1016/j.cden.2010.06.015
0011-8532/10/$ – see front matter © 2010 Elsevier Inc. All rights reserved.

dental.theclinics.com

> **Box 1**
> **Characteristics of an ideal local anesthetic**
>
> 1. Administration of the agent is nonirritating
> 2. The anesthetic has little or no allergenicity
> 3. A rapid onset and adequate duration of anesthesia
> 4. Anesthesia is completely reversible
> 5. Minimal systemic toxicity
> 6. Anesthesia is selective to nociception (pain) pathways

anesthetic agents in dentistry, have a 50-year history of effectiveness and safety in providing regional anesthesia for dental therapies. Practitioners prefer the amide local anesthetic agents to the ester agents (ie, procaine and propoxycaine) because amides produce profound surgical anesthesia more rapidly and reliably, with fewer sensitizing reactions than ester anesthetics. The availability of various dental formulations of amide agents (**Table 1**) that provide anesthesia of varying duration has dramatically improved patient care, permitting the development of many of the sophisticated surgical outpatient procedures that are now available in dentistry.[1]

Variations in the clinical characteristics of the local anesthetic agents can be attributed to differences in chemical properties of their molecular structures. An anesthetic's dissociation constant (pKa) determines the pH at which the drug's ionized (charged) and nonionized (uncharged) forms are in equal concentrations. This value is critical for effective anesthesia because the uncharged form of a local anesthetic molecule is essential to permit diffusion across lipid nerve sheaths and cell membranes.

Table 1
Local anesthetic formulations

Anesthetic Agent	Brand Names	Formulations Available in Dental Cartridges	Duration of Anesthesia
Articaine	Ultracaine, Septocaine, Articadent, Zorcaine	4% Articaine, 1:100,000 epinephrine	Medium
		4% Articaine, 1:200,000 epinephrine	Medium
Bupivacaine	Marcaine, Vivacaine	0.5% Bupivacaine, 1:200,000 epinephrine	Long
Lidocaine	Xylocaine, Octocaine, Lignospan, Alphacaine	2% Lidocaine, 1:100,000 epinephrine	Medium
		2% Lidocaine, 1:50,000 epinephrine	Medium
		2% Lidocaine plain	Ultrashort
Mepivacaine	Carbocaine, Polocaine, Scandonest	3% Mepivacaine plain	Short
		2% Mepivacaine, 1:20,000 levonordefrin	Medium
Prilocaine	Citanest, Citanest Forte	4% Prilocaine plain	Short
		4% Prilocaine, 1:200,000 epinephrine	Medium

Conversely, only the charged form can dissolve in water and diffuse through extracellular fluid and intracellular cytoplasm. Therefore, an agent's pKa is the most important factor in determining its diffusion properties and subsequently, the rate of onset. Procaine, with a pKa of 8.9, is 98% ionized at a normal tissue pH of 7.4. After procaine injection, most of the molecules exist in its charged state at normal pH and is therefore unable to cross cell membranes. The onset of anesthesia using procaine and other ester local anesthetics is thus unacceptably prolonged. Amide anesthetics having pKa values in the range of 7.6 to 8.0 have less of the drug in an ionized state, diffuse through tissue more readily, and have acceptably rapid onset times.[2–4]

The lipid solubility characteristics of a local anesthetic best predict its potency. Procaine is one of the least lipid-soluble and least potent local anesthetics, whereas bupivacaine is highly lipid soluble and most potent. Protein binding characteristics are a primary determinant of the duration of anesthesia. Agents that attach to protein components of nerve membranes are less likely to diffuse from the site of action and enter the systemic circulation. Lidocaine's short duration and bupivacaine's long duration of action are due, in part, to their distinctly different protein binding characteristics.[2,5]

It is clear that lipid solubility, ionization, and protein binding properties contribute to the clinical characteristics of local anesthetics. However, factors such as the site of injection, drug and vasoconstrictor concentration, volume of injection, and inherent vasodilating properties of the anesthetic also influence the clinical performance of a local anesthetic.

Local Anesthetics: Current Practice

Because anesthesia induced using ester anesthetics is less effective than with amides, and because ester anesthetics have a higher incidence of allergic reactions, dental anesthetic formulations containing ester agents are no longer marketed. Lidocaine remains the predominant local anesthetic agent used in the United States. In Canada, formulations of articaine have surpassed lidocaine in popularity, thus becoming the most frequently used dental anesthetic. A survey of US oral surgeons regarding their preferences for local anesthetic agents found bupivacaine, a long-acting local anesthetic, to be commonly administered to manage postoperative pain. Formulations used by less than 2% of the surveyed oral surgery practitioners included mepivacaine with 1:20,000 levonordefrin (Neo-Cobefrin), lidocaine with 1:50,000 epinephrine, 3% mepivacaine plain, and 4% prilocaine plain (**Table 2**).[6]

Until 1989, a combination of ester anesthetics, procaine and propoxycaine, was available in dental cartridges. This formulation was a combination of 0.4% propoxycaine (Ravocaine) and 2% procaine (Novocain) with 1:20,000 levonordefrin as a vasoconstrictor. As stated earlier, ester anesthetics are generally less effective than amides because they have poor diffusion properties. Procaine is a potent vasodilator and is not effective if used without a vasoconstrictor. The metabolism of esters is through hydrolysis by the plasma and tissue esterases, yielding para-aminobenzoic acid (PABA) and diethylamino alcohol. PABA seems to be the allergen associated with procaine's significant allergenicity. The concern regarding patient reporting of allergy to local anesthetics is addressed in an accompanying article by Speca and colleagues elsewhere in this issue.

Lidocaine hydrochloride

Lidocaine was introduced into practice in the 1950s and, because of its excellent efficacy and safety, has become the prototypic dental local anesthetic in North America. Besides having excellent anesthetic efficacy, lidocaine has limited allergenicity, with

Table 2
Local anesthetics administered for third molar extraction

Local Anesthetic Formulation	Frequency (%)
2% Lidocaine, 1:100,000 epinephrine	70.4
0.5% Bupivacaine, 1:200,000 epinephrine	11.3
4% Articaine, 1:100,000 epinephrine	7.3
4% Prilocaine, 1:200,000 epinephrine	3.1
2% Mepivacaine, 1:20,000 levonordefrin	1.9
2% Lidocaine, 1:50,000 epinephrine	1.8
3% Mepivacaine	0.7
4% Prilocaine	0.2

fewer than 20 confirmed cases of serious allergic anaphylactic reactions (ie, anaphylactoid) reported in the last 50 years. Given the frequent use of local anesthesia in dentistry (500,000–1,000,000 injections a day throughout the United States and Canada), the rare incidence of serious life-threatening hypersensitivity reactions associated with lidocaine is an extremely important clinical advantage.

Lidocaine is formulated in cartridges as 2% lidocaine with 1:50,000 epinephrine, 2% lidocaine with 1:100,000 epinephrine, and 2% lidocaine plain. The 2% lidocaine with 1:100,000 epinephrine formulation is considered the gold standard when evaluating the efficacy and safety of newer anesthetics.

Mepivacaine hydrochloride
Mepivacaine has an important role in dental anesthesia because it has minimal vasodilating properties and can therefore provide profound local anesthesia without being formulated with a vasoconstrictor such as epinephrine or levonordefrin (see **Table 1**). The availability of a 3% mepivacaine formulation without a vasoconstrictor is a valuable addition to a dentist's armamentarium. It is available in dental cartridges as 3% mepivacaine plain or 2% mepivacaine with 1:20,000 levonordefrin.

Mepivacaine plain is often reported to have a shorter duration of soft tissue anesthesia, making it potentially useful in pediatric dentistry in which children are known to chew their lips after dental procedures. However, one investigation suggests that although pulpal durations of mepivacaine plain are shorter than that of 2% lidocaine with epinephrine, duration of soft tissue anesthesia for mepivacaine and lidocaine with epinephrine are nearly identical.[7]

Alternatively, shortening of the duration of soft tissue anesthesia after completion of a dental procedure has been shown using the α-adrenergic receptor antagonist phentolamine. Local anesthesia reversal, a recent advancement in dental anesthesia therapeutics, is addressed in an article by Hersh and Lindemyer elsewhere in this issue.

Prilocaine hydrochloride
Prilocaine, like mepivacaine, is not a potent vasodilator and can provide excellent oral anesthesia with or without a vasoconstrictor. It is available in preparations of 4% prilocaine plain and 4% prilocaine with 1:200,000 epinephrine. The formulation containing epinephrine has anesthetic characteristics similar to 2% lidocaine with 1:100,000 epinephrine. The 4% prilocaine plain formulation provides a slightly shorter duration of surgical anesthesia. Prilocaine plain solution in dental cartridges has a somewhat less acidic pH. Although not confirmed by clinical trials, there is some indication that prilocaine causes less discomfort on injection.[8]

One of prilocaine's metabolic products has been associated with the development of methemoglobinemia. Methemoglobinemia has also been reported with overdoses of the topical anesthetic, benzocaine. The significance of this adverse reaction is addressed in an article by Trapp and Will elsewhere in this issue.

Articaine hydrochloride
Similar to most dental anesthetics available to the dental practitioner, articaine is classified as an amide anesthetic. However, the molecular structure of articaine is somewhat unique, containing a thiophene (sulfur-containing) ring and an ester side chain. As articaine is absorbed from the injection site into the systemic circulation, it is rapidly inactivated via hydrolysis of the ester side chain to articainic acid. Consequently, articaine has the shortest metabolic half-life (estimated to be between 27–42 minutes) of the anesthetics available in dentistry.[9,10] Formulations containing 4% articaine hydrochloride with 1:100,000 epinephrine and 4% articaine with 1:200,000 epinephrine are available in dental cartridges. Studies evaluating mandibular block and maxillary infiltration anesthesia have generally found that onset time, duration, and anesthetic profundity of articaine are comparable to that of 2% lidocaine with 1:100,000 epinephrine.[11–16] The relative efficacy of lidocaine and articaine formulations is thoroughly reviewed in an article by Paxton and Thome elsewhere in this issue.

Articaine does not seem to have a greater allergenicity than other available amide anesthetic agents, probably because the ester metabolite is not the allergen PABA. Reports of toxicity reactions after the use of articaine for dental anesthesia are extremely rare. The rapid inactivation of articaine by plasma esterases may explain the apparent lack of overdose reactions reported after its administration.

Articaine and prilocaine have been associated with inferior alveolar and lingual nerve paresthesias. This controversial topic is addressed in an article by Moore and Haas elsewhere in this issue.

There is a developing clinical research literature supporting the claim that articaine has superior diffusion properties and that anesthesia can be induced after buccal infiltration in the mandible. The efficacy of articaine to provide mandibular pulpal anesthesia after buccal infiltration is critically reviewed in an article by Meechan elsewhere in this issue.

Bupivacaine hydrochloride
In the last few decades, the long-acting amide local anesthetic bupivacaine has found a place in dentists' armamentarium. This long-acting agent plays a valuable role in the overall management of surgical postoperative pain associated with dental care.[6] The molecular structure of bupivacaine (1-butyl-2',6'-pipecoloxylidide) is identical to mepivacaine except for a butyl (4 carbon) substitution of the methyl (1 carbon) group at the amino terminus of the molecule. The addition of a butyl group to the chemical structures of mepivacaine provides enhanced lipid solubility and protein binding properties.[17,18]

Although bupivacaine may provide adequate surgical anesthesia, it is most useful for postoperative pain management.[19,20] Clinical trials have shown that bupivacaine, having an elevated pKa of 8.1, has a slightly longer onset time than conventional amide anesthetics. Onset times and profundity are optimized when preparations of bupivacaine include epinephrine.[5,21]

A combination strategy for managing postoperative pain using a nonsteroidal anti-inflammatory drug before surgery and a long-acting anesthetic may provide maximum patient comfort.[22] The management of postoperative and chronic pain using long-acting local anesthetics is the focus of a review article by Gordon and Dionne elsewhere in this issue.

TOXICITY REACTIONS ASSOCIATED WITH LOCAL ANESTHESIA

A dentist's ability to safely administer local anesthesia is essential for dental practice. Local anesthetic solutions used in North America for dental anesthesia are formulated with several components: an amide local anesthetic (ester local anesthetic drugs are no longer available in dental cartridges), an adrenergic vasoconstrictor, and a sulfite antioxidant. In susceptible patients, any of these components may induce systemic, dose-dependent, adverse reactions. Although extremely rare, allergic and hypersensitivity reactions to local anesthetics and sulfites may occasionally occur (see the article by Speca and colleagues elsewhere in this issue for further exploration of this topic). Signs and symptoms of the various adverse reactions associated with local anesthetics, such as methemoglobinemia, are quite distinctive, permitting rapid diagnosis and treatment. A critical review of acquired methemoglobinemia is provided in an article by Trapp and Will elsewhere in this issue. Significant cardiovascular stimulation can occur after rapid administration of agents containing an adrenergic vasoconstrictor.

Serious reactions are extremely infrequent and when treated properly, they are unlikely to result in significant morbidity or mortality. The most serious and life threatening of adverse reactions are toxicities caused by relative excessive dosing of the local anesthetic or vasoconstrictor. These reactions are preventable with proper patient assessment and dosage calculations.

When the anesthetic agent contained in a dental cartridge diffuses away from the site of injection, it is absorbed into the systemic circulation where it is metabolized and eliminated. The doses needed for local anesthesia in dentistry are usually minimal, and systemic effects after absorption of the drug are quite uncommon. However, if an inadvertent vascular injection occurs, if repeated injections are administered, or if relatively excessive volumes are used in pediatric dentistry, then blood levels of a local anesthetic may become significantly elevated. The addition of epinephrine to local anesthetic formulations can significantly reduce the absorption of the anesthetics.

Toxicity Reactions to Excessive Local Anesthetic Dose

Initially, excitatory reactions to local anesthetic overdose are seen, such as tremors, muscle twitching, shivering, and clonic-tonic convulsions.[23–25] These initial excitatory reactions are thought to be disinhibition phenomena resulting from selective blockade of small inhibitory neurons within the limbic system of the central nervous system (CNS).[2] Whether this initial excitatory reaction is apparent or not, a generalized CNS depression with symptoms of sedation, drowsiness, lethargy, and life-threatening respiratory depression follows if blood concentrations of the local anesthetic agent continue to increase. With extremely high toxic doses, myocardial excitability and conductivity may also be depressed, particularly with the highly lipid-soluble long-acting local anesthetic bupivacaine.[26] Cardiac toxicity to local anesthetic overdose is most often manifested as ectopic cardiac rhythms and bradycardia. With an extreme local anesthetic overdose, cardiac contractility is depressed and peripheral vasodilation occurs, leading to significant hypotension.

Compliance with local anesthetic dosing guidelines is the first and most important strategy for preventing this adverse event. Dosing calculations used to avoid systemic reactions to local anesthetics are dependent on the agent administered and the patient's body weight (**Table 3**). True dose-dependent toxicity reactions

Table 3
MRDs of injectable local anesthetics

Agents (Brand Name)	Concentration of Local Anesthetic		Concentration of epi/levo	Maximum Dosing		Maximum Number of Cartridges		
	mg/mL[a]	mg/cartridge[b]	mg/Cartridge[c]	Adult MRD (mg)	MRD/lb[d] (mg/lb)	Adults[e]	50 lb Child	25 lb Child
2% Lidocaine, 1:100,000 epi	20	36	0.018	500	3.3	13.8	4.6	2.3
2% Lidocaine, 1:50,000 epi	20	36	0.036	500	3.3	13.8	4.6	2.3
2% Lidocaine plain	20	36	—	300	2.0	8.3	2.8	1.4
4% Articaine, 1:100,000 epi	40	72	0.018[e]	500	3.3	6.9	2.3	1.1
4% Articaine, 1:200,000 epi	40	72	0.009[e]	500	3.3	6.9	2.3	1.1
3% Mepivacaine	30	54	—	400	2.6	7.4	2.5	1.2
2% Mepivacaine,1:20,000 levo	20	36	0.09	400	2.6	11.1	3.7	1.8
4% Prilocaine	40	72	—	600	4.0	8.3	2.8	1.4
4% Prilocaine, 1:200,000 epi	40	72	0.009	600	4.0	8.3	2.8	1.4
0.5% Bupivacaine,1:200,000 epi	5	9	0.009	90	0.6	10	NR	NR

All cartridges are assumed to contain approximately 1.8 mL.
Abbreviations: epi, epinephrine; levo, levonordefrin; MRD, maximum recommended dose; NR, not recommended.
[a] Calculation for drug concentration. For example, 2% lidocaine solution = 2 g/100 mL = 2000 mg/100 ml = 20 mg/mL.
[b] Calculation of mg/cartridge. For example, 2% lidocaine: 20 mg/mL × 1.8 mL/cartridge = 36 mg/cartridge.
[c] Calculation of mg/cartridge of epinephrine: for example, 1:100,000 = 1 g:100,000 mL = 1000 mg:100,000 mL = 0.01 mg/mL. A 1.8-mL cartridge contains 0.018 mg of epi.
[d] Calculation of weight-based MRD: for example, 500 mg for a 150-lb adult = 500 mg/150 lb = 3.3 mg/lb.
[e] Calculation of maximum number of cartridges: for example, for lidocaine/epi, the adult MRD for lidocaine/epi is 500 mg; 500 mg/36 mg per cartridge = 13.8 cartridges.

to local anesthetics are most frequently reported in pediatric patients.[23–25] A typical case report of a local anesthetic toxicity reaction in pediatric dentistry is as follows:

A healthy five-year-old female patient, weighing 36 lb. was scheduled for multiple extractions. The child received N2O/O2 sedation via a nasal mask, followed by maxillary and mandibular injections of five cartridges of 3% mepivacaine (270 mg). Ten minutes later the child experienced "stiffening and shaking" of all extremities that lasted ten seconds. Two more convulsive episodes occurred and cardiopulmonary arrest ensued. Transport to a local hospital and resuscitation measures were unsuccessful. Death occurred four days later.[27]

When administering local anesthetics to children, the dose must be lowered because of the child's smaller size. Clark rule predicts that this adjustment of dosing for children should be calculated as a fraction of the child's body weight (ie, child's dose = [child's weight/adult weight] × [adult dose]). In the case report presented earlier, the child's dose should have been lowered by the fraction 36 lb/150 lbs (ie, 24%). Toxicity reactions in children may occur more frequently because a child's lesser body weight does not represent a proportionate decrease in orofacial anatomy. The mandible and maxilla of a child weighing 36 lb is only 50% to 60% the size of an adult (weighing 150 lb); therefore, there is an apparent need to use relatively larger volumes when inducing local anesthesia in pediatric dental patients. The consequence of this disparity is that local anesthetic toxicity reactions occur more frequently in children. In addition, systemic drug interactions involving local anesthetics and other CNS-depressant drugs used for pediatric sedation are more likely to occur in children.[23,24]

The local anesthetic formulation of 3% mepivacaine plain seems to be associated with a disproportionate number of local anesthetic toxicity reports.[23–25,27–29] This toxicity may be due to the absence of a vasoconstrictor, thereby allowing more rapid systemic absorption of the anesthetic. In addition, the higher concentration of the drug used in its anesthetic formulation (3%) may result in the administration of larger relative doses. Pharmacokinetic studies by Goebel and colleagues[30,31] have demonstrated that peak anesthetic blood levels of 3% mepivacaine occur more rapidly and exceed that of an equal volume of 2% lidocaine with 1:100,000 epinephrine by approximately 3-fold after maxillary infiltration injections (**Fig. 1**).[30,31]

The ability of vasoconstrictors to limit the initial increase and the ultimate peak of local anesthetic drug levels is illustrated in **Fig. 1**. A higher peak serum concentration can be noted after administration of lidocaine plain than with lidocaine with epinephrine. Consequently, the maximum recommended dose (MRD) for lidocaine plain is less (300 mg for an adult) than for lidocaine with epinephrine (500 mg for an adult). Mepivacaine is a local anesthetic agent with less vasodilating properties than lidocaine. Consequently, the differences in serum levels between the mepivacaine formulations with and without a vasoconstrictor are less pronounced.

The 3% mepivacaine formulation is often chosen for children because it is considered to have a shorter duration of soft tissue anesthesia, thereby limiting severe lip biting and oral trauma seen in children after dental local anesthesia. However, the results of a double-blind randomized trial have found that onset time, peak effects, and duration of soft tissue anesthesia after mandibular block injections of 2% lidocaine with 1:100,000 epinephrine, 3% mepivacaine plain, or 4% prilocaine plain were very similar.[7] The selection of anesthetic formulations that do not contain a vasoconstrictor, such as 3% mepivacaine, may not be a significant clinical advantage for children.

The determination of MRDs for children receiving local anesthetics is complicated by the conflicting published dosage recommendations found in the literature and the

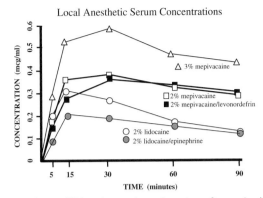

Fig. 1. Serum concentrations of lidocaine and mepivacaine after a single cartridge of each agent administered with a vasoconstrictor and without a vasoconstrictor. Open circles represent 2% lidocaine plain; closed circle, 2% lidocaine with 1:100,000 epinephrine; open squares, 2% mepivacaine plain; close squares, 2% mepivacaine with 1:20,000 levonordefrin; and open triangles, 3% mepivacaine plain. (*Data from* Goebel WM, Allen G, and Randall F. Circulating serum levels of mepivacaine after dental injection. Anesth Prog 1978;25:52–6; and Goebel WM, Allen G, and Randall F. The effect of commercial vasoconstrictor preparations on the circulating venous serum level of mepivacaine and lidocaine. J Oral Med 1980;35:91–6.)

various units involved in the calculation (milligram, percentage, cubic centimeter, milliliter, kilogram, pound, cartridges). The MRDs for dental local anesthetics published in the American Dental Association's guide to dental therapeutics as derived from manufacturers' package inserts are possibly the most current authoritative sources.[1] These values are summarized in **Table 3**. These recommendations permit the use of largest volume for lidocaine with epinephrine and smallest volume for mepivacaine and articaine. In addition, to prevent oral trauma after dental anesthesia, the long-acting local anesthetic bupivacaine is generally not indicated for young children.[32]

The maximum volume of 3% mepivacaine plain for an anesthetic injection (7.4 cartridges for a 150 lb adult) and the maximum volume of 4% articaine with epinephrine (6.9 cartridges for a 150 lb adult) are the most restrictive of any local anesthetics used in dentistry. In comparison, the maximum volume for 2% lidocaine with epinephrine (14 cartridges for a 150 lb adult) permits the greatest volume to be administered safely. In children, the formulation of 2% lidocaine with 1:100,000 epinephrine is the least likely to cause toxicity reactions, if multiple injections are required.

A simplified alternative for calculating maximum safe doses of local anesthesia has been established resulting in the most conservative guidelines that can be applied to all anesthetic formulations used in dentistry (**Table 4**). These guidelines, "the Rule of 25" state that for healthy patients, a dentist may safely use 1 cartridge of any marketed local anesthetic for every 25 lb of patient weight, that is, 1 cartridge for a patient weighing 25 lb, 3 cartridges for a patient weighing 75 lb, and 6 cartridges for a patient weighing 150 lb or greater.

Management of Local Anesthetic Overdose

Tonic-clonic convulsions are the most common manifestation of a true overdose situation. Local anesthetic–induced convulsions are usually transient. After a convulsive episode, loss of consciousness and severe prolonged respiratory depression is likely. Immediate treatment of this emergency should address both the convulsions and the potential respiratory depression. One must monitor vital signs (particularly respiratory

Table 4 Safe dose for local anesthetics: the Rule of 25[a]	
Body Weight in lbs (kg)	Number of Anesthetic Cartridges
25 (11.25)	1
50 (22.5)	2
75 (33.75)	3
100 (45)	4
125 (56.25)	5
150 (67.5)	6

[a] An easily remembered rule for determining a safe dose of dental local anesthetics in children is to use the "Rule of 25": 1 cartridge of any anesthetic formulation can be administered safely for every 25 lb of the child's body weight.

adequacy), protect the patient from injury, place the patient in supine position, and maintain the airway. If the patient is unconscious and in respiratory arrest, positive pressure oxygen ventilation is essential. Because local anesthesia–induced convulsions are usually transient, administration of an anticonvulsant, such as intravenous diazepam, 5 to 10 mg, is rarely required.

Toxicity Reactions to Excessive Vasoconstrictors Dose

Epinephrine and levonordefrin are the 2 catecholamine vasoconstrictors formulated with local anesthetic agents in dental cartridges. As shown in **Fig. 1**, the use of a vasoconstrictor can improve the safety of the formulation by slowing the systemic absorption of the local anesthetic and decreasing the peak blood levels of the anesthetic. There is minimal stimulation of the cardiovascular system after submucosal injection of 1 or 2 cartridges of anesthetic containing epinephrine or levonordefrin. However, when excessive amounts of these adrenergic vasoconstrictors are administered, or when the agents are inadvertently administered intravascularly, cardiovascular stimulation, with clinically significant increases in blood pressure and heart rate, can occur. For example, the administration of 7 cartridges of 4% articaine with 1:100,000 epinephrine has been found to increase the heart rate on an average by 9 beats per minute (bpm) (from 69 to 78 bpm) and to increase systolic blood pressure by 6 mm Hg (from 125 to 131 mm Hg).[10]

The small amount of epinephrine in a dental cartridge was once thought to be incapable of significantly increasing epinephrine blood levels after local anesthetic administration. Most of the cardiovascular stimulation reported after local anesthesia administration was thought to be due to patient fear and anxiety or the pain of injection. However, studies have found that the epinephrine in as little as 2 cartridges of 1:100,000 formulations can significantly increase circulating epinephrine levels. Lipp and colleagues[33] administered 2 mL of 4% articaine containing tritium-labeled epinephrine (1:100,000) to determine the extent to which the increase in total epinephrine plasma levels was due to the administered tritium-labeled epinephrine. With submucosal injections (16 subjects), the total epinephrine levels increased from a baseline level of 200 pg/mL to a peak level of 631 pg/mL at 7 minutes (**Fig. 2**). The increase in total epinephrine levels was mostly due to the injected tritium-labeled epinephrine. Because of the apparent inadvertent intravascular local anesthetic injections in 4 subjects, a rapid increase in epinephrine levels to a mean peak level of 2645 pg/mL was seen within a minute of their injections. Although this increase was

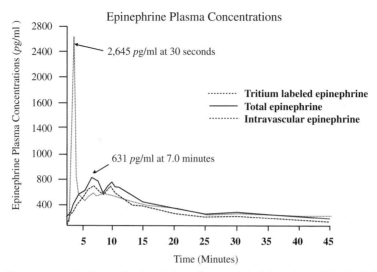

Fig. 2. Plasma concentrations of epinephrine after the administration of 2 mL of 4% articaine containing tritiated epinephrine (1:100,000). Epinephrine levels measured in the 4 patients who inadvertently received intravascular injections are shown (*dotted line*). Tritiated epinephrine levels (*dashed line*) and total epinephrine concentrations (*solid line*) representing subjects receiving submucosal injections are also shown. (*From* Lipp M, Dick W, Daubländer M, et al. Exogenous and endogenous plasma levels of epinephrine during dental treatment under local anesthesia. Reg Anesth 1993;18(1):6–12; with permission.)

short lived, some of these patients were found to have significant cardiovascular stimulation indicated by tachycardia and extrasystoles. It is clear that very large volumes or inadvertent intravascular injections can produce clinically significant cardiovascular responses. Using anesthetic formulations containing no or limited concentrations of vasoconstrictors, using a slow injection technique, and aspirating carefully and repeatedly are the common recommendations to prevent rapid systemic absorption of epinephrine and levonordefrin.

A patient's medical health history that indicates significant cardiovascular impairment may indicate limiting the use of vasoconstrictors. Although vasoconstrictors are rarely contraindicated, the potential stimulation of the cardiovascular system after intravascular injections should guide the dental practitioners to avoid vasoconstrictor-containing formulations if possible. A common recommendation, when a vasoconstrictor is required for a dental treatment and when there is a medical history that suggests a need for caution, is to limit the dose of epinephrine to 0.04 mg.[34] This dose reduction can be achieved by limiting the total anesthetics used to one of the following:

- One cartridge of an anesthetic containing 1:50,000 epinephrine
- Two cartridges of an anesthetic containing 1:100,000 epinephrine
- Four cartridges of an anesthetic containing 1:200,000 epinephrine.

In addition, practitioners must be alert to drug interactions when using local anesthetics containing the vasoconstrictors epinephrine and levonordefrin. Earlier reports suggest that vasoconstrictors should be used with caution in patients taking nonselective β-adrenoreceptor blockers, tricyclic antidepressants, cocaine, and α-adrenergic blockers.[35] Patients taking nonselective β-adrenergic antagonists such as propranolol may experience exaggerated systemic vasoconstrictive responses to epinephrine or levonordefrin.[17] This drug interaction is critically reviewed in article by Hersh and Giannakopoulos elsewhere in this issue.

Local anesthetic administration using agents containing vasoconstrictors may also be a concern among patients who are pregnant. A review of this potential risk and treatment recommendations for this special population is presented in another article by Fayans and colleagues elsewhere in this issue.

SUMMARY

The amide local anesthetic agents currently available in dentistry are extremely safe and effective. The availability of various formulations of lidocaine, mepivacaine, prilocaine, articaine, and bupivacaine permits a practitioner to select agents that can meet treatment requirements. Many advances in local anesthesia therapeutics and armamentarium have become available to the dental practitioner in recent years. Through careful selection of agents and proper adjustment of dosing, most serious adverse reactions associated with dental local anesthetic agents can be prevented.

REFERENCES

1. Yagiela J. Injectable and topical local anesthetics. In: ADA/PDR guide to dental therapeutics. 5th edition. Chicago: American Dental Association Publishing Co; 2009. p. 11–3.
2. Covino BG, Vassallo HG. Local anesthetics: mechanisms of action and clinical use. New York: Grune & Stratton; 1976.
3. Moore PA. Manual of local anesthesia in dentistry. 4th edition. Rochester (NY): Eastman-Kodak Co; 1996.
4. Haas DA. An update on local anesthetics in dentistry. J Can Dent Assoc 2002;68 (9):546–51.
5. Moore PA. Bupivaciane: a long-lasting local anesthetic for dentistry. Oral Surg 1984;58:369–74.
6. Moore PA, Nahouraii HS, Zovko J, et al. Dental therapeutic practice patterns in the U.S. I: anesthesia and sedation. Gen Dent 2006;54(2):92–8.
7. Hersh EV, Hermann DG, Lamp CL, et al. Temporal assessment of soft tissue anesthesia following mandibular block injection. J Am Dent Assoc 1995;126: 1531–5.
8. Wahl MJ, Overton D, Howell J, et al. Pain on injection of prilocaine plain vs. lidocaine with epinephrine: a prospective double-blind study. J Am Dent Assoc 2001; 132:1396–401.
9. Oertel R, Rahn R, Kirch W. Clinical pharmacokinetics of articaine. Clin Pharmacokin 1997;33(6):417–25.
10. Hersh EV, Giannakopoulos H, Levin LM, et al. The pharmacokinetics and cardiovascular effects of high-dose articaine with 1:100,000 and 1:200,000 epinephrine. J Am Dent Assoc 2006;137(11):1562–71.
11. Malamed SF, Gagnon S, Leblanc D. Efficacy of articaine: a new amide local anesthetic. J Am Dent Assoc 2000;131(5):635–42.
12. Donaldson D, James-Perdok L, Craig BJ, et al. A comparison of Ultracaine DS (articaine HCl) and Citanest forte (prilocaine HCl) in maxillary infiltration and mandibular nerve block. J Can Dent Assoc 1987;53(1):38–42.
13. Lemay H, Albert G, Helie P, et al. Ultracaine in conventional operative dentistry. J Can Dent Assoc 1984;50(9):703–8.

14. Haas DA, Harper DG, Saso MA, et al. Comparison of articaine and prilocaine anesthesia by infiltration in maxillary and mandibular arches. Anesth Prog 1990;37(5):230–7.
15. Moore PA, Boynes SG, Hersh EV, et al. Dental anesthesia using 4% articaine 1:200,000 epinephrine: two controlled clinical trials. J Am Dent Assoc 2006;137 (11):1572–81.
16. Moore PA, Delie RA, Doll B, et al. Hemostatic and anesthetic efficacy of 4% articaine HCl with 1:200,000 epinephrine and 4% articaine HCl with 1:100,000 epinephrine when administered intraorally for periodontal surgery. J Periodontol 2007;78(2):247–53.
17. Aberg G, Dhuner KG, Sydnes G. Studies on the duration of local anesthesia: structure/activity relationships in a series of homologous local anesthetics. Acta Pharacol Toxicol (Copenh) 1977;41:432–43.
18. Tucker T, Mather LE. Clinical pharmacokinetics of local anesthetics. Clin Pharmacokinet 1979;4:241–78.
19. Moore PA, Dunsky JL. Bupivacaine anesthesia: a clinical trial for endodontic therapy. Oral Surg 1983;55:176–9.
20. Trieger N, Gillen GH. Bupivacaine anesthesia and postoperative analgesia in oral surgery. Anesth Prog 1979;20:23–7.
21. Laskin JL, Wallace WR, DeLeo B. Use of bupivacaine hydrochloride in oral surgery—a clinical study. J Oral Surg 1977;35:25–9.
22. Dionne RA, Wirdzek PR, Fox PC, et al. Suppression of postoperative pain by the combination of a nonsteroidal anti-inflammatory drug, flurbiprofen and a long-acting local anesthetic, etidocaine. J Am Dent Assoc 1984;108:598–601.
23. Goodson JM, Moore PA. Life-threatening reactions following pedodontic sedation: an assessment of narcotic, local anesthetic and antiemetic drug interaction. J Am Dent Assoc 1983;107:239–45.
24. Moore PA, Goodson JM. Risk appraisal of narcotic sedation for children. Anesth Prog 1985;32:129–39.
25. Reynolds F. Adverse effects of local anesthetics. Br J Anaesth 1987;59:78–95.
26. Liu PL, Feldman HS, Giasi R, et al. Comparative CNS toxicity of lidocaine, etidocaine, bupivacaine, and tetracaine in awake dogs following rapid intravenous administration. Anesth Analg 1983;62:375–9.
27. Hersh EV, Helpin ML, Evans OB. Local anesthetic mortality: report of case. J Dent Child 1991;58:489–91.
28. Virts BE. Local anesthesia toxicity review. Pediatr Dent 1999;21:375.
29. Moore PA. Prevention of local anesthesia toxicity. J Am Dent Assoc 1992;123:60–4.
30. Goebel WM, Allen G, Randall F. Circulating serum levels of mepivacaine after dental injection. Anesth Prog 1978;25:52–6.
31. Goebel WM, Allen G, Randall F. The effect of commercial vasoconstrictor preparations on the circulating venous serum level of mepivacaine and lidocaine. J Oral Med 1980;35:91–6.
32. Moore PA. Long-acting local anesthetics: a review of clinical efficacy in dentistry. Comp Cont Dent Ed 1990;11:22–30.
33. Lipp M, Dick W, Daubländer M, et al. Exogenous and endogenous plasma levels of epinephrine during dental treatment under local anesthesia. Reg Anesth 1993; 18(1):6–12.
34. Little JW, Falace DA. Dental management of the medically compromised patient. 4th edition. St Louis (MO): Mosby; 1993.
35. Yagiela JA. Adverse drug interactions in dental practice: interactions associated with vasoconstrictors. Part V of a series. J Am Dent Assoc 1999;130(5):701–9.

The Use of Local Anesthetic Agents in Medicine

Steven Ganzberg, DMD, MS*, Kyle J. Kramer, DDS

KEYWORDS

• Local anesthetics • Dentistry • Medicine • Regional anesthesia

Local anesthetics are commonly used in both dentistry and medicine.[1–5] These drugs are similarly used in some office-based medical practices. For example, in dermatology local infiltration, which dentists commonly use in the maxilla, is provided for minor surgical procedures such as excisional biopsy of skin lesions. In ophthalmology a retrobulbar nerve block, similar to what a dentist would commonly provide for mandibular anesthesia, is used for local anesthesia of the globe. These are but 2 examples of minor medical procedures that can be performed by office-based physicians.

Anesthesiologists can also provide regional anesthesia for most surgical procedures, although for various reasons the use of general anesthesia is frequently preferred. Peripheral surgical procedures, such as many upper and lower extremity procedures, some head and neck surgery, and superficial abdominal procedures (eg, inguinal hernia) can be easily completed with local anesthesia with or without sedation. Even some major abdominal surgeries can be performed with the use of neuraxial anesthesia, such as local anesthesia applied around the spinal cord or epidural space. As opposed to anesthesiologist practice, the typical doses of local anesthetic administered for dental procedures are usually well below the levels associated with toxicity issues, such as altered consciousness, seizures, or unconsciousness. However, many of the regional anesthesia techniques discussed here require larger volumes of local anesthetic (up to 40–50 mL), far exceeding the volumes usually used in dentistry. As expected, toxicity complications are more common, requiring close monitoring during administration; rapid recognition of overdose symptoms; and prompt treatment, including immediate endotracheal intubation and advanced supportive measures, when indicated. Except for minor procedures, most physicians

Section of Anesthesiology, College of Dentistry, College of Medicine and Public Health, The Ohio State University, 305 West 12th Avenue, Columbus, OH 43210-1267, USA
* Corresponding author.
E-mail address: ganzberg.1@osu.edu

Dent Clin N Am 54 (2010) 601–610
doi:10.1016/j.cden.2010.06.001
0011-8532/10/$ – see front matter

dental.theclinics.com

who require complicated nerve blocks rely on anesthesiologists to administer the local anesthesia, usually in combination with some form of sedation, and at times, general anesthesia in the hospital operating room or ambulatory surgery center setting.

This article reviews the types and uses of local anesthesia in anesthesiology.

LOCAL ANESTHETICS USED IN MEDICINE

Both ester and amide local anesthetics are routinely used in medical practice (**Table 1**). The general pharmacology of these agents has been reviewed in the introductory article "Local anesthetics: pharmacology and toxicology" in this issue by Moore and Hersh. By far the most commonly used agents in office-based medical practice are the amides, specifically lidocaine (Xylocaine) and bupivacaine (Marcaine) with or without epinephrine. Examples of the commonly used ester local anesthetics include benzocaine (Hurricaine, Cetacaine), cocaine, procaine (Novocaine), chloroprocaine, and tetracaine (see **Table 1**). Some unique aspects of local anesthesia as used in medical practice are reviewed here.

Ester Local Anesthetics

The benzocaine molecule is very insoluble in water, and as such is indicated for topical applications in a spray or gel form. Benzocaine is used to provide topical anesthesia for a limited duration to nasal, oral, or orotracheal mucosa. One preparation in particular, Cetacaine, is a mixture that includes benzocaine, tetracaine, and butyl aminobenzoate (Butamben), which is an additional lipophilic ester local anesthetic. Cetacaine spray has historically been used to provide topical anesthesia to the oronasopharyngeal mucosa for procedures such as esophagogastroduodenoscopy, bronchoscopy, or "awake" endotracheal intubation, in which endoscopes are passed into the esophagus or trachea through the mouth or nose. However, Cetacaine, a topical anesthetic containing tetracaine, benzocaine, and butyl aminobenzoate, can cause methemoglobinemia, especially if administered in large quantities, which can occur with these procedures.

Cocaine, which was the first local anesthetic to be discovered, is still occasionally used clinically. However, it is restricted to topical use only, most commonly

Table 1						
Physiochemical and biologic properties of local anesthetics					
Agent	pKa	% Total Drug in Base Form at pH 7.4	Onset	Duration	Class
Benzocaine	3.5	100	Fast	Short	Ester
Mepivacaine	7.6	39	Fast	Moderate	Amide
Lidocaine	7.9	24	Fast	Moderate	Amide
Etidocaine	7.7	33	Fast	Long	Amide
Bupivacaine	8.1	17	Slow	Long	Amide
Tetracaine	8.6	14	Slow	Long	Ester
Procaine	8.9	3	Slow	Short	Ester
Chloroprocaine	9.1	2	Slow	Short	Ester

Data from Joyner MJ. Local anesthetics: mechanism of action. In: Faust RJ, Cucchiara RF, Rose SH, et al, editors. Anesthesiology review. 3rd edition. Philadelphia: Churchill Livingstone; 2002. p. 283; and Horlocker TT. Local anesthetic pharmacology. In: Faust RJ, Cucchiara RF, Rose SH, et al, editors. Anesthesiology review, 3rd edition. Philadelphia: Churchill Livingstone; 2002. p. 285.

administered as a 10% solution delivered with cotton pledgets, usually before nasal surgery or nasal endotracheal intubations. Because cocaine is the only local anesthetic with intrinsic vasoconstrictor properties, it would seem to be an ideal agent for this purpose. However, despite cocaine being a potent local anesthetic, its rare usage is most likely attributed to the high potential for complications involving the cardiovascular and sympathetic nervous systems. Systemically, cocaine inhibits the reuptake of norepinephrine, which causes stimulation of the sympathetic nervous system. In addition, cocaine sensitizes the myocardial cells to stimulation from norepinephrine or epinephrine release. Of particular concern are the cardiovascular side effects if administered concurrently with nonselective β-blockers. Use of nonselective β-blockers in conjunction with cocaine can lead to an unopposed alpha response, leading to hypertensive emergency.

Procaine is still occasionally used for spinal block or skin infiltration when a very short duration of action is preferred. Another commonly used ester is chloroprocaine, which has a rapid onset and low toxicity, making it an ideal drug for administration during labor and delivery for infiltration or more commonly via an epidural. It can also be administered for peripheral nerve blocks. Chloroprocaine is often avoided during spinal (intrathecal) injections because of reports of neural complications, including prolonged sensory and motor deficits, particularly when sodium metabisulfite is used as an antioxidant.

Tetracaine is the most commonly used ester local anesthetic administered for spinal blocks. When placed intrathecally, tetracaine has a rapid onset and produces a dense neural blockade. Used in conjunction with epinephrine, spinal blocks can last for 4 to 6 hours. Tetracaine is also supplied as a topical spray, often used to anesthetize the upper airway to help the patient tolerate naso-oropharyngeal endoscopic procedures. However, because of its rapid uptake, excessive topical use can lead to toxic reactions such as methemoglobinemia.

Amide Local Anesthetics

As in dentistry, amides are the most commonly used local anesthetics. In addition to lidocaine, mepivacaine (Carbocaine) and bupivacaine (Marcaine), all used in dentistry, ropivacaine (Naropin) and levobupivacaine (Chirocaine) are also used. In this section, when applicable, differences in uses or preparations in medical versus dental practice are highlighted.

Lidocaine has a rapid onset along with moderate potency and duration of action. Along with bupivacaine, it is the most commonly used local anesthetic. Whereas a 2% solution is the only available concentration in dental cartridges, single-dose and multidose vials are supplied in 0.5% to 4% solutions with or without epinephrine. In fact, 0.5% or 1% solutions are mostly used in medicine.

Although routinely administered for infiltration anesthesia and peripheral nerve blocks, within the last 20 years lidocaine has fallen out of favor with anesthesiologists for spinal blocks after multiple reports of complications involving lower back pain. Initially thought to be related to the use of highly concentrated lidocaine solutions, reports persisted of lower back pain lasting approximately 2 days, despite trials with lower concentrations of lidocaine.

Mepivacaine has a very similar clinical profile when compared with lidocaine. When administered in the epidural space, it provides a slightly longer duration of action. It is also frequently combined with longer-acting local anesthetics such as bupivacaine or ropivacaine during peripheral nerve blocks. This combination provides a quick-onset anesthetic that also has the benefits of a prolonged duration.

Bupivacaine, because of its higher log dissociation constant (pKa) of 8.1, has a somewhat slower onset than lidocaine. Its more prolonged duration of action is due to its increased lipophilicity and greater protein-binding properties. These properties make it a useful local anesthetic when delivered via peripheral and neuraxial blocks. Many clinicians believe that it is more predictable than tetracaine when administered for intrathecal or spinal blocks. Because of its slow onset of action, it is often used concurrently with a local anesthetic that has a more rapid onset when administered for peripheral nerve blocks. Of special concern is the cardiotoxicity of bupivacaine. If accidentally administered intravascularly, bupivacaine can cause cardiac dysrhythmias and ultimately, cardiovascular collapse. This potentially life-threatening complication can only be treated with prompt intravenous administration of intralipid, a fat emulsion, which acts as a bupivacaine sink, causing a rapid decrease in bupivacaine concentration in the blood plasma. Levobupivacaine, the S-enantiomer of bupivacaine, is reported to have decreased cardiac and central nervous system toxicity.

Ropivacaine is a local anesthetic that is popular for use during peripheral nerve blocks because of the extended clinical half-life in addition to a predilection for sensory over motor nerves. However, it does not share the cardiac toxicity profile that is unique to bupivacaine. As such, clinicians often use ropivacaine for peripheral nerve blocks, especially if larger doses are needed to cover multiple areas.

Etidocaine has a long duration of action similar to that of bupivacaine. However, because its lower pKa is closer to physiologic pH, the onset of anesthesia is noticeably quicker. Also, etidocaine produces a denser motor blockade than bupivacaine, which can be beneficial if skeletal muscle relaxation is desired in addition to anesthesia.

LOCAL ANESTHESIA TECHNIQUES IN MEDICINE
Primary Surgical Anesthesia

As in dentistry, infiltration and localized peripheral nerve blocks are the more common techniques for administration of local anesthetics in medicine. Nerve block techniques are often used as the sole anesthetic technique in the medicine for a large variety of surgical procedures, just as in dentistry. Nerve blocks serve as a useful alternative for patients who would otherwise be at a higher risk for complications of general anesthesia because of complex medical conditions. For example, a patient requiring an incision and drainage of an infected ankle fracture who has a compromised cardiac history may be at an increased risk for further cardiopulmonary complications if the surgery is performed under general anesthesia. The placement of a nerve block, with or without sedation, not only lowers the potential risk for additional systemic complications but also provides the patient and surgeon with a comfortable, reliable, high-quality anesthetic experience.

Infiltration Anesthesia

Similar to maxillary infiltration techniques used in dentistry, local anesthetics are delivered subcutaneously and allowed to diffuse into the surrounding tissue. This method provides adequate anesthesia for the overlying skin and subcutaneous structures. With the use of a longer needle and injecting while simultaneously withdrawing the needle, local anesthetic coverage to a larger area or field is achieved. Infiltration or field blocks are used frequently during carpal tunnel surgeries to anesthetize the nerves of the wrist or during ankle procedures to block the nerves of the ankle. Although useful, field blocks often require larger volumes of local anesthetic, especially if vasoconstrictors are not added.

Major regional nerve blocks

Regional nerve blocks are conceptually identical to the various nerve blocks used in dentistry, but larger nerves covering broader areas are targeted. For example, by delivering local anesthetic to the main nerve branches innervating the extremities, it is possible to provide adequate anesthesia to allow a patient to undergo an invasive arm or leg surgical procedure without any intraoperative pain. Anesthesiologists almost exclusively provide major regional anesthesia, and have additional equipment at their disposal that helps identify anatomic relationships and direct needle placement. These techniques include the use of electronic nerve stimulators, portable ultrasound machines, and even fluoroscopy. An electronic nerve stimulator emits small electrical stimuli that can elicit motor or sensory responses when delivered in the proximity of a nerve. By attaching the nerve stimulator to a special needle, anesthesiologists watch for a motor response and are then able to amplify that response by directing the needle closer to the nerve. Once the motor response is maximized, the local anesthetic is delivered through the needle, right at the level of the targeted nerve. This procedure helps to eliminate problems associated with missed blocks. Portable ultrasound machines are now used to visualize the anatomic structures so that the needle can be guided directly toward the targeted neural structures. Ultrasound machines are even capable of visualizing vascular structures, which helps reduce the likelihood of an intravascular injection. Similarly, the use of fluoroscopy, a conventional x-ray unit that relays immediate information from both static and moving images, allows for real-time visualization of both soft and hard tissue. With this technique, it is possible to inject medications directly at the level of specific nerve roots as they exit the spinal column with visualization of the needle and surrounding tissue simultaneously.

Specific regional nerve blocks: upper extremities

The main innervations of the upper extremities all arise from levels C5–C8 and T1. These nerves coalesce to form the brachial plexus shortly after exiting the intervertebral foramina. After intermingling within the brachial plexus, they extend distally to provide motor and sensory innervation to the shoulder, upper arm, forearm, and hand. There are several techniques that are used to provide anesthesia via deposition of local anesthetic along the distribution of the brachial plexus nerves. From the proximal aspect of the brachial plexus distally, the techniques include interscalene, supraclavicular, infraclavicular, axillary, and digit blocks (**Fig. 1**). Selection of the type of upper extremity block depends on what dermatomes or areas of the arm are involved in the surgery. As expected, deposition of local anesthetic at each specific nerve will provide anesthesia to all areas innervated distally from that site of injection. Upper extremity nerve blocks are easily placed; are usually fairly well tolerated by patients, requiring minimal sedation for comfort; and have a fairly low complication rate when performed by trained personnel, such as an anesthesiologist.

The Bier block (intravenous regional anesthesia) is a technique that is capable of providing dense anesthesia for a short duration. It can be used for surgical procedures involving the hand or forearm, such as carpal tunnel release. The method involves placing an intravenous catheter in the dorsum of the hand, exsanguinating the limb in a proximal direction from the fingers down to the forearm with an elastic wrap, and then inflating a tourniquet on the upper arm. After removing the elastic wrap, 40 to 50 mL of 0.5% lidocaine is slowly injected intravascularly through the catheter. After delivery of the anesthetic the catheter is removed; and adequate anesthesia is achieved within 10 minutes. The tourniquet is slowly deflated after completion of the surgical procedure, preventing a rapid surge of lidocaine back into the systemic

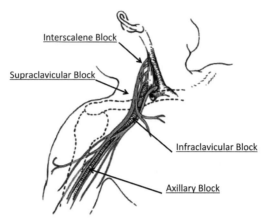

Fig. 1. Brachial plexus blocks. (*Adapted from* Morgan EG, Mikhail MS, Murray MJ, et al, editors. Clinical anesthesiology. 3rd edition. New York: McGraw-Hill; 2002. p. 330; with permission.)

circulation, thereby reducing the risk of anesthetic overdose and central nervous system symptoms.

Specific regional nerve blocks: lower extremities

Despite the nerves being less superficial and often more difficult to locate than those in the upper extremities, regional anesthesia remains a viable option for patients undergoing surgical procedures on their lower extremities. Surgical procedures involving the calf and thigh may require multiple injections because of the pathways of the nerves innervating the leg. The nerves supplying the leg arise from level L2–S3. Similar to the upper extremity nerves, the femoral (L2–L4), obturator (L2–L4), and lateral femoral (L1–L3) all join together to form the lumbar plexus. By injecting local anesthetic at the level of the lumbar plexus, it is possible to cover the anterior knee, thigh, and medial aspect of the foot. The remaining main nerve, the sciatic nerve (L4–S3), innervates the posterior aspect of the leg. To provide anesthesia to the entire leg, both sites would need coverage (**Fig. 2**).

NEURAXIAL TECHNIQUES

Neuraxial anesthesia involves the delivery of local anesthetics to the nerves within or immediately exiting the spinal cord (see **Fig 2**). This anesthesia consists of the nerves that are contained within the subarachnoid space, so-called spinal anesthesia, and those that transverse the epidural space. Depending on the site of delivery, the administered drugs will then interact with the spinal nerves within the spinal column or as they exit through the intervertebral foramina.

Spinal Technique

The subarachnoid, intrathecal, or spinal space exists between the pia and arachnoid mater within the spinal meninges. It extends superiorly through the foramen magnum and down to level S2 and the filum terminales. This anatomic space contains the spinal nerves, which terminate around level L1–L2, along with cerebral spinal fluid. Because this is a continuous space, any administered medication can potentially migrate well beyond the site of injection and involve additional levels of the spinal cord, or even the brain. Migration depends not only on the position of the patient but also on the

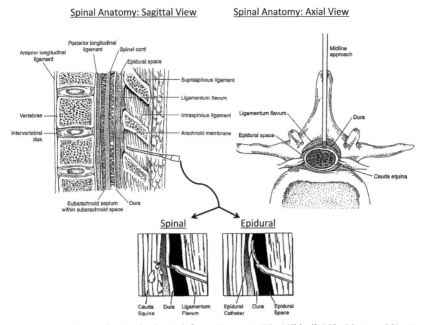

Fig. 2. Neuraxial anesthesia. (*Adapted from* Morgan EG, Mikhail MS, Murray MJ, et al, editors. Clinical anesthesiology. 3rd edition. New York: McGraw-Hill; 2002. p. 292 & 294; and Stoelting RK, Miller RD, editors. Basics of anesthesia. 4th edition. New York: Churchill Livingstone; 2000. p. 181; with permission.)

properties of the drug, such as baricity, and volume administered. Spinal blocks are frequently used for shorter surgical procedures involving the lower extremities or perianal region, such as hemorrhoidectomy. The benefits of a spinal block include a quick onset, high reliability, and minimal risk of drug toxicity. By injecting a small bolus of an opioid, such as fentanyl or morphine, with the local anesthetic into the lower lumbar spinal space, the anesthesiologist can completely anesthetize the patient from the waist down and also provide potent analgesia for the postoperative period.

Epidural Technique

Similar to the spinal block, the epidural technique also works directly on the spinal nerves, though not within the spinal cord. The epidural space extends vertically from the foramen magnum down to the sacral hiatus; however, it lies outside the spinal meninges. It is bound anteriorly by the posterior longitudinal ligament and posteriorly by the ligamentum flavum. Of importance, the lateral aspect of the epidural space is bound by the intervertebral foramina, which is where the spinal nerves exit the spinal canal. Delivery of local anesthetics creates a band of anesthesia that involves mainly the nerve roots at the levels adjacent to the epidural without blocking all the nerves inferiorly. Because the epidural space is actually a potential space, it has no important contents or structures. As such, it will easily accept not only medications but also the passage of flexible catheters through which drugs can be delivered continuously via a computer-programmed pump, which is the main advantage of this technique. Some of the benefits to epidural anesthesia include titration of the analgesic level, prolonged or continuous drug delivery, and flexible dosage schedules. Epidurals are most frequently placed for obstetric anesthesia or during peripheral vascular procedures on the lower extremities. For example, it is common for epidural catheters to be placed to help provide pain control for labor once the mother is dilated past 4 to 5 cm. Should the mother have to undergo a Caesarean section, the epidural can provide the sole anesthetic, allowing the mother to remain conscious during the procedure. An alternative technique would be placement of a spinal block prior to undergoing Caesarean section, but the downside is the inability to titrate postoperative pain control. However, in selected patients the combination of spinal and epidural techniques can be used when the advantages of both techniques are desired. The use of thoracic epidurals during invasive thoracic surgical procedures has greatly increased. The ability to selectively block the thoracic nerves and improve postoperative pain control following thoracotomies helps patients breathe much easier, preventing potential postoperative complications such as splinting, atelectasis, and pneumonia.

COMBINED GENERAL AND LOCAL ANESTHESIA

As discussed earlier, local anesthetics are versatile drugs that can serve as sole anesthetics if needed. However, it is common for anesthesiologists to combine their use with a general anesthetic technique. When used as a supplement, local anesthetics reduce and even eliminate the perception of the noxious stimuli (ie, pain) produced by the surgical procedure. This multifaceted approach helps reduce general anesthetic requirements, leading to the administration of smaller doses of systemically acting general anesthetic drugs, invariably reducing the risk of potential systemic complications and pharmacologic side effects. An example includes the placement of an upper extremity nerve block prior to general anesthesia for the repair of a humeral fracture. This technique is commonly used in dentistry, where regional anesthesia of the oral cavity is usually predictable. The method permits light general anesthesia to be administered, allowing rapid recovery and resulting in fewer adverse effects of systemically administered anesthetics.

POSTOPERATIVE ANALGESIA WITH LOCAL ANESTHETICS

In addition to serving as a sole anesthetic and a powerful adjunct to general anesthesia, local anesthetics are being increasingly used for postoperative analgesia. Local anesthetics are arguably the most effective postoperative analgesic. For example, bupivacaine is often injected subcutaneously along an incision after closure of an abdominal wound, effectively blocking any pain from the incisional site for several hours. This drug provides adequate analgesia that extends well into the immediate postoperative period, decreasing the amount of opioids required by patients in the postanesthesia care unit. High doses of opioids can cause a variety of postoperative complications ranging from nausea, vomiting, urinary retention, respiratory depression, and even respiratory arrest. By decreasing the opioid requirements with the use of local anesthetics, patients are kept comfortable with a lower risk of opioid side effects. In addition to incisional anesthesia, anesthesiologists often use peripheral techniques in combination with a small catheter and pump mechanism to provide continuous delivery of local anesthetic to the surgical area. In addition, the use of an ON-Q Pain Relief System (I-Flow Corp, Lake Forest, CA, USA) allows the patient to ambulate at home while wearing the self-contained pump system (**Fig. 3**) in a portable fanny pack. This device provides powerful pain control for several days following a surgical procedure without the patient having to remain in the hospital. It not only drastically reduces the opioid requirements for patients but also allows for

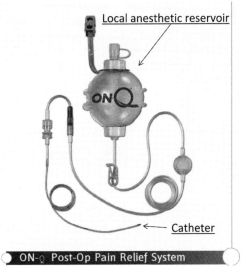

Local anesthetic reservoir

Catheter

ON-Q Post-Op Pain Relief System

Fig. 3. ON-Q Pain Relief System. (*Courtesy of* I-Flow Corp, a Kimberly-Clark Health Care company.)

a more rapid recovery period and/or early rehabilitation for orthopedic surgical patients.

SYSTEMIC USE OF LOCAL ANESTHETICS

Lidocaine has long been used intravenously as an emergency drug because of its ability to function as an arrhythmic agent. As a class Ib antiarrhythmic drug, it inhibits the opening of cardiac Na^+ channels, thus preventing the influx of Na^+ ions into conduction fibers and cardiac muscle. The intention is to cause a blockade or slowing of electrical conduction through ectopic ventricular pacemakers, thus correcting dysrhythmias such as ventricular tachycardia and preventricular contractions. Lidocaine is also used during the early phase of an acute myocardial infarction, although its outcome benefit is not clear. It has minimal effects on normal cardiac pacemakers at recommended doses, but targets rapidly firing ectopic pacemakers by using dependent block as in sensory nerves. However, once the therapeutic plasma level is surpassed, lidocaine begins causing nervous system side effects commonly resulting in parasthesias, seizures, and unconsciousness. Because lidocaine is metabolized by the liver, any patients with reduced hepatic blood flow or hepatic derangements are at particular risk for overdose.

Procainamide (Pronestyl, Procan, Procanbid) is the amide version of the ester anesthetic procaine. It is classified as a Ia antiarrhythmic drug useful for both supraventricular and ventricular arrhythmias. Hypotension and widening of the QRS complex are possible, rendering procainamide a second-line antiarrhythmic agent.

TOPICAL USE OF LOCAL ANESTHETICS

Lidocaine can be mixed with prilocaine, creating a mixture that melts very easily. This eutectic mixture of local anesthetics (with the brand name EMLA) serves as a useful topical anesthetic when applied as a cream directly to the skin and left for approximately 1 hour while covered with an adhesive dressing. Often used with pediatric patients, this technique usually provides adequate anesthesia to allow for pain-free placement of an intravenous catheter, or even a quick superficial surgical procedure.

For chronic pain management, lidocaine patches can be applied to large areas of skin surface where peripheral neuropathy has developed. These patches most commonly are used for postherpetic neuralgia that has a significant peripheral versus central component of pain transmission.

SUMMARY

Local anesthetics are some of the most versatile drugs available to medical and dental professionals. Although local anesthetics are mainly used to alleviate painful stimuli from surgical procedures, they can also be administered during specific medical emergencies. These drugs are capable of being administered by varying arrays of techniques ranging from topical to intravenous routes. Despite the almost exclusive use of amide local anesthetics in dentistry, esters remain as useful alternatives in the medical field.

REFERENCES

1. Curtis MJ, Pugsley MK. Drugs and the cardiovascular system. In: Page CP, Curtis MJ, Sutter MC, et al, editors. Integrated pharmacology. 2nd edition. New York: Mosby; 2002. p. 369–73.
2. Ries CR, Quastel DMJ. Drug use in anesthesia and critical care. In: Page CP, Curtis MJ, Sutter MC, et al, editors. Integrated pharmacology. 2nd edition. New York: Mosby; 2002. p. 356–9.
3. Faust RJ, Cucchiara RF, Rose SH, et al, editors. Anesthesiology review. 3rd edition. Philadelphia: Churchill Livingstone; 2002.
4. Morgan EG, Mikhail MS, Murray MJ, et al, editors. Clinical anesthesiology. 3rd edition. New York: McGraw-Hill; 2002.
5. Stoelting RK, Miller RD, editors. Basics of anesthesia. 4th edition. New York: Churchill Livingstone; 2000.

Long-Acting Local Anesthetics and Perioperative Pain Management

Sharon M. Gordon, DDS, MPH, PhD[a],*,
Anastasia V. Mischenko, DDS, MS[b], Raymond A. Dionne, DDS, PhD[c]

KEYWORDS

- Local anesthetics • Postoperative pain • Inflammation
- Bupivacaine • Lidocaine

Although the use of long-acting local anesthetics has become a useful therapeutic approach for managing peri- and postoperative pain, recent evidence reveals unexpected outcomes. This article reviews the clinical use of long-acting local anesthetics, presents current clinical research findings, and makes recommendations for their use.

STRATEGIES FOR PERIOPERATIVE PAIN MANAGEMENT USING LONG-ACTING LOCAL ANESTHETICS

Pharmacologic management of dental pain is accomplished through three general mechanisms: blocking the nociceptive impulse along the peripheral nerve, reducing nociceptive input from the site of injury, or attenuating the perception of pain in the central nervous system (CNS). These strategies can be combined to manage pain throughout the perioperative period.

Blocking Nociceptive Impulse

Stimulation of peripheral nerve endings and accumulation of chemical mediators both directly and indirectly activate nerve endings, resulting in pain. Input along trigeminal

This work was supported in part by a grant from the Foundation of the American Association of Endodontics.

[a] Department of Oral-Maxillofacial Surgery, Baltimore College of Dental Surgery, Dental School, University of Maryland, 650 West Baltimore Street, Room 6255, Baltimore, MD 21231, USA
[b] Department of Endodontics, Prosthodontics, and Operative Dentistry, Baltimore College of Dental Surgery, Dental School, University of Maryland, 650 West Baltimore Street, Room 4221, Baltimore, MD 21231, USA
[c] National Institute of Nursing Research, National Institutes of Health, 10 Center Drive, Room 2-1339, Rockville, MD 20892, USA
* Corresponding author.
E-mail address: sgordon@umaryland.edu

nerve pathways is routinely blocked for dental procedures by administering a local anesthetic in the vicinity of the nerve. The duration of pulpal anesthesia of local anesthetic agents such as lidocaine and articaine with epinephrine is from 1 to 2 hours after injection. If the procedure has initiated the cytokine cascade leading to inflammation, the offset of local anesthesia coincides with peak release of pain mediators such as prostaglandins and bradykinin.[1] Administration of a long-acting local anesthetic postpones the onset of sensation and thus the perception of postoperative pain.

Reducing Nociceptive Input from the Site of Injury

Recognition that locally released mediators can activate peripheral nerve endings suggests the therapeutic potential of interfering with the release or actions of these mediators. For example, cytokines and inflammatory mediators such as prostaglandin (PGE_2) not only directly signal peripheral nerve endings, they also instigate other inflammatory mediators such as bradykinin to directly activate peripheral nociceptors. Both the direct effects of PGE_2 to signal pain and its ability to magnify the response to other inflammatory mediators intensifies pain sensations.[2] Therefore, drugs that block PGE_2 synthesis or function after tissue injury are effective for reducing inflammatory pain. This information has an important practical application: pretreating patients with anti-inflammatory agents before or soon after dental surgery blocks cyclooxygenase (COX) enzymes before the initiation of tissue damage results in the synthesis of proinflammatory cytokines. This not only has immediate analgesic effects but also blocks the amplification of pain perception, which otherwise can result in increased and prolonged pain.[3–5] A well-documented strategy for blocking pain in the immediate postoperative period is the administration of anti-inflammatory drugs such as ibuprofen before or immediately after surgery, but before pain onset.[6]

Attenuating the Perception of Pain in the CNS

Once the nociceptive input reaches the CNS, the management of pain becomes more difficult because of the complex modulation and redundant pathways mediating transmission through the CNS. The CNS also reacts to nociceptive input with changes (called sensitization) that lead to the development of increased pain perception, called hyperalgesia, which can prolong pain and result in pain from stimuli that might otherwise not be perceived as painful. Inhibition of these processes has been demonstrated by the preventive use of anti-inflammatory drugs,[6–8] and these effects are additive if a combination of a nonsteroidal anti-inflammatory drug (NSAID) and long-acting local anesthetic is used to minimize immediate postoperative pain.[9]

LONG-ACTING LOCAL ANESTHETICS IN PERIOPERATIVE PAIN MANAGEMENT

It is necessary to maintain profound anesthesia when performing dental procedures, and many surgical procedures are lengthy, necessitating a longer duration of action. In addition to the intraoperative nociceptive barrage during the procedure, postoperative pain is a common occurrence following surgical dental procedures due to the resulting tissue injury leading to the release of proinflammatory mediators, cytokine signaling, and inflammatory cell infiltrate. Pain from the surgical incision and tissue manipulation occurs immediately, but gives way to inflammatory pain following inflammatory cell recruitment to the injured area over the course of several hours. Among the multitude of mediators involved in the acute phase response, proinflammatory cytokines such as tumor necrosis factor alpha (TNF-α) and interleukins (IL-1 β, IL-6, IL-8, and others) are known to play a key role in the inflammatory cascade.[10] It is also well documented that inflammatory mediators increase at the site of tissue injury after dental surgical procedures.[1,2] Increased expression of proinflammatory cytokines and induction of COX-2, which results in increased prostanoid production 2 to 4 hours after surgery contribute to sensitization, resulting in prolongation of pain.[2,10]

Pain from surgical treatments arises early in the postoperative period.[11] The pain following endodontic surgical root canal therapy usually reaches its highest peak on the day of surgery after the local anesthesia dissipates,[11,12] with abatement within 2 to 3 days.[13–15] Pain from periodontal surgery varies, with mucosal versus osseous procedures having less versus more pain, respectively.[16,17] Although pain experience after dental surgery is of relatively short duration compared with other surgical procedures, it can have a negative impact on patients' function and quality of life and negatively affect the perception of dental treatment.[18] Inadequate pain control also leads to prolonged recovery time and poorer patient outcomes.[4] Hence, effective management of postoperative pain is of utmost importance. Long-acting local anesthetics have been recommended for use in the perioperative period, as they are comparable in onset and efficacy to lidocaine, but because of their longer duration, attenuate pain for hours after the procedure, when acute pain is most intense.[12,19,20]

Several studies have indicated that administration of long-acting local anesthetics given either before or immediately following surgery can inhibit central sensitization leading to diminution of postoperative pain.[14–16] Of the long-acting local anesthetics that have been marketed in the United States (ropivacaine, etidocaine, and bupivacaine) currently only bupivacaine is available for use in dental cartridges. Ropivacaine is a relatively new amide agent and is used primarily for epidural blocks. A few studies have demonstrated its efficacy for dental procedures,[21–24] but it is not used routinely in dental practice because of lack of availability in dental cartridges. Similarly, etidocaine is no longer marketed in the United States.

Bupivacaine

Bupivacaine hydrochloride (1-butyl-2', 6'-pipeloloxylidide hydrochloride) is a long-acting local anesthetic similar in structure to mepivacaine. It is commercially available as Marcaine (Kodak [Eastman Kodak, Rochester, NY, USA]), and it is formulated in concentrations of 0.25%, 0.5%, and 0.75% with or without epinephrine 1:200,000. The 0.5% concentration of bupivacaine with 1:200,000 epinephrine is available in dental cartridges and is the long-acting local anesthetic most commonly used in dentistry.[25]

The pH of the solution depends on the vasoconstrictor. Bupivacaine solution without epinephrine has a pH of 6.0 to 6.5; with epinephrine, it has a pH of 3.5. Because of its increased lipid solubility and neuronal protein binding, bupivacaine induces local anesthesia lasting 2.5 to 3 times longer than lidocaine.[13,19,20] Lidocaine 2% with 1:100,000 epinephrine is a common anesthetic used in dental procedures and is regarded as a standard to which other local anesthetics are compared. When compared with lidocaine, bupivacaine has a relative potency value of approximately 4, meaning that 0.5% solution of bupivacaine is as effective in blocking nerve conduction as 2.0% solution of lidocaine.[26]

Because of its long-lasting effects, bupivacaine is frequently used for dental surgical procedures of long duration, or where inflammation and pain are expected postoperatively. A clinical practice to delay the onset of pain is the injection of bupivacaine at the end of the surgical procedure that was performed with 2% lidocaine with 1:100,000 epinephrine. Lidocaine is often employed to obtain anesthesia for the surgical procedure because of a significant lag in bupivacaine's onset time seen in some patients, a product of bupivacaine's slightly higher pKa. It has been shown that when bupivacaine is used at the end of a mandibular periodontal surgical procedure, it provides a significantly greater duration of anesthesia, a reduction in postoperative pain, and a decrease in the amount of opioid analgesics taken compared with the postoperative administration of lidocaine.[27] In the oral surgery model, a reduction in pain in the immediate postoperative period and a decrease in analgesic requirements were demonstrated when 0.5% bupivacaine was injected postoperatively in combination with general anesthesia, with an effect up to 48 hours.[14,15]

Local anesthetics block the generation and the conduction of nerve impulses by increasing the threshold for electrical excitation in the nerve, thus slowing or eliminating the propagation of the nerve impulse and reducing the rate of rise of the action potential. The efficacy, onset time, and duration of both bupivacaine and lidocaine have been well described for various clinical applications, as summarized in **Table 1**. After injection of bupivacaine for peripheral nerve block in people, peak blood levels of bupivacaine are reached in 30 to 45 minutes, with a half-life of 2.7 hours and an anesthetic duration of up to 7 hours depending on injection type.[26]

EMERGING EVIDENCE FOR BUPIVACAINE'S MOLECULAR MECHANISMS

Although local anesthetics have been used widely for decades, the interaction of local anesthetics with cellular function is a more recent focus of study. Local anesthetics have been shown to impede cellular proliferation.[28] Reports of lidocaine cellular toxicity are conflicting, however, with some studies showing cellular toxicity,[28] proliferation,[29] or wound healing,[30] and others showing no inflammatory[31,32] or an anti-inflammatory effect.[33] In particular, the toxic effects of bupivacaine are gaining recognition. In cell culture, the proliferation of tendon cells over a several-day period was reduced in a dose-dependant manner by a single exposure to bupivacaine, and collagen and glycosaminoglycan production were lower for all concentrations of bupivacaine compared with saline control.[34] Similarly, even brief exposure (15 minutes) of chondrocytes to 0.5% bupivacaine has been found to be cytotoxic,[35] and chondrocyte viability in human articular cartilage explants was reduced significantly by bupivacaine, but not ropivacaine or saline control after 30 minutes of exposure.[36,37]

Similarly, in animal studies, infusion of bupivacaine into the hip joint induced chondrolysis[38] and also has been shown to be myotoxic.[39–41] Neurotoxicity of local anesthetics additionally has been demonstrated in basic studies.[42,43] The neurotoxicity of local anesthetics, and in particular bupivacaine, mainly has been attributed to systemic exposure, and is greater for the marketed racemic formulation of bupivacaine.[44,45] Direct neurotoxicity to neurons, however, also has been observed for local anesthetics[42–47] and may be attributable to changes in calcium homeostasis[43] rather than sodium channel blocking mechanisms.[48]

Table 1 Comparison of anesthetic characteristics between lidocaine and bupivacaine for pulpal anesthesia using infiltration and mandibular block injection			
		2% Lidocaine 1:100,000 epi	0.5% Bupivacaine 1:200,000 epi
pH		4.5 (3.3 to 5.5)	4.0 (3.3–5.5)
pKa		7.9	8.1
Onset	Infiltration	<2 min	2–10 min
	Block	2–4 min	2–10 min
Duration	Infiltration	60 min	5–6 h
	Block	90 min	5–7 h

Abbreviation: epi, epinephrine.

Bupivacaine must be acidified to remain soluble, and this may be a source of its differential toxicity compared with other local anesthetics. In an ex vivo human blood cell culture assay, clinical grade bupivacaine and lidocaine in both medical and dental formulations were compared with the irritant lipopolysaccharide (LPS) as a positive control and physiologic saline (PBS) as an unstimulated negative control. Although bupivacaine had a lower pH in both sources of local anesthetics, levels were found to be within the manufacturer's reported pH range of 3.3 to 5.5 (**Table 2**). Cell stimulation experiments were performed with the agents unadjusted for pH and also adjusted to the same pH level as bupivacaine. PGE_2 was significantly elevated by bupivacaine and LPS as compared with the lidocaine and the unstimulated group (**Fig. 1**). These findings may be due to differences in pH or a higher cytotoxicity for bupivacaine compared with lidocaine. The pH adjustment experiments, however, showed significant differences between the positive and negative controls (LPS and PBS) in both adjusted and unadjusted samples, but the inflammatory effect of LPS remained proportionately increased. Thus, these small pH differences in local anesthetics are likely not the primary contributor to the inflammation produced as measured by PGE_2.[49]

A clinical study comparing bupivacaine with lidocaine showed bupivacaine induced a proinflammatory effect, resulting in upregulation of COX-2 gene expression and increased PGE_2 production, which resulted in increased postoperative pain at 48 hours following oral surgery.[5] Others also have noted this effect for bupivacaine in the surgical setting.[50,51] In a recent study, patients undergoing surgical endodontic treatment were randomly assigned to receive via infiltration either 2% lidocaine with 1:100,000 epinephrine or 0.5% bupivacaine with 1:200,000 epinephrine as a postoperative local anesthetic. Punch biopsies were taken before and immediately after surgery and at 48 hours to detect tissue expression of enzymes, cytokines, and inflammatory mediators as analyzed by microarray. There were no significant differences in gene expression between bupivacaine and lidocaine group at baseline; however, at 48 hours, the gene for matrix metallopeptidase 1 (MMP1) was significantly upregulated in the bupivacaine group tissues. There was also a trend for patients to report more pain in the bupivacaine group at 48 hours. Thus, at 48 hours following administration, bupivacaine upregulated MMP1, a protease product of the inflammatory cascade. This increase is associated with a trend for more postoperative pain report in this group at the same time point.[52]

This and other evidence[2,53] indicate that local anesthetics modulate inflammatory responses. The mechanism of chondrotoxicity has been attributed to nitric oxide synthase-2 activity, thus exacerbating the inflammatory processes through the production of nitric oxide.[54] Furthermore, it has been shown that calcium mobilization can lead to the activation of genes responsible for prostanoid production independent of the COX pathway.[55,56] Taken together, the influence of local anesthetics on local

Table 2
Comparison of local anesthetic pH by source

		pH	
		Measured	Package Insert
Bupivacaine with epinephrine	Medical vial	3.6 ± 0.05	3.3–5.5
1:200,000	Dental cartridge	3.9 ± 0.06	
Lidocaine with epinephrine	Medical vial	4.3 ± 0.06	3.3–5.5
1:200,000	Dental cartridge	3.6 ± 0.1	

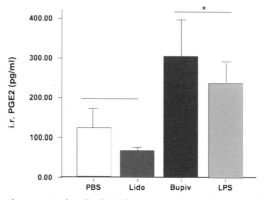

Fig. 1. Immunoreactive prostaglandin (PGE$_2$) concentrations for each of the conditions. As expected, PGE$_2$ was induced by lipopolysaccharide (LPS) at levels higher than physiologic saline (PBS) as the negative control. Lidocaine as a stimulant induced low PGE$_2$ levels similar to PBS, and these two were not significantly different. In contrast, bupivacaine induced high PGE$_2$ protein levels similar to LPS, and these two were not significantly different from each other. Both LPS and bupivacaine were statistically significant from PBS and lidocaine ($P<.001$).

tissue ion homeostasis may contribute to excitotoxicity and changes in cell signaling. In the environment of tissue injury, these processes may exacerbate the inflammatory process, leading to further tissue damage and increased pain.

Recent reports of tissue damage with prolonged intra-articular infusion of bupivacaine for management of postoperative pain focus attention on the potential for iatrogenic injury from clinical use of bupivacaine. Pain pumps used after arthroscopic joint surgery deliver controlled doses of drug directly to the joint. A study reported

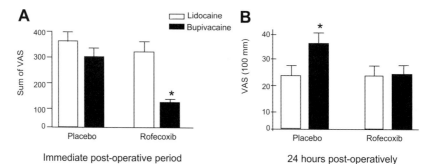

Fig. 2. (A) Sum of the pain intensity scores over the first 4 hours postoperatively for lidocaine and bupivacaine local anesthetics administered with either placebo or rofecoxib 50 mg administered an hour before surgery. where the sum of the visual analog scale (VAS) approximates the area under the curve (AUC) between 0 and 4 hours. Data are presented as mean plus or minus standard error of the mean; n = 25–31; * indicates $P<.01$ compared with the other treatment groups. (B) Pain intensity measured at 24 hours postoperatively for lidocaine and bupivacaine local anesthetics administered immediately preoperatively with either placebo or rofecoxib 50 mg administered 1 hour before surgery. Data are presented as mean plus or minus standard error of the mean; n = 25–31; * indicates $P<.05$ compared with the other treatment groups. Data at 48 hours were nearly identical and not shown.

intra-articular pain pump catheters, used most commonly with a combination of bupivacaine and epinephrine, are highly associated with postarthroscopic glenohumeral chondrolysis, leading to the US Food and Drug Administration issuing a warning stating

> "The infused local anesthetic drugs, the device materials, and/or other sources may have resulted in the development of chondrolysis."

These events have refocused attention on the local toxicity of bupivacaine and underscore the clinical applicability of the basic studies. Moreover, since bupivacaine with or without opioids is commonly used in arthroscopic surgery of the temporomandibular joint, these reports of toxicity are likely relevant to dental practice.

SUMMARY

Studies of bupivacaine for pain control have yielded conflicting results. One study found bupivacaine significantly reduced the postoperative pain experience only at 8 hours postoperatively with no effect on analgesic requirements,[55] while other studies demonstrated increased duration of analgesia up to 48 hours with reduced need for analgesic intake.[14–16] The explanation for this has been that the long duration of anesthesia due to bupivacaine diminishes postoperative pain over the first few hours and thereby reduces sensitization. More recent clinical studies,[5,51,52] however, suggest that bupivacaine also stimulates the inflammatory response, thus increasing the amount of postoperative pain at time of maximal inflammation (48 hours) in spite of decreased pain in the immediate postoperative period. Similarities between studies suggest that bupivacaine is effective for blocking pain during the surgical procedure and also conveys analgesia in the postoperative period up to 24 hours. Although pain increases between 24 and 48 hours at the point of maximal inflammation, addition of an NSAID[1,9] or COX-2 inhibitor[5] before or after surgery profoundly suppresses pain **(Fig. 2)**.

Taken together, the evidence suggests that bupivacaine instigates inflammation and exacerbates the inflammation from the tissue injury of the surgical procedure, leading to increased pain at later time points when inflammation peaks. This phenomenon, however, may be overcome by the addition of an anti-inflammatory agent. Thus, bupivacaine is useful during the intraoperative and immediate postoperative periods, and in combination with an anti-inflammatory drug, optimal perioperative pain control is achievable with minimal risk for tissue toxicity.

REFERENCES

1. Rozkowski MT, Swift JQ, Hargreaves KM, et al. Effect of NSAID administration on tissue levels of immunoreactive prostaglandin E2, leukotriene B4, and (S)-fluribiprofen following extraction of impacted third molars. Pain 1997;73:339–45.
2. Woolf CJ, Chong MS. Pre-emptive analgesia—treating postoperative pain by preventing the establishment of central sensitization. Anesth Analg 1993;77(2): 362–79.
3. Hietbrink F, Koenderman L, Rijkers G, et al. Trauma: the role of the innate immune system. World J Emerg Surg 2006;1:15.
4. Pape HC, Grimme K, Van Griensven M, et al. Impact of intramedullary instrumentation versus damage control for femoral fractures on immunoinflammatory parameters: prospective randomized analysis by the EPOFF Study Group. J Trauma 2003;55(1):7–13.

5. Gordon SM, Chuang BP, Wang XM, et al. The differential effects of bupivacaine and lidocaine on prostaglandin E2 release, cyclooxygenase gene expression and pain in a clinical pain model. Anesth Analg 2008;106(1):321–7.
6. Dionne RA, Cooper SA. Evaluation of preoperative ibuprofen on postoperative pain after impaction surgery. Oral Surg Oral Med Oral Pathol 1978;45: 851–6.
7. Kvist T, Reit C. Postoperative discomfort associated with surgical and nonsurgical endodontic retreatment. Endod Dent Traumatol 2000;16(2):71–4.
8. Seymour RA, Meechan JG, Blair GS, et al. Postoperative pain after apicoectomy. A clinical investigation. Int Endod J 1986;19(5):242–7.
9. Dionne RA, Wirdzek PR, Fox PC, et al. Suppression of postoperative pain by the combination of a nonsteroidal anti-inflammatory drug, flurbiprofen, and a long-acting local anesthetic, etidocaine. J Am Dent Assoc 1984;108:598–601.
10. Watkins LR, Maier SF, Gohler LE. Immune activation: the role of pro-inflammatory cytokines in inflammation, illness responses and pathological pain states. Pain 1995;63(3):289–302.
11. Tsesis I, Fuss Z, Lin S, et al. Analysis of postoperative symptoms following surgical endodontic treatment. Quintessence Int 2003;34(10):756–60.
12. Walton RE, Torabinejad M. Managing local anesthesia problems in the endodontic patient. J Am Dent Assoc 1992;123(5):97–102.
13. Moore PA, Dunsky JL. Bupivacaine anesthesia—a clinical trial for endodontic therapy. Oral Surg Oral Med Oral Pathol 1983;55(2):176–9.
14. Gordon SM, Brahim JS, Dubner R, et al. Attenuation of pain in a randomized trial by suppression of peripheral nociceptive activity in the immediate postoperative period. Anesth Analg 2002;95(5):1351–7.
15. Gordon SM, Dionne RA, Brahim J, et al. Blockade of peripheral neuronal barrage reduces postoperative pain. Pain 1997;70:209–15.
16. Kaurich MJ, Otomo-Corgel J, Nagy RJ, et al. Comparison of postoperative bupivacaine with lidocaine on pain and analgesic use following periodontal surgery. J West Soc Periodontol Periodontal Abstr 1997;45(1):5–8.
17. Truollos ES, Hargreaves KM, Butler DP, et al. Comparison of nonsteroidal anti-inflammatory drugs, ibuprofen and flurbiprofen, to methylprednisolone and placebo for acute pain, swelling, and trismus. J Oral Maxillofac Surg 1990;48: 945–52.
18. Gordon SM, DeFina V, Dionne RA, et al. Quality of life in patients experiencing acute and chronic pain. Presented at the Annual Meeting of the American Pain Society. Washington, DC, May, 2006.
19. Nespeca JA. Clinical trials with bupivacaine in oral surgery. Oral Surg Oral Med Oral Pathol 1976;42(3):301–7.
20. Moore PA. Bupivacaine: a long-lasting local anesthetic for dentistry. Oral Surg Oral Med Oral Pathol 1984;58(4):369–74.
21. El-Sharrawy E, Yagiela JA. Anesthetic efficacy of different ropivacaine concentrations for inferior alveolar nerve block. Anesth Prog 2006;53:3–7.
22. Kennedy M, Reader A, Beck M. Anesthetic efficacy of ropivacaine in maxillary anterior infiltration. Oral Surg Oral Med Oral Pathol Oral Radiol Endod 2001;91: 406–12.
23. Meechan JG. A comparison of ropivacaine and lidocaine with epinephrine for intraligamentary anesthesia. Oral Surg Oral Med Oral Pathol Oral Radiol Endod 2002;93:469–73.
24. Axelsson S, Isacsson G. The efficacy of ropivacaine as a dental local anaesthetic. Swed Dent J 2004;28:85–91.

25. Nahourali HS, ZorkosWisnieoski R. Dental therapeutic practice patterns in the US I: anesthesia and sedation. Gen Dent 2006;54(2):92–8.

26. Covino BG, Giddon DB. Pharmacology of local anesthetic agents. J Dent Res 1981;60(8):1454–9.

27. Curtis JW Jr, McLain JB, Hutchinson RA, et al. The incidence and severity of complications and pain following periodontal surgery. J Periodontol 1986; 57(10):637–42.

28. Matinsson T, Haegerstrand A, Dalsgard CJ, et al. Ropivacaine and lidocaine inhibit proliferation of nontransformed cultured adult human fibroblasts, endothelial cells, and keratinocytes. Agents Actions 1993;40:78–85.

29. Hirata M, Sakaguchi M, Mochida C, et al. Lidocaine inhibits tyrosine kinase activity of the epidermal growth factor receptor and suppresses proliferation of corneal epithelial cells. Anesthesiology 2004;100(5):1206–10.

30. Eriksson AS, Sinclair R. Leukocyte hydrogen peroxide production in a surgical wound in mice. The effects of an amide local aneasthetic. Inflammation 1996; 20(5):569–79.

31. Eroglu E, Eroglu F, Agalar F, et al. The effect of lidocaine/prilocaine cream on an experimental wound healing model. Eur J Emerg Med 2001;8(3):199–201.

32. Drucker M, Cardenas E, Arizti P, et al. Experimental studies on the effect of lidocaine on wound healing. World J Surg 1998;22(4):394–7.

33. Lahav M, Levite M, Bassani L, et al. Lidocaine inhibits secretion of IL-8 and IL-1beta and stimulates secretion of IL-1 receptor antagonist by epithelial cells. Clin Exp Immunol 2002;127:226–33.

34. Scherb MB, Seung-Hwan H, Coumeya JP, et al. Effect of bupivacaine on cultured tenocytes. Orthopedics 2009;32:26–30.

35. Chu CR, Izzo NJ, Papas NE, et al. In vitro exposure of 0.5% bupivacaine is cytotoxic to bovine articular chondrocytes. Arthroscopy 2006;22:693–9.

36. Pere P, Watanabe H, Pitkanen M, et al. Local myotoxicity of bupivacaine in rabbits after continuous supraclavicular brachial plexus block. Reg Anesth 1993;18: 304–7.

37. Takahashi S. Local anesthetic bupivacaine alters function of sarcolasmic reticulum and sarcolemnal vesicles from rabbit masseter muscle. Pharmacol Toxicol 1994;75:119–28.

38. Piper SL, Kim HT. Comparison of ropivacaine and bupivacaine toxicity in human articular chondrocytes. J Bone Joint Surg Am 2008;90:986–91.

39. Guttu RL, Page DG, Laskin DM, et al. Delayed healing of muscle after injection of bupivicaine and steroid. Ann Dent 1990;49(1):5–8.

40. Orimo S, Hiyamuta E, Arahata K, et al. Analysis of inflammatory cells and complement C3 in bupivacaine-induced myonecrosis. Muscle Nerve 1991;14(6):515–20.

41. Park CY, Park SE, Oh SY, et al. Acute effect of bupivacaine and ricin mAb 35 on extraocular muscle in the rabbit. Curr Eye Res 2004;29:293–301.

42. Yamashita A, Matsumoto M, Matsumoto S et al. A comparison of the neurotoxic effects on the spinal cord of tetracaine, lidocaine, bupivacaine, and ropivacaine administered intrathecally in rabbits. Anesth Analg 97:512–9.

43. Gold MS, Reichling DB, Hampl KF, et al. Lidocaine toxicity in primary afferent neurons from the rat. J Pharmacol Exp Ther 1998;285:413–21.

44. Gristwood RW. Cardiac and CNS toxicity of levobupivacaine; strengths of evidence for advantage over bupivacaine. Drug Saf 2002;25:153–63.

45. Maganella C, Bruno V, Matrisciano F, et al. Comparative effects of levobupivacaine and racemic bupivacaine on excitotoxic neuronal death in culture and N-methyl-D-aspartate-induced seizures in mice. Eur J Pharmacol 2005;518:111–5.

46. Radwan I, Aito S, Goto F, et al. The neurotoxicity of local anesthetics on growing neurons: a comparative study of lidocaine, bupivacaine, mepivacaine, and ropivacaine. Anesth Analg 2002;94:319–24.

47. Johnson ME, Saenz JA, DaSilva AD, et al. Effect of local anesthetic on neuronal cytoplasmic calcium and plasma membrane lysis (necrosis) in a cell culture model. Anesthesiology 2002;97:1466–76.

48. Sakura S, Bollen AW, Ciriales R, et al. Local anesthetic neurotoxicity does not result from blockade of voltage-gated sodium channels. Anesth Analg 1995;81: 338–46.

49. Mischenko A, Letwin N, Hicks L, et al. Comparison of bupivacaine vs lidocaine on inflammatory regulation. International Association of Dental Research. Barcelona, Spain, July, 2010.

50. Buvanendran A, Kroin JS, Berger RA, et al. Upregulation of prostaglandin E2 and interleukins in the central nervous system and peripheral tissue during and after surgery in humans. Anesthesiology 2006;104(3):403–10.

51. Kroin JS, Buvanendran A, Watts DE, et al. Upregulation of cerebrospinal fluid and peripheral prostaglandin E2 in a rat postoperative pain model. Anesth Analg 2006;103(2):334–43.

52. Mischenko A, Wills K, Letwin N, et al. Bupivacaine increases PGE2 expression in vivo. Presented at the Annual Meeting of the American Association of Endodontists. Orlando, FL, April, 2009.

53. Chiang N, Schwab JM, Fredman G, et al. Anesthetics impact the resolution of inflammation. PLoS One 2008;3(4):e1879.

54. Gomoll AH, Kang RW, Wiliams JM, et al. Chondrolysis after continuous intra-articular bupivacaine infusion: an experimental model investigating chondrotoxicity in the rabbit shoulder. Arthroscopy 2006;22(8):813–9.

55. Bouloux GF, Punnia-Moorthy A. Bupivacaine versus lidocaine for third molar surgery: a double-blind, randomized, crossover study. J Oral Maxillofac Surg 1999;57(5):510–4 [discussion: 515].

56. Feinstein DL, Murphy P, Sharp A, et al. Local anesthetics potentiate nitric oxide synthase type 2 expression in rat glial cells. J Neurosurg Anesthesiol 2001;13: 99–105.

Infiltration Anesthesia in the Mandible

John G. Meechan, BDS, PhD, FDSRCS, FDSRCPS

KEYWORDS

- Infiltration anesthesia • Mandible • Regional block techniques
- Pulpal anesthesia

The gold-standard method of anesthetizing teeth in the lower jaw is by one of the regional block techniques, such as the Halstead, Gow-Gates,[1] or Akinosi[2] methods. An alternative is the mental and incisive nerve block. Regional blocks have several potential disadvantages when compared with infiltration anesthesia. The advantages of infiltration anesthesia are listed in **Box 1**. In addition, the complications of local anesthesia, such as intravascular injection and nerve damage, are principally associated with regional block techniques. This association is not surprising because blood vessels are more likely to be associated with nerve trunks and deeper injections. Similarly, nerve trunks are more often damaged either by physical or chemical agents during regional block techniques. Another factor to consider is the finding that injections, such as inferior alveolar nerve blocks, are not equally successful for all teeth. The most susceptible are the premolars followed by the molars and then the mandibular anterior teeth (**Fig. 1**).[3,4] This susceptibility may be the result of an inability to counter collateral nerve supply, as may happen in the midline where structures receive bilateral nerve supply.

Of course, techniques, such as periodontal ligament (intraligamentary), intraosseous, and intrapulpal methods, may be used in the mandible; however, these are generally considered to be supplementary methods.[5] These methods also have complications that are best avoided. Intraligamentary anesthesia produces damage to the tooth root, periodontium, and alveolar bone,[6,7] although in the main these are reversible. It was previously mentioned that teeth vary in their susceptibility to inferior alveolar nerve blocks. A similar state of affairs exists with periodontal ligament anesthesia; lower incisor teeth are the most difficult to anesthetize with this method,[8,9] probably as the result of few perforations in the cribriform plate of the dental socket in this region.[8] This paucity of perforations inhibits the flow of solution from the periodontal ligament into the cancellous bone. Intraosseous anesthesia can cause

School of Dental Sciences, Newcastle University, Framlington Place, Newcastle Upon Tyne, England NE2 4BW, UK
E-mail address: j.g.meechan@newcastle.ac.uk

Dent Clin N Am 54 (2010) 621–629
doi:10.1016/j.cden.2010.06.003
0011-8532/10/$ – see front matter © 2010 Elsevier Inc. All rights reserved.

> **Box 1**
> **Advantages of infiltration anesthesia compared to regional block**
>
> - Technically simple
> - More comfortable for patients
> - Provides hemostasis where it is needed
> - Counters collateral supply in many cases
> - Avoids damage to nerve trunks
> - Less chance of intravascular injection
> - Safer in patients with bleeding diatheses
> - Reduced chances of needle stick injury
> - Preinjection topical masks needle penetration discomfort

systemic effects because this route is analogous to the intravenous delivery in relation to entry of local anesthetic and vasoconstrictor into the circulation.[10] In addition, it is possible to produce physical damage to tooth roots during intraosseous anesthesia.[11] Intrapulpal anesthesia has obvious limited indications.

INFILTRATION ANESTHESIA

Infiltration anesthesia is the technique of choice in the upper jaw. It provides pulpal anesthesia by diffusion into the cancellous bone via the thin cortical plate of the maxillary alveolus. The thicker cortical plate of the mandible is considered to be a barrier to such diffusion in the lower jaw. Nevertheless a thick cortical plate is not always a barrier to local anesthetic diffusion. Evidence of this is the efficacy of the anterior middle superior alveolar (AMSA) technique in the palate where solution is deposited in the mucosa of the hard palate in the mid-premolar region halfway between the gingival margin and the midline.[12] This technique can provide anesthesia of the pulps of the maxillary premolar, canine, and incisor teeth. The solution gains access to the

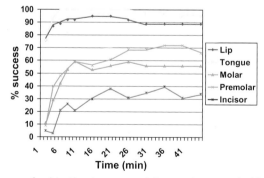

Fig. 1. The incidences of subjective tongue and lip numbness and objective pulpal anesthesia of first molar, first premolar, and lateral incisor teeth after the injection of 2.0 mL of 2% lidocaine with 1:80,000 epinephrine as an inferior alveolar nerve block. The premolar is the most readily anesthetized of the teeth; the lateral incisor shows the poorest efficacy. (*Data from* Kanaa MD, Meechan JG, Corbett IP, et al. Efficacy and discomfort associated with slow and rapid inferior alveolar nerve block injection. J Endodont 2006;32:919–23.)

cancellous space via perforations in the palatal bone. The mandibular cortex has perforations. The mandibular and mental foramina are obvious examples; however, other holes are present especially in the lingual aspect of the incisor region. Regional block techniques, such as the infraorbital and maxillary nerve blocks, can be used but infiltration is preferred in the maxilla because it is simple and effective. Thus it seems reasonable to assume that where both infiltration and regional blocks are effective the former is preferred. In addition to being a technically simple procedure, two major advantages that infiltration anesthesia provides are the countering of collateral supply and the provision of localized hemostasis.

INFILTRATION ANESTHESIA IN THE MANDIBLE

Infiltration may be used in the mandible either to supplement other methods, such as regional block anesthesia, or as a primary technique.

Infiltration as a Supplementary Technique in the Mandible

Several studies have looked at the use of mandibular infiltration as a means of supplementing inferior alveolar nerve block injections. In an investigation of 331 subjects having regional block anesthesia in the mandible, Rood[13] recorded 79 failures of pulpal anesthesia. This author used infiltration of 2% lidocaine with 1:80,000 epinephrine to overcome failure in these 79 individuals. A supplemental infiltration of 1.0 mL on the buccal aspect resulted in successful anesthesia in 70 of the 79 subjects. Seven of the other 9 subjects achieved successful anesthesia following further infiltration on the lingual aspect.

Haase and colleagues[14] compared the effect of a supplemental infiltration of 1.8 mL of either 2% lidocaine or 4% articaine both with 1:100,000 epinephrine in the buccal sulcus in the mandibular first molar region on the efficacy of an inferior alveolar block with 4% articaine and 1:100,000 epinephrine. Using a double-blind, randomized crossover design these investigators reported that the articaine supplemental infiltration significantly increased anesthetic efficacy for the mandibular first molar compared with the lidocaine infiltration (88% vs 71% anesthetic success, respectively).

In a similar investigation, Kanaa and colleagues[15] looked at the effect of a supplemental infiltration of 1.8 mL of 4% articaine with 1:100,000 epinephrine in the buccal sulcus in the mandibular first molar region on the success of an inferior alveolar nerve block of 2% lidocaine with 1:80,000 epinephrine in a randomized, double-blind crossover investigation. These investigators noted an increase in the incidence of pulpal anesthesia in mandibular teeth following the supplementary articaine infiltration compared with a dummy infiltration (needle penetration only) in the same region (92% and 56% anesthetic success for first molar anesthesia, respectively). In this last study the significant increase in efficacy was apparent not only in the first molar (where the infiltration was performed) but also in the first premolar and lateral incisor teeth. In the premolar teeth the supplementary articaine infiltration produced a success rate of 89% compared with 67% for the inferior alveolar nerve block alone; for the lateral incisor the success rates were 78% after the supplementary infiltration compared with 19% with the regional block alone. This finding demonstrates an effect on the nerve trunk within the inferior alveolar canal and not merely diffusion through to the apices of the first molar tooth. Whether this is the result of direct diffusion into the canal at the site of injection or spread along to the mental foramen and entry at that point is not possible to determine, but this is being investigated in another trial, unpublished at the time of writing.

Matthews and colleagues[16] investigated the efficacy of a buccal infiltration of 1.8 mL of 4% articaine with 1:100,000 epinephrine in pulpitic teeth that had failed to succumb to an inferior alveolar nerve block. The supplemental injection allowed pain-free treatment in 57% of the subjects in whom the original block failed. The investigators state that this modest rate of success means that a buccal infiltration of 4% articaine with 1:100,000 epinephrine cannot be guaranteed to provide anesthesia in teeth with pulpitis.

Rosenberg and colleagues[17] also looked at the use of supplementary buccal injections of either 4% articaine or 2% lidocaine (both with 1:100,000 epinephrine) to overcome failed inferior alveolar nerve blocks in subjects suffering from irreversible pulpitis. These investigators measured pain scores at various points throughout treatment and found no significant difference in the change in pain scores between the two supplemental solutions.

Similarly, Aggarwal and colleagues[18] looked at the use of supplemental infiltrations to improve the efficacy of inferior alveolar nerve block injections in subjects with irreversible pulpitis. Inferior alveolar nerve block alone was successful in 33% of subjects; a supplemental buccal and lingual infiltration of 2% lidocaine with 1:200,000 epinephrine increased success to 47%; and similar supplemental buccal and lingual infiltrations with 4% articaine containing 1:200,000 epinephrine was successful in 67% of cases, which was significantly better than the lidocaine infiltrations.

Fan and colleagues[19] compared the intraligamentary injection of 0.4 mL of 4% articaine with 1:100,000 epinephrine with a buccal infiltration of the same dose of this solution as supplementary injections following an inferior alveolar nerve block in subjects suffering from irreversible pulpitis in the mandibular first molar. Both methods produced similar success rates (83% and 81%, respectively).

Infiltration as a Primary Technique in the Mandible

The use of infiltration anesthesia as a primary technique for anesthesia of the mandibular teeth has been investigated. Some studies have reported infiltration to be effective for many treatments in the mandibular deciduous dentition.[20,21] The following discussion relates solely to the use of mandibular infiltration techniques for the permanent dentition in adults.

Incisor and canine region

It was previously mentioned that both regional block anesthesia and intraligamentary anesthesia were poor in providing anesthesia of the pulps of the mandibular incisor teeth. In this region the cortex is quite thin and might provide little resistance to infiltration. Three investigations have looked at the success of infiltration anesthesia for mandibular incisor teeth. Yonchak and colleagues[22] compared the efficacies of 1.8 mL of 2% lidocaine with 1:50,000 or 1:100,000 epinephrine injected buccally to the lower lateral incisor for anesthesia of the ipsilateral canine and the lateral and central incisors. They noted no difference in anesthetic efficacy between solutions and recorded successes in the range of 47% to 53% for the canine, 43% to 45% for the lateral incisor, and 60% to 63% for the central incisor. In addition, these investigators looked at the success of injection of 1.8 mL of the 1:100,000 preparation lingually to the lower lateral incisor and recorded 11% success for the canine, 50% for the lateral, and 47% for the central incisor. Meechan and Ledvinka[9] performed a similar investigation with 1.0 mL of 2% lidocaine containing 1:80,000 epinephrine and obtained 50% successful anesthesia of the mandibular central incisor when the local anesthetic was injected either buccally or lingually to the test tooth. In this last study, the success was increased to 92% when the dose of anesthetic was split between the buccal and lingual sides. A further randomized, double-blind crossover study comparing buccal versus buccal and lingual split dosing of 1.8 mL of 2% lidocaine with 1:100,000 epinephrine by Jaber and colleagues[23] confirmed the finding that the latter technique improved the efficacy of anesthesia for the lower central incisor tooth. In this last study, which used a larger dose than that employed by Meechan and Ledvinka,[9] the injection of 1.8 mL 2% lidocaine with 1:100,000 epinephrine provided successful anesthesia in 77% of volunteers after the buccal infiltration and 97% after the split buccal/lingual dose. This study also compared the use of 4% articaine to 2% lidocaine (both with 1:100,000 epinephrine) as an anesthetic for infiltration anesthesia in the anterior mandible. These investigators reported that 4% articaine was superior to 2% lidocaine in obtaining anesthesia of the pulps of the mandibular central incisor adjacent to the injection site and the contralateral lateral incisor following both buccal or buccal and lingual infiltrations. The success rate after articaine as a buccal injection was 94% at the lower central incisor and after the split buccal and lingual technique success for this tooth was 97%. For the contralateral lateral incisor the success rates with articaine were 61% as a buccal injection and 74% after the split buccal and lingual infiltrations compared with 36% and 42% with lidocaine.

Haas and colleagues[24,25] compared the buccal infiltration of 4% articaine and 4% prilocaine for anesthesia of mandibular canine teeth and reported no significant difference in efficacy. The success rates these investigators noted were 65% for articaine and 50% for prilocaine.

Fig. 2 shows the efficacies of different methods of anesthesia for mandibular incisor teeth using no response to maximum stimulation from an analytical pulp tester as the criterion for success in similar populations.[4,23,26] It can be seen from this graph that infiltration appears to be the method of choice for anesthesia of the mandibular incisors.

Molar region

Some of the studies previously cited suggested that the success of mandibular infiltration anesthesia was dependent upon the choice of anesthetic solution. Jaber and colleagues[23] showed that 4% articaine with 1:100,000 epinephrine was more successful than 2% lidocaine with 1:100,000 epinephrine in obtaining pulpal anesthesia of mandibular incisor teeth after infiltration. Similarly, Haase and colleagues[14]

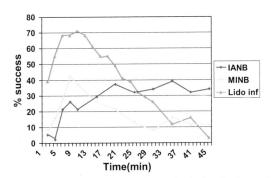

Fig. 2. The success of different methods of local anesthesia for the lower incisor teeth when using 2% lidocaine with epinephrine. Infiltration appears to be the method of choice. IANB, inferior alveolar nerve block; Lido Inf, buccal infiltration; MINB, mental and incisive nerve block. (*Data from* Refs.[4,23,26])

showed that 4% articaine with 1:100,000 epinephrine was more successful than 2% lidocaine with 1:100,000 in supplementing an inferior alveolar nerve block for mandibular first molar anesthesia. In addition, the studies of Meechan and Ledvinka[9] and Jaber and colleagues[23] suggested that the splitting of a dose between buccal and lingual infiltrations was more effective than either buccal or lingual alone. The influence of different local anesthetic solutions and dose splitting for mandibular first molar anesthesia following infiltrations in the mandible has been investigated in several studies.

Kanaa and colleagues[27] compared the infiltration of 1.8 mL of 2% lidocaine or 4% articaine (both with 1:100,000 epinephrine) for pulpal anesthesia of mandibular first molar teeth in a randomized, double-blind crossover volunteer study. These workers noted significantly greater efficacy for the articaine (64% success) compared with the lidocaine (39% success) solution. In an almost identical study, Robertson and colleagues[28] reported similar findings, again noting superior efficacy with the more concentrated solution. These investigators noted anesthesia was successful in 87% of volunteers when 4% articaine was injected compared with 57% success with 2% lidocaine. Similarly, Abdulwahab and colleagues[29] noted that 4% articaine with 1:100,000 epinephrine was more successful than 2% lidocaine with 1:100,000 epinephrine for pulpal anesthesia when infiltrated in the buccal sulcus in the mandibular first molar region. These last investigators reported success rates for first molar anesthesia of 39% with the articaine solution compared with 17% with lidocaine. Their success was lower than those of Kanaa and colleagues[27] and Robertson and colleagues,[28] probably because a smaller volume (0.9 mL) was used. It is not clear whether or not these results represent a greater inherent ability of articaine to diffuse through bone or simply reflect the use of a more concentrated anesthetic solution. It is apt, however, to point out that no significant differences were noted in the comparison of two different anesthetics (articaine and prilocaine) at the same concentration performed by Haas and colleagues.[24,25]

Meechan and colleagues[30] compared the effect of splitting a 1.8 mL dose of 2% lidocaine with epinephrine between buccal and lingual infiltrations to a buccal dose only and noted no difference in the incidence or pattern of pulpal anesthesia in mandibular first molar teeth (32% vs 39%, respectively). Similarly, Corbett and colleagues[31] compared splitting a 1.8 mL dose of 4% articaine between buccal and lingual sides and found no benefit compared with the same dose injected on the buccal side only for pulpal anesthesia of mandibular first molars (68% vs 65% rates of successful anesthesia, respectively). Thus, contrary to the case with mandibular incisor anesthesia, there appears to be no benefit in splitting a dose between buccal and lingual sides in the mandibular first molar region. Whether or not that is the case for teeth more posteriorly positioned in the mandible, where the apices approximate the lingual side, has not been determined and is worthy of investigation.

Comparisons of Infiltration and Regional Nerve Blocks

Two human, healthy-volunteer investigations have compared the efficacies of inferior alveolar nerve blocks to mandibular buccal infiltrations of 4% articaine with epinephrine for pulpal anesthesia of mandibular first molars. Jung and colleagues[32] compared the buccal infiltration of 1.7 mL of 4% articaine with 1:100,000 epinephrine to an inferior alveolar nerve block with the same volume of the same solution and reported no significant difference in success between methods; success rates for first mandibular molars were 54% and 43%, respectively. These investigators noted that onset of anesthesia was quicker following the infiltration technique. Corbett and colleagues[31] compared the infiltration of 1.8 mL of 4% articaine with 1:100,000 epinephrine to an inferior alveolar nerve block of 2.0 mL of 2% lidocaine with 1:80,000 epinephrine and, like Jung and colleagues,[32] noted no difference in success between regimens (70% and 56%, respectively). These last investigators noted no significant difference in onset time of anesthesia between methods.

SUMMARY

Infiltration is the method of choice in the mandibular incisor region.

Infiltration anesthesia can produce pulpal anesthesia for adult dentition teeth in the mandible in some volunteers.

Four percent articaine with epinephrine is superior to 2% lidocaine with epinephrine for infiltration techniques in the mandible in healthy volunteers.

Splitting an anesthetic dose between the buccal and lingual sides improves pulpal anesthesia in mandibular incisor teeth compared with buccal injection alone.

There is no advantage to splitting the dose between buccal and lingual sides in the first molar region.

A supplemental buccal infiltration of 4% articaine increases the efficacy of an inferior alveolar nerve block in volunteers.

Supplemental buccal infiltration has a modest effect on increasing the efficacy of inferior alveolar nerve blocks in patients with irreversible pulpitis.

The buccal infiltration of 4% articaine with epinephrine is as effective as an inferior alveolar block with the same solution or 2% lidocaine with epinephrine for mandibular first molar pulpal anesthesia in some volunteers.

REFERENCES

1. Gow-Gates GA. Mandibular conduction anaesthesia: a new technique using extraoral landmarks. Oral Surg Oral Med Oral Pathol 1973;36:321–8.
2. Akinosi JO. A new approach to the mandibular nerve block. Br J Oral Surg 1977; 15:83–7.
3. Hinkley SA, Reader A, Beck M, et al. An evaluation of 4% prilocaine with 1:200,000 epinephrine and 2% mepivacaine with 1:20,000 levonordefrin compared to 2% lidocaine with 1:100,000 epinephrine for inferior alveolar nerve block. Anesth Prog 1991;38:84–9.
4. Kanaa MD, Meechan JG, Corbett IP, et al. Efficacy and discomfort associated with slow and rapid inferior alveolar nerve block injection. J Endod 2006;32: 919–23.
5. Meechan JG. Supplementary routes to local anaesthesia. Int Endod J 2002;35: 885–96.
6. Brannstrom M, Nordenvall K-J, Hedstrom KG. Periodontal tissue changes after intraligamentary anaesthesia. ASDC J Dent Child 1982;49:417–23.
7. Walton RE, Garnick JJ. The periodontal ligament injection: histologic effects on the periodontium in monkeys. J Endod 1982;8:22–6.
8. White JJ, Reader A, Beck M, et al. The periodontal ligament injection: a comparison of the efficacy in human maxillary and mandibular teeth. J Endod 1988;14: 508–14.
9. Meechan JG, Ledvinka JI. Pulpal anaesthesia for mandibular central incisor teeth: a comparison of infiltration and intraligamentary injections. Int Endod J 2002;35:629–34.
10. Lilienthal B, Reynolds AK. Cardiovascular responses to intraosseous injections containing catecholamines. Oral Surg Oral Med Oral Pathol 1975;40:574–83.

11. Coggins R, Reader A, Nist R, et al. Anesthetic efficacy of the intraosseous injection in maxillary and mandibular teeth. Oral Surg Oral Med Oral Pathol 1996;81: 634–41.

12. Friedman MJ, Hochman MN. The AMSA injection: a new concept for local anesthesia of maxillary teeth using a computer-controlled injection system. Quintessence Int 1998;29:297–303.

13. Rood JP. The analgesia and innervation of mandibular teeth. Br Dent J 1976;140: 237–9.

14. Haase A, Reader A, Nusstein J, et al. Comparing anesthetic efficacy of articaine versus lidocaine as a supplemental buccal infiltration of the mandibular first molar after an inferior alveolar nerve block. J Am Dent Assoc 2008;139:1228–35.

15. Kanaa MD, Whitworth JM, Corbett IP, et al. Articaine buccal infiltration enhances the effectiveness of lidocaine inferior alveolar nerve block. Int Endod J 2009;42: 238–46.

16. Matthews R, Drum M, Reader A, et al. Articaine for supplemental buccal mandibular infiltration anesthesia in patients with irreversible pulpitis when the inferior alveolar nerve block fails. J Endod 2009;35:343–6.

17. Rosenberg PA, Amin KG, Zibari Y, et al. Comparison of 4% articaine with 1:100,000 epinephrine and 2% lidocaine with 1:100,000 epinephrine when used as a supplemental anesthetic. J Endod 2007;33:403–5.

18. Aggarwal V, Jain A, Kabi D. Anesthetic efficacy of supplemental buccal and lingual infiltrations of articaine and lidocaine after an inferior alveolar nerve block in patients with irreversible pulpitis. J Endod 2009;35:925–9.

19. Fan S, Chen W, Pan C, et al. Anesthetic efficacy of inferior alveolar nerve block plus buccal infiltration or periodontal ligament injections with articaine in patients with irreversible pulpitis in the mandibular first molar. Oral Surg Oral Med Oral Pathol Oral Radiol Endod 2009;108(5):e89–93.

20. Oulis CJ, Vadiakis GP, Vasilopoulou A. The effectiveness of mandibular infiltration compared to mandibular block anesthesia in treating primary molars in children. Pediatr Dent 1996;18:301–5.

21. Sharaf AA. Evaluation of mandibular infiltration versus block anesthesia in pediatric dentistry. ASDC J Dent Child 1997;64:276–81.

22. Yonchak T, Reader A, Beck M, et al. Anesthetic efficacy of infiltrations in mandibular anterior teeth. Anesth Prog 2001;48:55–60.

23. Jaber A, Al-Baqshi B, Whitworth J, et al. The efficacy of infiltration anesthesia for adult mandibular incisors. J Dent Res 2009;88. Special issue A, [abstract 702].

24. Haas DA, Harper DG, Saso MA, et al. Comparison of articaine and prilocaine anesthesia by infiltration in maxillary and mandibular arches. Anesth Prog 1990;37:230–7.

25. Haas DA, Harper DG, Saso MA, et al. Lack of differential effect by Ultracaine (articaine) and Citanest (prilocaine) in infiltration anaesthesia. J Can Dent Assoc 1991;57:217–23.

26. Whitworth JM, Kanaa MD, Corbett IP, et al. Influence of injection speed on the effectiveness of incisive/mental nerve block: a randomised controlled double blind study in adult volunteers. J Endod 2007;33:1149–54.

27. Kanaa MD, Whitworth JM, Corbett IP, et al. Articaine and lidocaine mandibular buccal infiltration anesthesia: a prospective randomised double-blind cross-over study. J Endod 2006;32:919–23.

28. Robertson D, Nusstein J, Reader A, et al. The anesthetic efficacy of articaine in buccal infiltration of mandibular posterior teeth. J Am Dent Assoc 2007;138: 1104–12.

29. Abdulwahab MN, Boynes SG, Moore PA, et al. The efficacy of six local anesthetic formulations used for posterior mandibular buccal infiltration anesthesia. J Am Dent Assoc 2009;140:1018–24.
30. Meechan JG, Kanaa MD, Corbett IP, et al. Pulpal anaesthesia for mandibular permanent first molar teeth: a comparison of buccal and buccal plus lingual infiltration injections. Int Endod J 2006;39:764–9.
31. Corbett IP, Kanaa MD, Whitworth JM, et al. Articaine infiltration for anesthesia of mandibular first molars. J Endod 2008;34:514–8.
32. Jung I-Y, Kim J-H, Kim E-S, et al. An evaluation of buccal infiltrations and inferior alveolar nerve blocks in pulpal anesthesia for mandibular first molars. J Endod 2008;34:11–3.

Phentolamine Mesylate for Accelerating Recovery from Lip and Tongue Anesthesia

Elliot V. Hersh, DMD, MS, PhD[a,b,]*, Rochelle G. Lindemeyer, DMD[c]

KEYWORDS

- Phentolamine mesylate • Dental local anesthesia • Epinephrine
- Levonordefrin • Lip and tongue numbness
- Local anesthetic reversal

Phentolamine mesylate, marketed under the proprietary name OraVerse, was granted Food and Drug Administration (FDA) approval on May 12, 2008 with an indication for the reversal of soft tissue anesthesia (lip and tongue numbness) and the associated functional deficits resulting from a local dental anesthetic containing a vasoconstrictor.[1,2] This approved FDA indication does not include the use of this drug in children younger than 6 years or weighing less than 15 kg (33 lb) because of a lack of research in this younger age group.[1] Phentolamine was originally developed for the treatment of hypertension and is still used off-label to treat hypertensive crises (characterized by catecholamine excess) by administering an intravenous bolus dose of 5 to 15 mg.[3] Such hypertensive emergencies include drug (indirect sympathomimetics such as pseudoephedrine) and food interactions (those containing tyramine) with monoamine oxidase inhibitors, cocaine toxicity, and amphetamine overdose.[4,5] The

Disclosure: Dr Hersh is a member of the Clinical Advisory Board of Novalar Pharmaceuticals, the manufacturer of OraVerse. Novalar has also partially sponsored several continuing education courses that Dr Hersh has presented.

[a] Department of Oral Surgery and Pharmacology, University of Pennsylvania School of Dental Medicine, 240 South 40th Street, Philadelphia, PA 19104-6030, USA

[b] Office of Regulatory Affairs, University of Pennsylvania, 240 South 40th Street, Philadelphia, PA 19104-6030, USA

[c] Department of Preventive and Restorative Sciences, University of Pennsylvania School of Dental Medicine, 240 South 40th Street, Philadelphia, PA 19104 6030, USA

* Corresponding author. Department of Oral Surgery and Pharmacology, University of Pennsylvania School of Dental Medicine, 240 South 40th Street, Philadelphia, PA 19104-6030.

E-mail address: evhersh@pobox.upenn.edu

current FDA-approved intravenous and intramuscular formulation of phentolamine is indicated for the prevention and treatment of dermal necrosis resulting from the venous extravasation of the vasoconstrictor norepinephrine (which is used as a pressor agent in patients with severe hypotension) and for the diagnosis and treatment of severe hypertension in patients with pheochromocytoma (a rare tumor of the adrenal medulla that secretes excessive epinephrine and norepinephrine).[5,6] Recommended intravenous and intramuscular dosages are 5 to 10 mg in adults and 1 to 3 mg in children.[6] For dental local anesthetic reversal, the drug is packaged in a standard dental cartridge containing only 0.4 mg phentolamine mesylate in 1.7 mL of solution and is injected submucosally at the end of the dental procedure using the same location, volume, and injection technique as the previous local anesthetic injection.[1]

QUALITY-OF-LIFE ISSUES REGARDING LINGERING SOFT TISSUE ANESTHESIA IN DENTAL PATIENTS

One of the shortcomings of dental local anesthetic agents, especially those used for routine restorative and scaling procedures that produce minimal postprocedural pain and are usually completed in less than an hour, is that the duration of soft tissue anesthesia (numbness to the lip and tongue) typically lasts for 3 to 5 hours.[7,8] With mandibular block injections, lip anesthesia tends to persist longer than tongue anesthesia.[7,9]

In adult dental patients, the major complaints concerning this residual anesthesia after leaving the dental office are difficulty speaking, smiling, drinking, and eating, plus a fear of drooling in public.[9,10] Residual sensations of numbness after leaving the dental office have also been shown to provoke moderate to extreme emotions of dislike in the vast majority of adult and adolescent restorative patients.[11] In children, prolonged soft tissue anesthesia can lead to inadvertent biting and mutilation of the lips, tongue, and cheeks.[12] The results of one prospective study in 320 children revealed that 18% of children younger than 4 years, 16% of children between 4 and 7 years, and 13% of children between 8 and 11 years displayed postprocedural soft tissue trauma after receiving mandibular block injections.[13] Lip biting injuries following local anesthetic injections are often misdiagnosed as bacterial infections and may result in unnecessary hospitalizations and unnecessary antibiotic administration.[14]

PHARMACOLOGY OF PHENTOLAMINE

Phentolamine is classified as a nonselective α-adrenergic blocking agent, that is, it opposes the effects of norepinephrine and epinephrine on tissues containing α_1- and α_2-adrenergic receptors. In particular, the smooth muscles of many vascular beds, including those beneath the oral mucosa, contain α-receptors (predominantly α_1), and the ultimate effect of α-receptor blockade is vasodilation. At relatively high dosages (5–10 mg) that are used in conditions of local and systemic catecholamine excess, parenteral phentolamine produces a profound blood pressure lowering effect.[3] This hypotensive action plus the ability of phentolamine to block prejunctional α_2-autoreceptors on neuronal membranes can produce tachycardia both due to baroreceptor reflex mechanisms and an enhanced release of neuronal norepinephrine, which then stimulates β_1-adrenergic receptors in the heart.[15,16]

In contrast, oral submucosal injections of phentolamine at dosages that have been studied in phase 2 and 3 randomized, controlled clinical trials and subsequently approved by the FDA (0.2 mg–0.8 mg) have not been associated with significant cardiovascular changes, most notably hypotension or tachycardia, when compared with either placebo or sham injections.[9,10,12] Previous to these trials, an open-label phase 1 study revealed that peak blood levels after administration of 1 cartridge of intravenous phentolamine alone (0.4 mg) was approximately 8 times higher than when the same dose was administered via an intraoral supraperiosteal infiltration injection over the maxillary first molar 30 minutes after a single cartridge of 2% lidocaine with 1:100,000 epinephrine was injected into the same site (10.98 vs 1.34 ng/mL). When 2 cartridges (0.8 mg or 3.4 mL) of intraoral phentolamine were administered into the same sites as 2 previous mandibular block and maxillary infiltration injections of lidocaine with epinephrine (4 cartridges or 7.2 mL total), an approximate doubling of peak phentolamine blood levels (2.73 ng/mL) was seen compared with the infiltration of a single phentolamine cartridge (1.34 ng/mL). From a safety standpoint, neither the submucosal doses nor the intravenous dose of phentolamine (which could be delivered clinically in the dental office via an inadvertent intravascular injection) produced hypotension at a rate greater than the infiltration administration of 4 cartridges of 2% lidocaine with 1:100,000 epinephrine alone.[17] Because there are no published studies describing peak phentolamine blood levels after medical intravenous dosing (5–10 mg), direct pharmacokinetic comparisons with the intravenous or submucosal administration of only 0.4 to 0.8 mg used for dental local anesthetic reversal cannot be made. However, if it is assumed that the intravenous pharmacokinetics of phentolamine with respect to peak blood levels remains relatively linear, 5 to 10 mg of intravenous phentolamine would result in 12.5-fold greater blood levels (137 ng/mL–274 ng/mL) than that produced by the intravenous administration of 0.4 to 0.8 mg (11–22 ng/mL) and approximately 100-fold greater blood levels than 1 or 2 nonintravenous submucosal injections of 0.4 mg phentolamine (1.34–2.73 ng/mL). Thus, the low blood levels achieved with dental dosing, even when administered intravenously, in all likelihood accounted for the lack of untoward cardiovascular effects reported in this and subsequent clinical trials.

As illustrated in **Fig. 1**, vasodilation induced by a subsequent phentolamine injection results in a more rapid redistribution of the local anesthetic away from the injection site compared with an injection of the local anesthetic solution alone. The lower

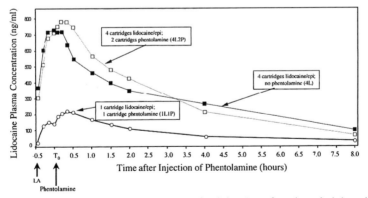

Fig. 1. Plasma concentration versus time curves for lidocaine after the administration of 1 cartridge of 2% lidocaine with 1:100,000 epinephrine followed 30 minutes later with 1 cartridge of phentolamine (1L1P, *open circles*), 4 cartridges of 2% lidocaine with 1:100,000 epinephrine followed 30 minutes later with 2 cartridges of phentolamine (4L2P, *open squares*), and 4 cartridges of 2% lidocaine with 1:100,000 epinephrine followed by no phentolamine (4L, *closed squares*). Lidocaine (LA) was administered 30 minutes prior (-0.5 hours) to phentolamine administration (T_0 hours). (*From* Moore PA, Hersh EV, Papas AS, et al. Pharmacokinetics of lidocaine with epinephrine following local anesthesia reversal with phentolamine mesylate. Anesth Prog 2008;55(2):45; with permission.)

concentration-time curve in this figure clearly shows a small but distinct second peak in lidocaine plasma concentrations immediately after the administration of 1 cartridge of phentolamine at the site of a previous lidocaine with epinephrine injection. Likewise, a second small peak was also produced when 4 cartridges of 2% lidocaine with 1:100,000 epinephrine was followed 30 minutes later by the injection of 2 cartridges of phentolamine into the same intraoral sites. In essence, the administration of phentolamine is antagonizing the α-adrenergic effects of epinephrine. A second peak in plasma levels was not observed when 4 cartridges of 2% lidocaine with 1:100,000 epinephrine was not followed by 2 phentolamine injections. From a safety standpoint, maximum plasma concentrations were only increased from 716.67 ng/mL with lidocaine plus epinephrine alone to 799.82 ng/mL when 4 cartridges of lidocaine with epinephrine were followed by phentolamine.[17] This increase is still at least 5-fold less than lidocaine blood levels of 4500 ng/mL, which have been reported to be associated with early systemic local anesthetic toxicity.[8]

PIVOTAL PHASE 2 AND PHASE 3 EFFICACY AND SAFETY TRIALS

The 4 pivotal clinical trials that are described involved healthy individuals in need of nonsurgical routine dental care consisting of simple restorative procedures, a single crown preparation, or a periodontal maintenance procedure requiring local anesthesia in combination with a vasoconstrictor in 1 quadrant of the mouth. The injection technique had to produce profound lip anesthesia and adequate pain control, which had to be achieved using 1 or 2 cartridges of local anesthetic. In all trials, bupivacaine with 1:200,000 epinephrine was not evaluated because its main use is to help control postsurgical pain via its prolonged duration of soft tissue and periosteal anesthesia.[18]

Trial 1 was a phase 2, double-blind, randomized, placebo-controlled (using the phentolamine vehicle) study in 122 subjects between the ages of 10 and 65 years.[10] Participants received 1 or 2 cartridges (as needed for pain control) of local anesthetic with vasoconstrictor before dental treatment in either the maxillary or mandibular arch. The local anesthetic solutions that were used included 2% lidocaine with 1:100,000 epinephrine, 4% articaine with 1:100,000 epinephrine, 4% prilocaine with 1:200,000 epinephrine, or 2% mepivacaine with 1:20,000 levonordefrin randomized in an equal allocation scheme. Immediately after treatment, an equal number of phentolamine 0.4 mg cartridges or phentolamine vehicle cartridges (to the previous local anesthetic volume) were injected in a 1:1 ratio. The primary efficacy end point was the median time to normal lip sensation recovery after the administration of study drug using a standardized lip tapping procedure, whereby lip sensation was rated as numb (no feeling), feeling pins and needles (tingling), or normal. For procedures performed in the lower arch, tongue and chin tapping procedures were used to evaluate sensory recovery of these tissues. Safety was assessed by recording spontaneously observed or reported adverse events, intraoperative Holter monitoring of cardiac rhythm, periodic recording of vital signs, and recording pain at the study drug injection site using a Heft-Parker 170-mm visual analog scale (VAS).[19] The median time to the return of normal sensation of the lip in subjects who received phentolamine was 50 minutes in the maxillary arch and 101 minutes in the mandibular arch compared with 155 minutes and 150 minutes, respectively, in the placebo group ($P<.0001$ in both arches in favor of phentolamine). This translated into a 68% acceleration in median recovery time in the maxillary arch and a 33% acceleration in median recovery time in the mandibular arch for lip anesthesia in the phentolamine group compared with placebo. The median time to recovery of normal sensation in the chin and tongue was also significantly more rapid ($P<.01$) in the phentolamine group (80.5 and

73.5 minutes, respectively) than the placebo group (140 and 105 minutes, respectively). There were no serious adverse events observed in this study with a similar number of what was judged to be treatment-related adverse events reported in the phentolamine (n = 57) and placebo groups (n = 50). Most of these events were mild in severity. Tachycardia was the most frequently recorded adverse event, occurring in 22 individuals in the phentolamine group and 25 individuals in the placebo group. During the first 8 hours after study drug administration, the phentolamine-treated subjects reported an average pain rating of weak (30 and 32.5 mm) and the placebo-treated patients reported an average pain rating of faint (4 and 2 mm) in the maxilla and mandibular injection sites, respectively, as measured on the Heft-Parker VAS. Although these differences were statistically significant ($P<.05$), they were not considered clinically meaningful and may have represented the more rapid dissipation of anesthesia in the phentolamine group.

Trials 2 and 3 were pivotal phase 3 trials in adults and adolescents with an age range of 12 to 92 years and used the same types of patients, local anesthetic and phentolamine dosages, and lip and tongue tapping sensory assessments as in trial 1.[9] Lidocaine with epinephrine was administered to approximately two-thirds of the subjects, whereas the other one-third was divided among those receiving articaine with epinephrine, prilocaine with epinephrine, or mepivacaine with levonordefrin. Trial 2 (n = 244) was performed in the mandibular arch, and trial 3 (n = 240) was performed in the maxillary arch. Instead of using a placebo vehicle injection, a sham injection was used, whereby the plastic shield covering the local anesthetic needle was kept in place and pressed against the tissues by a single unblinded investigator at each research center, with a visual barrier covering the eyes of the research subjects. All subsequent measures of phentolamine or sham efficacy and safety were made by blinded investigators. In addition to the sensory assessments, subjects completed a soft tissue anesthesia recovery (STAR) questionnaire and a functional assessment battery (FAB) before the injection of local anesthetic, before the injection of phentolamine or sham, immediately after the injection of phentolamine or sham, and at various time points through 5 hours postadministration of phentolamine or sham. The STAR questionnaire measured the subject's perception of altered function, sensation, and appearance. The FAB included measurements of smiling, speaking, presence or absence of drooling, and the ability to drink 3 ounces of water at various times during the study.[20,21] A researcher and the subject rated each of these functional assessments as normal or abnormal. Safety measures included recordings of systolic and diastolic blood pressure and pulse and measurements of pain at various time points, including immediately after the local anesthetic injection and immediately after the sham or active phentolamine injection, using the Heft-Parker VAS.

The primary efficacy end point for trials 2 and 3 was the median time to recovery of normal lip sensation based on the subjects' reports of numbness every 5 minutes while they performed the standardized lip palpation procedures. Secondary end points included median time to return to a score of zero derived from the STAR questionnaire; median time to return to normal on the FAB of smiling, speaking, drooling, and drinking; and, in the mandibular study (trial 2), the time to return of normal tongue sensation using the standardized tongue palpation method.

As displayed in **Fig. 2**, the median time to recovery of normal lower lip sensation in trial 2 was 70 minutes (95% confidence interval [CI], 65–80 minutes) for subjects in the phentolamine group and 155 minutes (95% CI, 140–165 minutes) for subjects in the sham group ($P<.0001$). The effect of phentolamine was an 85-minute reduction (54.8%) in median time to recovery of normal lower lip sensation. In addition, subjects

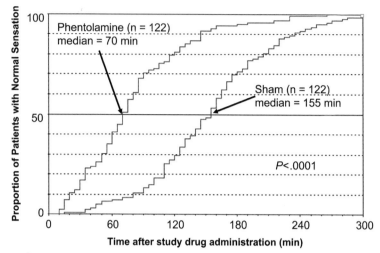

Fig. 2. Median time to return of normal lip sensation in the mandibular arch in adults and adolescents as assessed via subjects using a standardized finger palpation procedure. Recovery curves for phentolamine mesylate and sham groups are shown in Kaplan-Meier time-to-event analysis plots. (*From* Hersh EV, Moore PA, Papas AS, et al. Reversal of soft tissue local anesthesia with phentolamine mesylate in adolescents and adults. J Am Dent Assoc 2008;139(8):1086; with permission.)

in the phentolamine group were more likely to recover normal sensation in the lower lip during the early periods after injection of the study drug than were subjects in the sham group. Within the first 30 minutes, 21 subjects in the phentolamine group (17.2%) achieved normal lip sensation compared with only 1 subject in the sham group (0.8%). By 60 minutes, 50 subjects in the phentolamine group (40.9%) had achieved normal sensation compared with 9 subjects in the sham group (7.4%). By 90 minutes, 86 subjects in the phentolamine group (70.5%) compared with only 36 subjects in the sham group (13.1%) had achieved normal lip sensation. At 2 hours, 99 subjects in the phentolamine group (81.1%) and 36 subjects in the sham group (29.5%) had attained normal lip sensation. Only 23 subjects in the phentolamine group (18.9%) required more than 2 hours to achieve normal sensation in the lower lip compared with 86 subjects in the sham group (70.5%). **Fig. 3** illustrates the return of normal tongue sensation in subjects in the mandibular study. The median times to recovery of normal sensation in the tongue were 60 and 125 minutes for subjects in the phentolamine and sham groups, respectively. The effect of phentolamine was a 65-minute reduction (52%) in median time to recovery of normal sensation for subjects in the phentolamine group compared with subjects in the sham group (P<.0001). Subjects in the phentolamine group recovered at earlier times throughout the study. In addition, median recovery times on the STAR questionnaire and FAB were significantly more rapid (P<.001) for this group than the sham group (90 and 60 minutes vs 150 and 120 minutes, respectively).

As displayed in **Fig. 4**, the median time to recovery of normal sensation in the upper lip in trial 3 was 50 minutes (95% CI, 45–60 minutes) for subjects in the phentolamine group and 133 minutes (95% CI, 115–145 minutes) for subjects in the sham group (P<.0001). The effect of phentolamine was an 82.5-minute reduction (62.3%) in median time to recovery of normal upper lip sensation for subjects in the phentolamine group compared with subjects in the sham group. Subjects in the phentolamine group

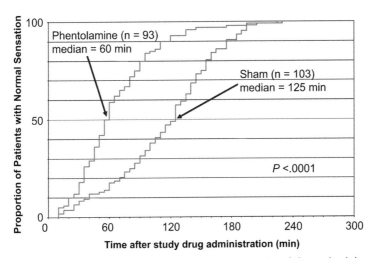

Fig. 3. Median time to return of normal tongue sensation in adults and adolescents as assessed via subjects using a standardized finger palpation procedure. Recovery curves for phentolamine mesylate and sham groups are shown in Kaplan-Meier time-to-event analysis plots. The sample sizes for this analysis differ from those of the lip, as not all subjects had numb tongues immediately before the study drug was administered. (*From* Hersh EV, Moore PA, Papas AS, et al. Reversal of soft-tissue local anesthesia with phentolamine mesylate in adolescents and adults. J Am Dent Assoc 2008;139(8):1087; with permission.)

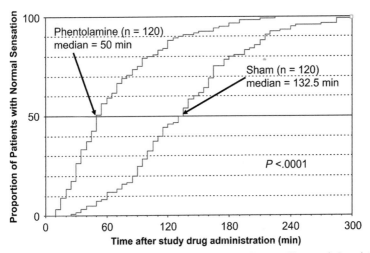

Fig. 4. Median time to return of normal lip sensation in the maxillary arch in adults and adolescents as assessed via subjects using a standardized finger palpation procedure. Recovery curves for phentolamine mesylate and sham groups are shown in Kaplan-Meier time-to-event analysis plots. (*From* Hersh EV, Moore PA, Papas AS, et al. Reversal of soft-tissue local anesthesia with phentolamine mesylate in adolescents and adults. J Am Dent Assoc 2008;139(8):1087; with permission.)

were more likely than subjects in the sham group to recover normal sensation in the upper lip during the early periods after injection of the study drug (see **Fig. 4**). Within the first 30 minutes, 32 subjects in the phentolamine group (26.7%) achieved normal sensation compared with only 2 subjects in the sham group (1.7%). By 60 minutes, 71 subjects in the phentolamine group (59.2%) had achieved normal sensation compared with only 14 subjects in the sham group (11.7%). By 90 minutes, 90 subjects in the phentolamine group (75.0%) had achieved normal sensation compared with 30 subjects in the sham group (25.0%). At 2 hours, 106 subjects in the phentolamine group (88.4%) had attained normal sensation compared with only 55 subjects in the sham group (45.8%). Fourteen subjects in the phentolamine group (11.6%) required more than 2 hours to achieve normal sensation in the upper lip. In the sham group, 65 subjects (54.2%) required more than 2 hours to achieve normal sensation in the upper lip. As in trial 2 (the mandibular study), median recovery times on the STAR questionnaire and FAB in the phentolamine group were significantly more rapid ($P<.001$) than in the sham group (60 and 60 minutes vs 120 and 105 minutes, respectively). In both the mandibular and maxillary studies, function (the ability to smile, speak, drink, and not drool) seemed to recover more rapidly than sensation (as assessed by the combined lip and tongue palpation procedures) or the perception of impairment as measured on the STAR questionnaire.[10]

A subgroup breakdown of the analyses for lip sensation recovery is shown in **Table 1**. Phentolamine seemed to work equally well in both arches, for all local anesthetic solutions and for all age groups, with 2 exceptions. In the maxillary arch, for adolescents 12 to 17 years old, the median acceleration in recovery was only 23% compared with sham, and for 4% prilocaine with 1:200,000 epinephrine in the same arch, there was no improvement compared with sham. The apparent discrepancy in these results was most likely because of the small sample sizes (n = 24 and n = 27 respectively) in each group and the large variability and potential error inherent with analyzing small sample sizes.[22,23] There was no significant difference in the incidence or severity of adverse events between phentolamine and sham in either trial. Mean systolic and diastolic blood pressure and pulse rates were nearly identical for both

Table 1
Percentage reduction in the median duration of lip numbness of phentolamine-treated patients compared with sham in the various age and anesthetic subgroups

Subgroup	Mandible % Reduction	Maxilla % Reduction
Age (y)		
12–17 (n = 31, 24)[a]	63	23
18–64 (n = 186, 188)	52	62
≥65 (n = 27, 28)	50	62
Local Anesthetic Type[b]		
Lidocaine (n = 163, 159)	54	63
Articaine (n = 28, 27)	48	69
Prilocaine (n = 27, 27)	37	0
Mepivacaine (n = 26, 27)	43	46

[a] The numbers in parentheses indicate the total number of patients enrolled in each subgroup in the mandibular and the maxillary study, respectively.
[b] Anesthetic and vasoconstrictor combinations used were 2% lidocaine with 1:100,000 epinephrine, 4% articaine with 1:100,000 epinephrine, 4% prilocaine with 1:200,000 epinephrine, and 2% mepivacaine with 1:20,000 levonordefrin.

treatments throughout the duration of both studies. Of particular note, 2 measurements of standing blood pressures and pulse performed at 5 and 10 to 20 minutes after the phentolamine or sham injections did not provoke any signs of postural hypotension, which is a common side effect with the medical usage of α-adrenergic blocking drugs.[15] Also of note was that mean pain scores as measured on the 170-mm Heft-Parker VAS of the phentolamine injection (11 mm in the mandible and 7 mm in the maxilla) could not be clinically differentiated from the sham injection (5 mm in both arches). All these values represent faint pain, and many subjects perceived no pain at all, probably because the patients were still numb at the time of the phentolamine or sham injections. Of the 77 adverse events reported in the mandibular study, blinded researchers judged 55 to be related to the injection of the study drug (32 adverse events in 19.7% of subjects in the phentolamine group and 23 adverse events in 16.4% of subjects in the sham group). In the maxillary study, a similar percentage of subjects in both groups reported having treatment-related adverse events (13.3% in the phentolamine group and 10% in the sham group). The most frequently reported adverse events in the mandibular and maxillary studies were injection site pain (6.6% and 6.7%, respectively, for the phentolamine group; 5.7% and 1.7%, respectively, for the sham group), postprocedural pain (3.3% and 1.7%, respectively, for the phentolamine group; 4.9% and 2.5%, respectively, for the sham group), and headache (3.3% and 1.7%, respectively, for the phentolamine group; 1.6% and 0.8%, respectively, for the sham group).

Trial 4 was a phase 2 trial completed in 152 pediatric subjects aged 4 to 11 years who received half or a single cartridge of 2% lidocaine with 1:100,000 epinephrine in either the mandibular or maxillary arch followed at the end of the procedure with an equal volume of phentolamine (0.2–0.4 mg) or a sham injection in a 2:1 ratio. Children who were 4 or 5 years old were only evaluated for safety, whereas those who were 6 years or older were also evaluated for efficacy if they were trainable in the lip and tongue palpation techniques.[12] The degree of intraoral pain was assessed by using the Wong-Baker FACES Pain Rating Scale. This scale is made up of 6 circular faces progressing from very happy to crying, which are scored 0 (no hurt) to 5 (hurts worst).[24] Safety comparisons between phentolamine and sham were in fact the primary outcome measures for this study.

There were no serious adverse events recorded in this pediatric trial; 14 subjects had adverse events in the phentolamine group and 7 subjects had adverse events in the sham group. In fact the 1 report of severe injection site pain occurred in a sham-treated subject. The most frequently reported treatment-related adverse events were injection site pain (5 subjects with phentolamine and 3 subjects with sham) and increased blood pressure (2 subjects with phentolamine and 2 subjects with sham). All adverse events resolved within 48 hours. Of special interest was that the highest Wong-Baker FACES scores were obtained immediately after the local anesthetic injection, with a mean score of 0.8 for the phentolamine group and 0.9 for the sham group. Immediately after the phentolamine or sham injections, mean pain scores in both groups were approximately 0.3, which means that most subjects perceived no pain during the active phentolamine injection. With respect to efficacy, the pediatric subjects in the phentolamine group reported a median time to recovery of normal lip sensation of 60 minutes, whereas the median time to recovery in the sham group was 135 minutes ($P < .0001$), which represented a 75-minute or 55.6% acceleration in recovery times for phentolamine over sham. Likewise, for the tongue in subjects who had received mandibular block injections, a 67.5-minute or 60% reduction in median time to recovery occurred in the phentolamine-treated subjects compared with sham ($P = .0003$).

SUMMARY AND FUTURE RESEARCH

Phentolamine seems to be safe and effective in reducing soft tissue local anesthetic recovery time in adults and children as young as 6 years.[9,10,12] Limited data support a favorable safety profile in children as young as 4 years.[12] A pivotal phase 4 (postmarketing) trial in 2- to 5-year-old children is planned in the near future in an attempt to further establish safety and efficacy in this age group. A previously published study of 22 dental patients between the ages of 13 and 75 years reported that 19 (86%) had a moderate dislike and 3 (14%) had an extreme dislike for the length of numbness following routine restorative procedures.[11] Extrapolating data from this very small sample size, it can be predicted that several adults and adolescents would potentially opt for a phentolamine reversal injection after routine nonsurgical local anesthesia. However, the current cost per cartridge is somewhat high, and some dentists are reluctant to pass the full cost of the drug on to the patient. The pediatric dental community and general dentists who treat young children seem most enthusiastic about the introduction of phentolamine for local anesthetic reversal. Although the median reduction in recovery time of the lip and tongue is typically an hour or more and some patients recover sensation and function even earlier (see **Figs. 2–4; Fig. 5**), it remains to be seen if this translates into a lower incidence of lip and tongue mutilation in a busy pediatric dental practice. It would also be worth studying the ability of phentolamine to hasten the soft tissue recovery following injections of 3% mepivacaine and 4% prilocaine plain. These solutions are often used in patients with hypertension or cardiovascular disease but still possess durations of lip and tongue anesthesia that are similar to lidocaine with 1:100,000 epinephrine.[7,8] Many clinicians still do not realize this, and excessive dosing of these plain solutions in pediatric dental patients because of their lower maximum recommended doses on a volume basis, is a prescription for disaster.[25–27]

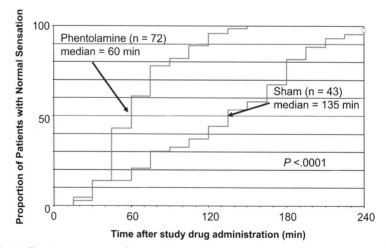

Fig. 5. Median time to return of normal lip sensation in pediatric patients aged 6 to 11 years in both the mandibular and maxillary arches as assessed via subjects using a standardized finger palpation procedure. Recovery curves for phentolamine mesylate and sham groups are shown in Kaplan-Meier time-to-event analysis plots. (*Adapted from* Tavares M, Goodson JM, Studen-Pavolich D, et al. Reversal of soft-tissue anesthesia with phentolamine mesylate in pediatric patients. J Am Dent Assoc 2008;139(8):1102; with permission.)

REFERENCES

1. OraVerse Package Insert. Available at: http://www.novalar.com/assets/pdf/package_inset_jan09.pdf. Accessed August 20, 2009.
2. Malamed SF. Phentolamine mesylate for the reversal of residual soft-tissue anesthesia. Available at: http://www.ineedce.com/coursereview.aspx?url=1597%2fPDF%2fPhentolaminerev.pdf&scid=13942. Accessed July 15, 2009.
3. Chobanian AV, Bakris GL, Black HR, et al. Seventh report of the Joint National Committee on Prevention, Detection, Evaluation, and Treatment of High Blood Pressure. Hypertension 2003;42:1206–52.
4. Elliott WJ. Clinical features in the management of selected hypertensive emergencies. Prog Cardiovasc Dis 2006;48:316–25.
5. Rhoney D, Peacock WF. Intravenous therapy for hypertensive emergencies: part 1. Am J Health Syst Pharm 2009;66(15):1343–52.
6. Phentolamine mesylate for injection package insert. Available at: http://www.bedfordlabs.com/BedfordLabsWeb/products/inserts/PHT-P01.pdf. Accessed August 20, 2009.
7. Hersh EV, Hermann DG, Lamp CJ, et al. Assessing the duration of mandibular soft tissue anesthesia. J Am Dent Assoc 1995;126(11):1531–6.
8. Malamed SF. Handbook of local anesthesia. 5th edition. St Louis (MO): Mosby Inc; 2004.
9. Hersh EV, Moore PA, Papas AS, et al. Reversal of soft-tissue local anesthesia with phentolamine mesylate in adolescents and adults. J Am Dent Assoc 2008;139(8):1080–93.
10. Laviola M, McGavin SK, Freer GA, et al. Randomized study of phentolamine mesylate for reversal of local anesthesia. J Dent Res 2008;87(7):635–9.
11. Rafique S, Fiske J, Banerjee A. Clinical trial of an air-abrasion/chemomechanical operative procedure for the restorative treatment of dental patients. Caries Res 2003;37(5):360–4.
12. Tavares M, Goodson JM, Studen-Pavolich D, et al. Reversal of soft-tissue anesthesia with phentolamine mesylate in pediatric patients. J Am Dent Assoc 2008;139(8):1095–104.
13. College C, Feigal R, Wandera A, et al. Bilateral versus unilateral mandibular block anesthesia in a pediatric population. Pediatr Dent 2000;22(6):453–7.
14. Chi D, Kanellis M, Himadi E, et al. Lip biting in a pediatric dental patient after dental local anesthesia: a case report. J Pediatr Nurs 2008;23(6):490–3.
15. Starke K. Presynaptic α-autoreceptors. Rev Physiol Biochem Pharmacol 1987;107:73–146.
16. Piacik MT, Abel PW. Adrenergic blocking drugs. In: Yagiela JA, Dowd FJ, Neidle EA, editors. Pharmacology and therapeutics for dentistry. 5th edition. St Louis (MO): Elsevier Mosby; 2004. p. 113–24.
17. Moore PA, Hersh EV, Papas AS, et al. Pharmacokinetics of lidocaine with epinephrine following local anesthesia reversal with phentolamine mesylate. Anesth Prog 2008;55(2):40–8.
18. Moore PA, Nahouraii HS, Zovko JG, et al. Dental therapeutic practice patterns in the U.S. II. Analgesics, corticosteroids, and antibiotics. Gen Dent 2006;54(3):201–7.
19. Heft M, Parker SR. An experimental basis for revising the graphic rating scale for pain. Pain 1984;19(2):153–61.
20. Fisher HB, Logemann JA. The Fisher-Logemann Test of Articulation Competence. Boston: Houghton Mifflin; 1971.

21. DePippo KL, Holas MA, Reding MJ. Validation of the 3-oz water swallow test for aspiration following stroke. Arch Neurol 1992;49(12):1259–61.

22. Bates BT, Dufek JS, Davis HP. The effect of trial size on statistical power. Med Sci Sports Exerc 1992;24(9):1059–65.

23. Wong WK, Furst DE, Clements PJ, et al. Assessing disease progression using a composite endpoint. Stat Methods Med Res 2007;16(1):31–49.

24. Wong DL, Baker CM. Pain in children: comparison of assessment scales. Pediatr Nurs 1988;14(1):9–17.

25. Hersh EV, Helpin ML, Evans OB. Local anesthetic mortality: report of case. ASDC J Dent Child 1991;58(6):489–91.

26. Moore PA. Preventing local anesthetic toxicity. J Am Dent Assoc 1992;123(9): 60–4.

27. Goodson JM, Moore PA. Life-threatening reactions after pedodontic sedation: an assessment of narcotic, local anesthetic, and antiemetic drug interaction. J Am Dent Assoc 1983;107(2):239–45.

Efficacy of Articaine Formulations: Quantitative Reviews

Kellie Paxton, DMD, MS[a],*, David E. Thome, DDS[b]

KEYWORDS

• Articaine • Carticaine • Local anesthesia • Efficacy

In 1969, carticaine hydrochloride, with a chemical code name of Hoe 40 045, was synthesized as the first amide-type drug with a lipophilic thiophene ring and an additional ester side chain (**Fig. 1**). Carticaine became available for clinical use in Germany in 1976, and in 1984 was renamed *articaine*.[1] In 2000, the US Food and Drug Administration (FDA) approved the use of 4% articaine with epinephrine 1:100,000, and with epinephrine 1:200,000 in 2006.[2]

Articaine has been commonly compared with its predecessor, lidocaine hydrochloride (**Fig. 2**). Since its introduction in 1948, lidocaine has maintained a status as the most widely used local dental anesthetic in most countries.[1] Proven efficacy with low allergenicity and toxicity over long-term clinical use and research have confirmed the value and safety of this drug. Thus, it became the gold standard to which all new local anesthetics are compared.[1] Several injectable lidocaine formulations have been approved by the FDA for dental applications: 2% without vasoconstrictor, 2% with epinephrine 1:50,000, and 2% with epinephrine 1:100,000.[2] The 2% lidocaine with 1:100,000 epinephrine formulation continues to be the most commonly used local anesthetic agent for routine dental procedures in the United States.[1]

Despite the gold standard status of lidocaine, numerous reports and editorials have supported and recognized the use of articaine. An editorial in the *Journal of the American Dental Association* acknowledged that articaine "has garnered a majority of the dental market in many of the countries in which it is available."[3] Another editorial quoted a drug company's marketing approach, "Articaine has become the most popular local anesthetic for dentists wherever it has been introduced."[4]

In a 1993 survey based in Ontario, Canada, dentists reported articaine with epinephrine 1:200,000 was used 19.9% of the time, articaine with epinephrine 1:100,000 was

[a] Private Endodontic Practice, Executive Endodontics of Weston, 2711 Executive Park Drive, Suite 1, Weston, FL 33331, USA
[b] Private Pediatric Dental Practice, Westside Orthodontics and Pediatric Dentistry, 16223 Miramar Parkway, Miramar, FL 33027, USA
* Corresponding author.
E-mail address: paxtonkellie@yahoo.com

Dent Clin N Am 54 (2010) 643–653
doi:10.1016/j.cden.2010.06.005
0011-8532/10/$ – see front matter © 2010 Elsevier Inc. All rights reserved.

Articaine

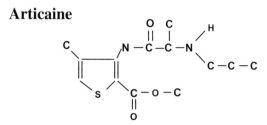

Fig. 1. Chemical structure of the local anesthetic articaine.

used 17.9% of the time, and lidocaine with epinephrine 1:100,000 was used 23.4% of the time.[5] In a 2007 follow-up survey based in Ontario, Canada, dentists reported articaine with epinephrine 1:200,000 was used 27.04% of the time, articaine with epinephrine 1:100,000 was used 17.16% of the time, and lidocaine with epinephrine 1:100,000 was used 37.31% of the time.[6] In a survey from Germany, 911 dentists reported the use of articaine 90% of the time and lidocaine 2% of the time.[7] Another survey representing 541 dentists in Germany indicated routine administration of articaine 72% of the time and lidocaine 13% of the time.[8]

Articaine's superior reputation has been primarily based on clinicians' opinion that it may possess enhanced diffusion properties and better anesthetic efficacy. In a standard textbook of local anesthesia, articaine was described as having potency 1.5 times that of lidocaine, faster onset, and increased success rate, with dentists reporting that they "don't miss as often."[1] A review article on articaine clinical pharmacology reported, "In dentistry, articaine is the drug of choice in the vast majority of literature."[9] Isen[10] claimed "enhanced action of articaine over other local anesthetics" based on the molecule having more lipid-soluble abilities across the nerve membrane. Many of these claims may have been based on speculation because most of the literature has failed to support these claims.

Reports of articaine's superiority were mainly founded on the notion that its thiophene ring bestows enhanced performance. This feature has been credited with providing increased lipid solubility and protein binding, two properties theoretically related to increased anesthetic efficacy.[1,10] Lipid solubility is an intrinsic quality of local anesthetic potency. This quality is essential for penetration of the anesthetic through the lipid nerve membrane and subsequent diffusion into surrounding tissues.[1] In a clinical study evaluating this concept, alveolar blood levels were measured post-extraction for anesthetic concentrations (and their byproducts). After the injection of 2 ml of either 4% articaine or 2% lidocaine, both with epinephrine 1:100,000, a significant two-fold higher mean of articaine was observed in alveolar blood. The rationale for this "better diffusion" after injection was based on the higher descent of concentration derived from articaine.

Lidocaine

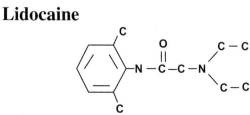

Fig. 2. Chemical structure of the local anesthetic lidocaine.

Therefore, superior anesthetic diffusion properties of articaine were not confirmed in the research.[11]

The degree of anesthetic molecules binding to the nerve membrane was suggested to dictate the duration of the anesthetic effect. The more secure a bond is, the slower the anesthetic is released from the receptor sites in the sodium channels and the greater the duration of the anesthetic effect. As determined by Courtney and colleagues,[12] mere lipid solubility of a local anesthetic did not determine the action on the ionic channels. Instead, Uihlein[13] determined that binding properties of the local anesthetic agent to plasma proteins have a greater correlation to action on ionic channels than does lipid solubility.

The first clinical trial in dentistry testing the efficacy of articaine was conducted in Denmark in 1972 by Winther and Nathalang.[14] Comparisons were made of 2% articaine with and without epinephrine 1:200,000, 2% lidocaine with and without epinephrine 1:200,000, and other anesthetic compounds. The results showed that articaine with epinephrine was significantly superior to lidocaine with epinephrine (and to the other anesthetic compounds) with respect to "frequency, extent and duration of analgesia."

Muschaweck and Rippel[15] conducted an early investigation of the pharmacology and toxicology of articaine (0.05%–0.5% solutions) in animal experiments, with lidocaine (0.05%–0.5% solutions) as a comparison. This investigation found that when compared with lidocaine, articaine had 1.5 times higher anesthetic activity in conduction anesthesia infiltration, "markedly superior" efficacy in infiltration anesthesia, equivalent efficacy in topical anesthesia, and similar low toxicity to local tissues.

In a multicenter trial conducted on 1325 subjects (aged 4–80 years) comparing the safety and efficacy of 4% articaine and 2% lidocaine, both with epinephrine 1:100,000, both agents demonstrated clinically effective and appropriate local anesthesia during general dental procedures.[16–18]

A LITERATURE REVIEW OF ARTICAINE AND LIDOCAINE

To date, 27 publications have reported on clinical trials comparing the anesthetic efficacy of 4% articaine with 2% lidocaine, both with epinephrine 1:100,000 in dental applications.[17–43] Although differences between these formulations were not consistently reported, a common trend is seen for articaine to outperform the gold standard lidocaine in dental applications. However, statistically speaking, results were divided regarding the anesthetic efficacy of the two anesthetic agents. Overall, 12 of these publications[21,22,26,29–35,40,43] reported a statistically significant difference between the anesthetic agents, whereas 12 other studies[17–20,23–25,27,28,37,39,42] found no statistical significant difference. Two studies reported a contrast in statistical significance between these anesthetic agents, depending on the tooth type analyzed.[38,41] One study did not statistically analyze the results; however, the outcome data followed the trend for articaine to be somewhat better than lidocaine.[36] In more recent publications, articaine efficacy has been tested when used as a supplemental anesthetic or in supplemental injection techniques.[37,40,44–51]

A QUANTITATIVE META-ANALYSIS COMPARING ARTICAINE AND LIDOCAINE

Because of the disparity in the results of published clinical trials, and because many studies lacked sufficient subject numbers to independently support a difference of statistical significance, the anesthetic efficacy of articaine is unclear. Using meta-analysis to quantitatively synthesize results from multiple clinical studies comparing 4% articaine with 2% lidocaine, both with epinephrine 1:100,000, a statistical comparison was performed.

The details of this quantitative review were published online in 2008 as one of the author's master's thesis.[52] The methods and results are summarized later. These specific formulations (anesthetic and epinephrine) were selected based on their frequent dental use in both clinical and research arenas. The primary outcome of interest was a comparison of anesthetic success achieved from the anesthetic agents as defined independently in each study.

A literature search to locate all published research was initially performed. The MeSH database, the National Library of Medicine's controlled vocabulary indexing system, was used to search the following terms closely related to this study: *carticaine*, *articaine*, *lidocaine*, *lignocaine*, *local anesthetics*, and *dental anesthesia*. It was concluded that the most appropriate and exhaustive Medical Subject Heading terms for the purpose of searching PubMed were *carticaine* and *lidocaine*. Searching PubMed, the National Library of Medicine's text-based search and retrieval system for biomedical literature, through January 2008 using the combination of MeSH terms *carticaine* and *lidocaine* produced 76 publications. Through limiting the literature to human studies, the 76 articles were reduced to 64. Abstracts or manuscripts were obtained and analyzed for these 64 studies.

Starting with these 64 identified articles, the first group of exclusions included 19 studies based on nondental topics. Of the remaining 45 dental-related articles, 10 were either review or editorial publications and therefore excluded. Furthermore, 14 articles could be eliminated because they reported on local anesthesia topics other than efficacy, such as allergic reactions, tissue reactions, anxiety, injection pain, systemic factors, complications, or nerve injury. One study only evaluated the efficacy of articaine and did not include lidocaine. Four studies evaluated both anesthetic agents, but the specified concentrations of one or both agents were not tested.

At this point, the remaining 16 articles were all clinical trials comparing the specific anesthetic agents of interest in dental applications. Supplemental anesthesia, with only lidocaine given initially, was reported in one publication. Because no comparison of initial anesthetic administration was made, this study was excluded. Further exclusions included two studies comparing the anesthetic agents of interest; however, randomization was not reported in one, and the methodology and results were unclear in another. Another publication was excluded because it reported data included in a previously included publication. After this level of exclusion, 12 original articles remained of human randomized clinical studies evaluating the dental anesthetic efficacy of both 4% articaine and 2% lidocaine, both with epinephrine 1:100,000, as initial local anesthetics. To exhaust the search for publications fulfilling the criteria stated earlier, cross-citations of these 12 studies were explored.

The final step in determining inclusion was the availability of sufficient information for analytic evaluation. For four of the 12 studies, it was necessary to seek supplemental data to include these studies in the proposed meta-analytic comparisons. The shortcomings of these four studies pertained to the lack of information relating to absolute determination of anesthetic success and failure in subjects. In particular, the information necessary for this meta-analysis included the number of experimental applications with absolute anesthetic success and absolute anesthetic failure with percentage calculations and *P* values. The results of three of the studies reported timeline comparisons of anesthetic onset and duration only. No outcome data were available to calculate a percentage of anesthetic success and failure. Another study only reported the mean, median, and range of visual analog scale scores for each anesthetic agent given. Thus, the results failed to define or report anesthetic success in terms of subjects who were pain-free.

Although not reported, the supplemental data necessary for this meta-analysis would most likely have been recorded during the course of each study. Reasonable effort was made to contact the authors of these four studies to obtain the necessary supplemental information. Adequate unpublished data were successfully obtained from Costa and colleagues[21] and Oliveira and colleagues.[25] Therefore, 10 studies could be included in this meta-analysis (**Table 1**). Inclusion criteria specified randomized clinical trials with clear determination of anesthetic efficacy with respect to initial administration of these two anesthetic agents in dental applications, resulting in total 1146 subjects and 1395 anesthetic administrations.[52,53]

As indicated in **Table 1**, two of these studies[22,26] reported significantly superior performance of articaine compared with lidocaine based on achievement of pulpal anesthetic success; a third study reported a suggestive result ($P = .057$).[23] In four additional studies,[19,20,24,28] the observed rate of anesthetic success was greater for articaine, although not significantly so. The performance of the two anesthetic agents was identical in the remaining three studies.[21,25,27]

As shown in **Fig. 3**, the combined estimate of the difference obtained using a random effects meta-analytic model was associated with an estimated 9.21% greater proportion of anesthetic success with articaine than with lidocaine (95% CI, 2.56%–15.58%), providing evidence of articaine superiority.[52,53]

A QUANTITATIVE META-ANALYSIS COMPARING TWO ARTICAINE FORMULATIONS

The clinical research literature includes several studies comparing different formulations of articaine. A multicenter trial determined the anesthetic efficacy of 4% articaine with epinephrine 1:100,000, epinephrine 1:200,000, and without epinephrine. The results of the trials showed that 4% articaine formulated with either epinephrine 1:100,000 or 1:200,000 had equivalent success rates for inducing pulpal anesthesia; however, statistically significant differences were observed in anesthetic success between the nonepinephrine and epinephrine-containing groups.[54] Other clinical trials in dentistry involving a comparison of the anesthetic efficacy of 4% articaine with epinephrine 1:100,000 and 1:200,000[21,23,27,29–32,43,54–63] have generally reported

Table 1
Differences in percentages of anesthetic success with confidence intervals

Study	Study Type	n[a]	Difference in Percentages	95% CI (Lower %, Upper %)
Berlin et al[19]	CO	102	11.77%	(−5.59%, 29.12%)
Costa et al[21]	CO	40	0%	(−14.80%, 14.80%)
Kanaa et al[22]	CO	62	25.81%	(5.93%, 45.68%)
Mikesell et al[24]	CO	114	8.77%	(−10.70%, 28.25%)
Oliveira et al[25]	CO	40	0%	(−14.80%, 14.80%)
Robertson et al[26]	CO	120	30.0%	(15.02%, 44.98%)
Ruprecht and Knoll-Kohler[27]	CO	20	0%	(−29.60%, 29.60%)
Claffey et al[20]	IS	72	14.7%	(−18.15%, 21.08%)
Khoury et al[23]	IS	771	6.37%	(−0.11%, 12.85%)
Sierra Rebolledo et al[28]	IS	54	14.17%	(−10.41%, 38.75%)

CO, crossover design in which each subject received two experimental administrations, one with articaine and one with lidocaine; IS, independent sample design in which each subject was randomized to an experimental group receiving either articaine or lidocaine.
[a] Number of experimental administrations.

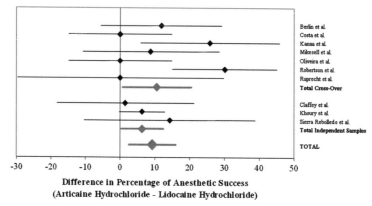

Fig. 3. Forest plot: point estimates and associated 95% CIs for the difference in the percentage of anesthetic success achieved with the two experimental administrations (4% articaine, 1:100,000 epinephrine vs 2% lidocaine, 1:100,000 epinephrine), and combined point estimates of the treatment differences and the associated 95% CIs overall and by study design. *Data from* Paxton K. Anesthetic efficacy of articaine hydrochloride versus lidocaine hydrochloride: a meta-analysis [master's thesis]. The University of Iowa; 2008; and Paxton KR, Dawson DV, Drake DR, et al. Anesthetic efficacy of articaine hydrochloride versus lidocaine hydrochloride: a meta-analysis. J Dent Res 2008;87(Spec Iss B):0025.

similar anesthetic success rates between these local anesthetics. When a difference was seen, the epinephrine 1:100,000 tended to outperform epinephrine 1:200,000, but without statistical significance.

As a follow-up assessment to the authors' lidocaine versus articaine meta-analysis, they performed a similar quantitative review of clinical studies comparing 4% articaine with epinephrine 1:100,000 and epinephrine 1:200,000.[64] The primary outcome of interest was a comparison of anesthetic success achieved from the anesthetic agents as defined independently in each study. Inclusion criteria included randomized clinical trials in humans, with a clear determination of anesthetic efficacy with respect to initial administration of these two anesthetic formulations in dental applications. As shown in

Table 2
Differences in percentages of anesthetic success with confidence intervals

Study	Study Type	n[a]	Difference in Percentages	95% CI (Lower %, Upper %)
Costa et al[21]	CO	40	0	(−14.8%, 14.8%)
Moore et al[57]	CO	84	0	(−7.05%, 7.05%)
Raab et al[55]	CO	52	0	(−11.38%, 11.38%)
Ruprecht and Knoll-Kohler[27]	CO	20	0	(−29.60%, 29.60%)
Santos et al[58]	CO	100	10	(−1.19%, 21.19%)
Tofoli et al[56]	CO	40	0	(−14.8%, 14.8%)
Khoury et al[23]	IS	771	2.62	(−3.66%, 8.90%)

CO, crossover design in which each subject received two experimental articaine administrations, one with epinephrine 1:100,000 and one with epinephrine 1:200,000; IS, independent sample design in which each subject was randomized to an experimental group receiving articaine with either epinephrine 1:100,000 or epinephrine 1:200,000.
[a] Number of experimental administrations.

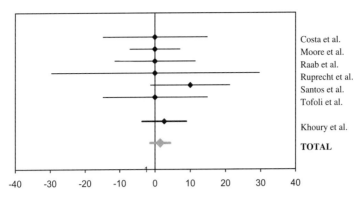

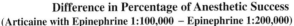

Difference in Percentage of Anesthetic Success
(Articaine with Epinephrine 1:100,000 − Epinephrine 1:200,000)

Fig. 4. Forest plot: point estimates and associated 95% CIs for the difference in the percentage of anesthetic success achieved with the two experimental articaine administrations (4% articaine, 1:100,000 epinephrine versus 4% articaine 1:200,000 epinephrine), and combined point estimates of the treatment differences and the associated 95% CIs overall. *From* Paxton KR, Dawson DV, Hill JR, et al. Articaine hydrochloride and epinephrine concentration: a meta-analysis. J Dent Res 2009;88(Spec Iss A):280; with permission.

Table 2, seven randomized clinical trials met the inclusion criteria, involving 958 subjects and 1126 anesthetic administrations.[64]

Fig. 4 shows the individual and total differences in anesthetic success between the epinephrine groups. Individually, in five of the studies,[21,27,55–57] the observed rate of anesthetic success was equal for both epinephrine concentrations based on achievement of pulpal anesthetic success. In two studies, the performance of epinephrine 1:100,000 was greater than that of epinephrine 1:200,000, although not significantly so.[23,58] The overall result for anesthetic success based on meta-analysis using the Fisher method showed no evidence that articaine with epinephrine 1:100,000 had statistically superior efficacy (*P*>.9) relative to epinephrine 1:200,000.[64]

SUMMARY

The combination of studies in these meta-analyses contributed power and multiplicity in the quest to compare the local anesthetic efficacy of articaine, with respect to its available epinephrine concentrations and compared with the gold standard, lidocaine. Despite the variability of outcomes in the literature, meta-analysis showed a significant difference between articaine and lidocaine, suggesting an advantage, at least in some clinical situations, to the use of articaine. When articaine with epinephrine 1:100,000 and 1:200,000 were compared, no significant difference was found.[52,53,64]

By principle, these meta-analyses included more subjects than any single constituent study comparing the anesthetic agents, providing greater power to investigate the relationship between the anesthetic agents. However, when comparing all studies included for both meta-analyses, many inconsistencies were observed. Subsequently, the meta-analytic results are broadly based on studies being conducted independently, with different geographic locations, populations, contexts, clinical conditions, and definitions of anesthetic success.

The limitations of these meta-analyses are acknowledged, the most important of which are the numerous sources of heterogeneity in study design, injection type, study population, target teeth, and, very importantly, definition of outcome. These limitations are further complicated by the lack of standardization in reporting. Nonetheless, these results seem to support the potential advantage to be gained from further systematic evaluation, particularly under more standardized conditions, which would enhance the ability to more definitively quantitate any increase in efficacy of articaine, and to delineate the conditions under which it pertains.

REFERENCES

1. Malamed SF. Handbook of local anesthesia. 5th edition. St Louis (MO): CV Mosby; 2004.
2. Center for Drug Evaluation and Research. Approved drug products with therapeutic equivalence evaluations. 27th edition. Washington, DC: U.S. Food and Drug Administration; 2007.
3. Schertzer ER Jr. Articaine vs. lidocaine. J Am Dent Assoc 2000;131:1242–3.
4. Weaver JM. Articaine, a new local anesthetic for American dentists: will it supersede lidocaine? Anesth Prog 1999;46:111–2.
5. Haas DA, Lennon D. Local anesthetic use by dentists in Ontario. J Can Dent Assoc 1995;61:297–304.
6. Gaffen AS, Haas DA. Survey of local anesthetic use by Ontario dentists. J Can Dent Assoc 2009;75:649.
7. Daublander M, Muller R, Lipp MD. The incidence of complications associated with local anesthesia in dentistry. Anesth Prog 1997;44:132–41.
8. Jakobs W. Status of dental anesthesia in Germany. Anesth Prog 1989;36: 210–2.
9. Vree TB, Gielen MJ. Clinical pharmacology and the use of articaine for local and regional anaesthesia. Best Pract Res Clin Anaesthesiol 2005;19:293–308.
10. Isen DA. Articaine: pharmacology and clinical use of a recently approved local anesthetic. Dent Today 2000;19:72–7.
11. Oertel R, Richter K, Weile K, et al. A simple method for the determination of articaine and its metabolite articainic acid in dentistry: application to a comparison of articaine and lidocaine concentrations in alveolus blood. Methods Find Exp Clin Pharmacol 1993;15:541–7.
12. Courtney KR, Kendig JJ, Cohen EN. The rates of interaction of local anesthetics with sodium channels in nerve. J Pharmacol Exp Ther 1978;207:594–604.
13. Uihlein M. [Analytical investigations with the local anesthetic ultracain (HOE 045)]. (author's transl). Prakt Anaesth 1974;9:152–7 [in German].
14. Winther JE, Nathalang B. Effectivity of a new local analgesic Hoe 40 045. Scand J Dent Res 1972;80:272–8.
15. Muschaweck R, Rippel R. [A new local anesthetic (carticaine) from the thiopene-series]. Prakt Anaesth 1974;9:135–46 [in German].
16. Malamed SF, Gagnon S, Leblanc D. Articaine hydrochloride: a study of the safety of a new amide local anesthetic. J Am Dent Assoc 2001;132:177–85.
17. Malamed SF, Gagnon S, Leblanc D. A comparison between articaine HCl and lidocaine HCl in pediatric dental patients. Pediatr Dent 2000;22:307–11.
18. Malamed SF, Gagnon S, Leblanc D. Efficacy of articaine: a new amide local anesthetic. J Am Dent Assoc 2000;131:635–42.
19. Berlin J, Nusstein J, Reader A, et al. Efficacy of articaine and lidocaine in a primary intraligamentary injection administered with a computer-controlled local anesthetic delivery system. Oral Surg Oral Med Oral Pathol Oral Radiol Endod 2005;99:361–6.

20. Claffey E, Reader A, Nusstein J, et al. Anesthetic efficacy of articaine for inferior alveolar nerve blocks in patients with irreversible pulpitis. J Endod 2004;30:568–71.
21. Costa CG, Tortamano IP, Rocha RG, et al. Onset and duration periods of articaine and lidocaine on maxillary infiltration. Quintessence Int 2005;36:197–201.
22. Kanaa MD, Whitworth JM, Corbett IP, et al. Articaine and lidocaine mandibular buccal infiltration anesthesia: a prospective randomized double-blind cross-over study. J Endod 2006;32:296–8.
23. Khoury F, Hinterthan A, Schurmann J, et al. Clinical comparative study of local anesthetics. Random double blind study with four commercial preparations. Dtsch Zahnarztl Z 1991;46:822–4.
24. Mikesell P, Nusstein J, Reader A, et al. A comparison of articaine and lidocaine for inferior alveolar nerve blocks. J Endod 2005;31:265–70.
25. Oliveira PC, Volpato MC, Ramacciato JC, et al. Articaine and lignocaine efficiency in infiltration anaesthesia: a pilot study. Br Dent J 2004;197:45–6.
26. Robertson D, Nusstein J, Reader A, et al. The anesthetic efficacy of articaine in buccal infiltration of mandibular posterior teeth. J Am Dent Assoc 2007;138:1104–12.
27. Ruprecht S, Knoll-Kohler E. [A comparative study of equimolar solutions of lidocaine and articaine for anesthesia. A randomized double-blind cross-over study]. Schweiz Monatsschr Zahnmed 1991;101:1286–90 [in German].
28. Sierra Rebolledo A, Delgado Molina E, Berini Aytis L, et al. Comparative study of the anesthetic efficacy of 4% articaine versus 2% lidocaine in inferior alveolar nerve block during surgical extraction of impacted lower third molars. Med Oral Patol Oral Cir Bucal 2007;12:E139–44.
29. Szabo G, Gaspar L, Divinyi T. Recent clinical experiences with Ultracain preparations versus different lidocains. Z Stomatol 1988;85:235–8.
30. Szabo G, Divinyi T, Klenk G, et al. [Comparative clinical and experimental studies on the anesthetics on Ultracaine D-S and Ultracaine D-S forte]. Fogorv Sz 1983;76:267–70 [in Hungarian].
31. Szabo G, Gaspar L, Divinyi T. [Comparative clinical and experimental study of the anesthetics Ultracaine D-s and Ultracaine D-s forte (II)]. Fogorv Sz 1985;78:274–6 [in Hungarian].
32. Szabo G, Divinyi T. [Comparison of Ultracain D-S and Ultracain D-S forte]. Stomatol DDR 1987;37:301–4 [in German].
33. Anisimova EN, Zorian EV, Shugailov IA. [The characteristics of the action of Carpule-delivered local anesthetics and their combinations with vasoconstrictors (a preliminary report)]. Stomatologiia (Mosk) 1997;76:25–9 [in Russian].
34. Anisimova EN, Zorian EV, Shugailov IA. [The action of Carpule-delivered local anesthetics and their combinations with vasoconstrictors]. Stomatologiia (Mosk) 1998;77:19–22 [in Russian].
35. Petrovskaia LP, Maksimovskii I, Grinin VM. [Comparative efficiency of local anesthetics from the group of complex amides during therapeutic stomatological interventions]. Stomatologiia (Mosk) 2002;81:38–41 [in Russian].
36. Bose W. [Introduction of anesthetics into the oral mucosa by iontophoresis]. Dtsch Zahnarztl Z 1991;46:806–9 [in German].
37. Rosenberg PA, Amin KG, Zibari Y, et al. Comparison of 4% articaine with 1:100,000 epinephrine and 2% lidocaine with 1:100,000 epinephrine when used as a supplemental anesthetic. J Endod 2007;33:403–5.
38. Evans G, Nusstein J, Drum M, et al. A prospective, randomized, double-blind comparison of articaine and lidocaine for maxillary infiltrations. J Endod 2008;34:389–93.

39. Sherman MG, Flax M, Namerow K, et al. Anesthetic efficacy of the Gow-Gates injection and maxillary infiltration with articaine and lidocaine for irreversible pulpitis. J Endod 2008;34:656–9.

40. Haase A, Reader A, Nusstein J, et al. Comparing anesthetic efficacy of articaine versus lidocaine as a supplemental buccal infiltration of the mandibular first molar after an inferior alveolar nerve block. J Am Dent Assoc 2008;139:1228–35.

41. Srinivasan N, Kavitha M, Loganathan CS, et al. Comparison of anesthetic efficacy of 4% articaine and 2% lidocaine for maxillary buccal infiltration in patients with irreversible pulpitis. Oral Surg Oral Med Oral Pathol Oral Radiol Endod 2009; 107:133–6.

42. Tortamano IP, Siviero M, Costa CG, et al. A comparison of the anesthetic efficacy of articaine and lidocaine in patients with irreversible pulpitis. J Endod 2009;35:165–8.

43. Abdulwahab M, Boynes S, Moore P, et al. The efficacy of six local anesthetic formulations used for posterior mandibular buccal infiltration anesthesia. J Am Dent Assoc 2009;140:1018–24.

44. Aggarwal V, Jain A, Kabi D. Anesthetic efficacy of supplemental buccal and lingual infiltrations of articaine and lidocaine after an inferior alveolar nerve block in patients with irreversible pulpitis. J Endod 2009;35:925–9.

45. Fan S, Chen WL, Pan CB, et al. Anesthetic efficacy of inferior alveolar nerve block plus buccal infiltration or periodontal ligament injections with articaine in patients with irreversible pulpitis in the mandibular first molar. Oral Surg Oral Med Oral Pathol Oral Radiol Endod 2009;108:e89–93.

46. Matthews R, Drum M, Reader A, et al. Articaine for supplemental buccal mandibular infiltration anesthesia in patients with irreversible pulpitis when the inferior alveolar nerve block fails. J Endod 2009;35:343–6.

47. Fan S, Chen WL, Yang ZH, et al. Comparison of the efficiencies of permanent maxillary tooth removal performed with single buccal infiltration versus routine buccal and palatal injection. Oral Surg Oral Med Oral Pathol Oral Radiol Endod 2009;107:359–63.

48. Kanaa MD, Whitworth JM, Corbett IP, et al. Articaine buccal infiltration enhances the effectiveness of lidocaine inferior alveolar nerve block. Int Endod J 2009;42: 238–46.

49. Jung IY, Kim JH, Kim ES, et al. An evaluation of buccal infiltrations and inferior alveolar nerve blocks in pulpal anesthesia for mandibular first molars. J Endod 2008;34:11–3.

50. Uckan S, Dayangac E, Araz K. Is permanent maxillary tooth removal without palatal injection possible? Oral Surg Oral Med Oral Pathol Oral Radiol Endod 2006;102:733–5.

51. Bigby J, Reader A, Nusstein J, et al. Articaine for supplemental intraosseous anesthesia in patients with irreversible pulpitis. J Endod. 2006;32:1044–7.

52. Paxton K. Anesthetic efficacy of articaine hydrochloride versus lidocaine hydrochloride: a meta-analysis [master's thesis]. Iowa City (IA): The University of Iowa; 2008.

53. Paxton KR, Dawson DV, Drake DR, et al. Anesthetic efficacy of articaine hydrochloride versus lidocaine hydrochloride: a meta-analysis. J Dent Res 2008; 87(Spec Iss B):0025.

54. Moore PA, Boynes SG, Hersh EV, et al. The anesthetic efficacy of 4 percent articaine 1:200,000 epinephrine: two controlled clinical trials. J Am Dent Assoc 2006; 137:1572–81.

55. Raab WH, Muller R, Muller HF. [Comparative investigations of anesthetic activity of 2- and 4% articain]. Quintessenz 1990;41:1207–16 [in German].

56. Tofoli GR, Ramacciato JC, de Oliveira PC, et al. Comparison of effectiveness of 4% articaine associated with 1: 100,000 or 1: 200,000 epinephrine in inferior alveolar nerve block. Anesth Prog 2003;50:164–8.
57. Moore PA, Doll B, Delie RA, et al. Hemostatic and anesthetic efficacy of 4% articaine HCl with 1:200,000 epinephrine and 4% articaine HCl with 1:100,000 epinephrine when administered intraorally for periodontal surgery. J Periodontol 2007;78:247–53.
58. Santos CF, Modena KC, Giglio FP, et al. Epinephrine concentration (1:100,000 or 1:200,000) does not affect the clinical efficacy of 4% articaine for lower third molar removal: a double-blind, randomized, crossover study. J Oral Maxillofac Surg 2007;65:2445–52.
59. Dudkiewicz A, Schwartz S, Laliberte R. Effectiveness of mandibular infiltration in children using the local anesthetic Ultracaine (articaine hydrochloride). J Can Dent Assoc 1987;53:29–31.
60. Schroll K, Eskici A, Cartellieri W. [Clinical testing of the local anesthetic carticaine (Ultracain) in dental surgery]. Osterr Z Stomatol 1978;75:247–51 [in German].
61. Calderari G, Loiaconi G. Clinical stomatologic research with a new local anesthetic: Hoe 40045. Dent Cadmos 1979;47:14–23.
62. Lemay H, Albert G, Helie P, et al. Ultracaine in conventional operative dentistry. J Can Dent Assoc 1984;50:703–8.
63. Pavek V, Jandl P, Urban F Jr. New local anesthetic Ultracain. Cesk Stomatol 1981; 81:217–24.
64. Paxton KR, Dawson DV, Hill JR, et al. Articaine hydrochloride and epinephrine concentration: a meta-analysis. J Dent Res 2009;88(Spec Iss A):280.

Allergic Reactions to Local Anesthetic Formulations

Steven J. Speca, DMD*, Sean G. Boynes, DMD, MS,
Michael A. Cuddy, DMD

KEYWORDS

- Allergic reaction • Local anesthesia
- Type I anaphylactic response
- Type IV delayed hypersensitivity response

During the history of local anesthesia administration, a constant effort by chemists and scholars has been made to improve the efficacy and minimize adverse events associated with local anesthesia. Innovative products continue to replace agents that have inferior properties, and practice protocols are constantly being fine tuned to avert problematic practices. Because of this self-assessment within the respective health care fields, the potential for adverse events with currently marketed amide local anesthetics is extremely rare.[1] Dentists need to follow recommended doses, use a stress protocol, take thorough medical histories, aspirate before injections, and slowly disperse anesthetics during injection.[2] These procedures will help to avert many of the adverse events seen associated with local anesthesia, including allergic reactions.

Although an allergic response to a local anesthetic is remarkably rare, local anesthetics are capable of causing true allergic reactions. Clinicians need to be educated to properly treat and definitively diagnose a true allergic reaction. In the past, most allergic reactions to local anesthetics could be ascribed to procaine. The antigenicity of procaine, and other ester agents, is most often related to the para-aminobenzoic acid (PABA) component of ester anesthetics, a decidedly antigenic compound.[3] This finding, as well as procaine's poor efficacy and short duration, led to the development and eventual widespread use of the superior anesthetic lidocaine, an amide compound. The incidence of true allergies to amide local anesthetics is widely accepted to be well less than 1%[4]; unfortunately, poor understanding of adverse reactions to local anesthetic and poor availability of allergy testing, has resulted in unnecessary dental consequences.

Department of Anesthesiology, University of Pittsburgh School of Dental Medicine, G-87 Salk Hall, 3501 Terrace Street, Pittsburgh, PA 15261, USA
* Corresponding author.
E-mail address: drspeca@yahoo.com

Dent Clin N Am 54 (2010) 655–664
doi:10.1016/j.cden.2010.06.006
0011-8532/10/$ – see front matter © 2010 Elsevier Inc. All rights reserved.

dental.theclinics.com

ADVERSE EVENTS: DIFFERENTIATING ALLERGIC REACTIONS

Adverse reactions caused by fear or anxiety, inadvertent intravascular administration of local anesthetic, toxic overdose, intolerance, and idiosyncrasy could be mistaken for a true allergic response.[5] Toxic adverse reactions associated with local anesthetics are related to systemic exposure or local pharmacologic effect.[6] Clinicians need to be aware of potential precipitating factors such as needle phobias, chair position, liver or kidney failure, maximum recommended doses, proper safety protocols, and concomitant drug interactions. A thorough medical history is the simplest and most efficient method for the detection of risk factors that can lead to an adverse event.[7] Patient familiarity is imperative for a provider and will allow for rapid diagnosis and effective treatment when adverse events present.[8]

Anxiety plays a major role in dentistry. Scott and Hirchman[9] reported that a large portion of the US population becomes increasingly anxious in relation to dentistry. Psychogenic effects are the most numerous and common adverse events seen in a dental office. Because of the similarities, these psychogenic responses are often misdiagnosed as allergic reactions. In addition, needle phobias, panic attacks, and vasovagal syncope are all anxiety-related events with the potential to produce urticaria, edema, bronchospasm and unconsciousness. These reactions can present with a wide array of symptoms, including hyperventilation, nausea, vomiting, and alterations in heart rate or blood pressure.[10] Understanding the differences among allergic reactions from psychogenic reactions is important so that patients receive the appropriate care.[1,11]

THE ALLERGIC RESPONSE

Initially, the body's immune response system was thought to be purely protective; however, the dangerous potentials of severe allergic responses were eventually discovered. Hypersensitivities or allergies are abnormally vigorous immune responses, in which the immune system causes tissue damage as it fights off a perceived threat, or antigen, that would otherwise be harmless to the body.[12] There are different types of hypersensitivity reactions, which are best classified on the basis of the immunologic mechanism mediating the disease (**Table 1**).

ALLERGY-TESTING PROCEDURES

The history of a reported allergic reaction needs to be thoroughly evaluated and a clear sequence of the events documented. The drugs used, the onset of the reaction, signs and symptoms, and the duration of the event are very helpful in diagnosing a true allergic reaction. Most reported adverse reactions are psychogenic in nature and a smaller proportion of adverse responses can be attributed to avoidable intravascular injection. It is important not to prematurely label the patient as being allergic; the true nature of the problem should be investigated. If the reaction is acute and strongly suggestive of an allergic response, referral to an allergist is considered the standard of care.[13] As demonstrated in **Fig. 1**, the allergist will use skin prick tests (SPTs), interdermal or subcutaneous placement tests, and/or drug provocative challenge testing (DPT) procedures to aid in the identification of a safe local anesthetic for an individual patient.

An SPT is usually administered first. The SPT is performed by placing a drop of the test solution on the forearm and puncturing the skin through the liquid. If this test demonstrates a positive result, a wheal and flare should occur within 20 minutes.[14] If a systemic reaction occurs, appropriate treatment protocol for allergic reactions

Table 1
Classification of immunologically mediated hypersensitivity reactions

Type	Response Time	Associated Disorder	Mechanism
Type I – Anaphylactic	5–30 min	Anaphylaxis, bronchial asthma, urticaria	Mediators from IgE-sensitized mast cells cause increased vascular permeability, edema, and smooth muscle contraction
Type II – Cytotoxic	1–3 h	Autoimmune hemolytic anemia, erythroblastosis fetalis, Goodpasture's disease	IgG or IgM antibody reacting with cell surface or cell attached antigens results in cell destruction
Type III – Immune Complex	1–3 h	Arthus reaction, serum sickness, acute glomerulonephritis	Immune complexes (antigen-antibody complexes) activate complement, which attracts leukocytes; mediators released from these cells produce inflammation
Type IV – Cell-Mediated (Delayed)	8–12+ h	Tuberculosis, contact dermatitis, transplant rejection	Sensitized T lymphocytes reacting with antigens release lymphokines that produce cellular inflammation

should be followed. If the test was completed with a significantly diluted agent, and proved negative, then a more concentrated agent should be used.[15] If the SPT proves negative, it would be appropriate to follow with an intracutaneous or intradermal test in which a minute amount of the test solution is injected in the epidermis of the forearm and the site observed for 20 minutes for wheal or flare reactions. A DPT with the suspected drug is performed only if case history, skin test, and laboratory test give equivocal results.[16] Many allergists consider the DPT the gold standard in the diagnosis of

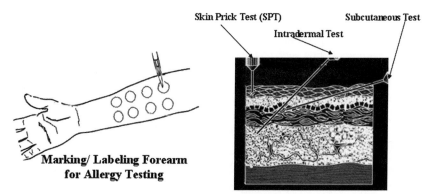

Fig. 1. Allergy testing procedures used for detection of hypersensitivity reactions to local anesthetics.

drug allergy; however, there is concern over the possible adverse consequences of the test.[17] Typically, the DPT uses the commercial preparation of the suspected allergen administered, ideally in the same way as it was given when the reaction occurred. Before performing any DPT, an individual risk-benefit evaluation should be accomplished and strict surveillance is needed with emergency protocols in place. Generally, the clinician should start with a low dose, carefully increasing the dosage with discontinuation of administration at the earliest appearance of any signs or symptoms.[17]

The patient should be provided the results of the testing with suggestions to minimize future risks. The success of this protocol is related to the rare instance of true allergic reaction to amide local anesthetics; however, the testing alleviates stress for the patient and doctor and it may permit the diagnosis of the truly rare instance of an amide allergy.[17]

ALLERGIC RESPONSE WITH DENTAL LOCAL ANESTHESIA
Allergic Reactions to Local Anesthetics

Although allergic reactions to local anesthetics are exceedingly rare, there are a large number of patients who claim allergy to these agents. This may be attributable to a misunderstanding on the part of the health practitioners, and patient, as to what constitutes allergy. The clinician must be able to differentiate among reactions to local anesthetics that are psychologically initiated, those related to dosage and toxicity, and those that are related to allergy. Skin manifestations of allergy should be used as key indicators of a true response, because an allergy is unlikely in their absence.[1] Corroboration with blood studies is also of value when hypersensitivity to local anesthetics is suspected. These blood studies are administered to differentiate between the 2 responses related to local anesthetics, type I and type IV reactions. Serum IgE (Type 1; Anaphylactic Reaction) levels are decreased within 1 hour after an allergic reaction has commenced. Following this initial decrease, there is a marked increase in the plasma concentration of IgE antibodies that remain elevated for 72 hours after an adverse response.[1] The complement system may also mediate a delayed allergic response with local anesthesia (Type IV; Cell-Mediated Reaction). Plasma samples showing consumption of complement proteins C3 and C4 are suggestive of allergy.[18]

In the early use of local anesthesia, most allergic reactions to local anesthetics could be attributed to procaine. The antigenicity of procaine, as well as other ester compounds, relates directly to its structural formula.[1] Because the ester agents are derivatives of PABA, this substance occurs as a metabolite following hydrolysis of the main compound. PABA is responsible for the allergic-type reactions observed.[19] It should be noted that susceptibility to procaine also implies hypersensitivity to structurally similar compounds such as tetracaine or chloroprocaine.[20] Therefore, all ester-linked local anesthetics are best avoided in patients with procaine allergy.[21]

Most investigators believe that true allergic reactions to amide local anesthetic agents are extremely rare; however, reports of suspected allergic, hypersensitivity, or anaphylactic responses to these local anesthetic compounds appear in literature.[19] Usually the diagnosis of such reaction is made when no obvious explanation is available for an adverse effect in a patient exposed to a local anesthetic drug; however, true allergic responses have been verified.[19] A true allergy diagnosis requires the formation of an antibody to an antigenic substance. To establish this diagnosis, an intracutaneous or pin-prick challenge with the allergen (amide anesthetic) should be performed by a specialist. Unfortunately, the reported evidence is limited in literature and the techniques used for diagnosis exhibit some variation and lack consistency in reporting.

Aldrete and Johnson[22] were among the first investigators to use the technique of intracutaneous testing to study patients with and without a presumptive history of local anesthetic allergy. Positive skin reactions were observed in 25 of 60 patients in the nonallergic group. In all cases, the cutaneous reaction followed injection of an ester-type anesthetic (procaine, tetracaine, chloroprocaine), whereas no reactions were observed after treatment with the amide-type agents (lidocaine, mepivacaine, prilocaine). In a more current evaluation, Gall and colleagues[23] evaluated 197 patients who reported a history of adverse allergic-type events after local anesthetic administration. Procaine was tested along with all of the currently marketed amide local anesthetics. Of the 197 patients, only 3 patients reacted after subcutaneous challenge with the causative drug (local anesthetics of the amide type). Although 1 patient showed a delayed-type response to mepivacaine, 2 patients had immediate-type reactions to articaine and lidocaine; however, in both cases no specific IgE antibody could be detected.

Haugen and Brown[24] reported a case of Type I hypersensitivity allergy to lidocaine hydrochloride. Within 15 minutes of the lidocaine injection, the patient complained of lightheadedness, and right periorbital swelling with noted wheezing were documented. Based on the patient's unusual response, an undiagnosed allergy to lidocaine was suspected. The patient was referred to an allergist for skin testing and a positive test to lidocaine was confirmed. An intradermal 1:10,000 dilution of lidocaine 1% produced a 4-mm skin wheal with flare. The saline solution control produced a negative result, and a histamine prick test produced a 7-mm wheal with flare. Although a rechallenge with lidocaine was not performed, a positive immediate hypersensitive reaction to lidocaine was strongly suggested based on the patient's history and positive intradermal skin test.

In an additional case report presented by Noormalin and colleagues,[16] a 7-year-old girl was diagnosed with a type I hypersensitivity to lignocaine (lidocaine) following a dental procedure. The child developed an ipsilateral facial swelling and was immediately administered intravenous antihistamine. The swelling subsided on the same day after the patient returned home with her parents. Because the swelling was at the site where local anesthesia was administered, it was postulated that the patient could have had a hypersensitivity reaction to 2% lignocaine HCL, oral lignocaine dental gel, or latex glove response. To reach a definitive diagnosis of allergy, an SPT was administered. The SPT revealed a positive reaction to pure 2% lignocaine HCL and lignocaine oral dental gel, whereas tests relating to latex were negative. The patient also developed urticaria after 10 minutes of performing the test. The authors did not proceed to intradermal testing because the SPT was positive and the child presented with urticaria. In addition, an immunoblot test demonstrated positive dot-blot reaction (IgE response) to both the 2% lignocaine and lignocaine oral gel.

Although most allergic reports in literature relate to the type I (anaphylactic) response, Fuzier and colleagues[25] evaluated 2 database systems to determine the incidence of both the type I and the type IV (delayed) response. The authors studied reports recorded in the French Pharmacovigilance database and the GERAP database over a 12-year period (1995 to 2006). For each report, Fuzier and colleagues[25] detailed the clinical features and skin tests used. A total of 16 reports were identified and lidocaine was the local anesthetic most often involved (11 of 16). Cutaneous symptoms were reported as the main features of allergic reactions with local anesthetics. Prick test, intradermal reaction, and challenge tests were used to confirm the diagnosis and type I (immediate) reactions were encountered in approximately 70% of the cases. Type IV delayed reactions were, therefore, noted 30% of the time.

Although true allergic reactions to local anesthetics are rare, some have been well documented. In addition, it has been noted that ester-type local anesthetics are more allergenic than amide-type; however, there are a significant number of reports of amide agents causing allergic reactions.[25] Cutaneous features, such as urticaria, pruritis, and erythema, are the most common features of local anesthetic hypersensitivity reactions. Furthermore, allergy to local anesthetics may be type I or type IV hypersensitivity reactions with the type I response more commonly reported in dentistry.[16,25]

Cross Reactivity among Amide Local Anesthetics

Cross reactivity among the amide family of local anesthetics was once thought not to exist; however, recent literature has demonstrated that cross-allergenicity may occur. The French Pharmacovigilance database and GERAP were studied to determine type I immediate and type IV delayed hypersensitivity reactions to local anesthetics, as well as cross reactivity between amide local anesthetics. The report found 11 immediate reactions with 6 having cross reactivity.[25] In addition, a case report of a 39-year-old man who attended an allergy unit in Spain presented with an immediate hypersensitivity reaction to mepivacaine and cross reactivity to lidocaine and ropivacaine but could tolerate bupivacaine and levo-bupivacaine. This patient was diagnosed by using prick tests and intradermal tests; challenge tests were not used citing ethical reasons.[13]

Allergic Reactions to Local Anesthetic Preservatives

Methylparaben

Methylparaben, a preservative commonly found in foods and cosmetics, was frequently used in amide anesthetic solutions to prevent contamination of the agent. Methylparaben is bacteriostatic and fungistatic, and has oxidant properties because of its phenol-like action, which acts by denaturation of proteins and by antimetabolite properties of p-hydroxybenzoic acid.[14] The structure of methylparaben is similar to PABA, a metabolite of procaine, which has been associated with a number of documented allergic reactions.[15,17] In 1984, the Food and Drug Administration (FDA) mandated methylparaben be removed from single-dose local anesthetic cartridges; since then the number of related allergic reactions has been almost nonexistent.[1]

Sulfites

Sulfites are commonly used to extend the shelf life of many injectable drugs, such as antibiotics and local anesthetics, as well as foods and wines. Sulfites are antioxidants that release sulfur dioxide, an active component, which may help stabilize epinephrine in local anesthetic solutions.[26] Most of the current dental anesthetics with vasoconstrictor contain the preservatives metabisulfite, sodium bisulfate, or potassium bisulfite. Metabisulfites may cause non–IgE-mediated hypersensitivity reactions, characterized by rhinitis, rash, headache, dyspnea, and cramping.[27] Koo and Dym[28] reported a type III hypersensitivity reaction in a 6-year-old boy anesthetized with lidocaine containing epinephrine. The child developed a delayed skin reaction following the injection that appeared as a leathery pigmented area, which is a similar feature seen in cutaneous necrotizing vasculitis. Metabisulfite was thought to be the primary cause of this reaction; however, because of potential scarring, no biopsy or further skin testing was done.[28] For definitive diagnosis, skin biopsy and histopathologic and immunopathologic testing should have been performed. Because of the existence of food allergy to sulfites, local anesthetics containing vasoconstrictor should be used cautiously or withheld in patients reporting food allergies associated with sulfites.[29] It is estimated 500,000 Americans have allergic reactions to sulfite-containing drugs. In 1986, the FDA reported 14 deaths linked to allergic reactions.[30] The history of sulfite allergy may be very misleading and skin tests are very inconsistent. Most reactions to sulfites are seen in individuals with asthma; reactions in those who do not have asthma are very rare.[31] Formulations not containing a vasoconstrictor, such as 3% mepivacaine or 4% prilocaine, do not contain sulfite preservative.

Latex Sensitivity

Dental cartridges contain latex stoppers and diaphragms, which can serve as potential allergens. Latex allergies can lead to type I and type IV hypersensitivity reactions. The type IV reaction is most commonly associated with the area of latex contact and usually presents as contact dermatitis. Estimates of the prevalence of allergy to latex allergens in the general population vary widely, from less than 1% to 6%.[32] Health care provider visits for contact dermatitis and other eczemas, which include atopic dermatitis, are approximately 7 million per year.[33]

Shojeil and Hass[34] conducted an evaluation of relevant publications from 1966 to 2001 to investigate evidence of latex allergies associated with medication vials or dental cartridges for dental local anesthesia. This review found evidence in the literature that latex allergens can be released into pharmaceutical solutions. However, the investigators concluded there were no reports of studies or cases implicating a dental cartridge as the cause of latex allergy. Even though there are no reports to date, it does not rule out the possibility of a future reaction. Fortunately, one of the major local anesthetic manufactures, in an attempt to reduce latex in health care, has recently developed latex-free dental cartridges.

Treatment of an Allergic Reaction

Overall, true allergic responses to local anesthetics may be localized or general, immediate in onset or delayed.[35] Most accounts of allergic reactions to amides or to the preservatives added to commercial dental local anesthetic solutions suggest that the type I (anaphylactoid) response is the most likely allergic reaction to produce a generalized effect in patients after intraoral injection.[36] Even though the incidence of true allergic reactions is very low, they do occur and anaphylaxis is the major concern and often takes treatment precedence over other situations.[14,37]

In anaphylaxis, a combination of the anesthetic antigen with antibodies bound to mast cells release specific mediators, such as basophils and neutrophils, which affect various tissues of the body. The common manifestations of anaphylaxis (erythema, pruritis, and urticaria) involve the skin and require a fundamental treatment method. Requiring a more concise treatment methodology, the most concerning manifestation of an anaphylactic reaction relates to smooth muscle contraction. This can lead to bronchial constriction in which death can occur from bronchial spasm or laryngeal edema.

Generally, the signs and symptoms involved with anaphylaxis will follow a progressive pattern that initiates with skin reactions and terminates with respiratory distress and cardiovascular depression.[38] In the event of generalized anaphylaxis, the signs will demonstrate a progressive pattern as follows[38,39]:

- Skin manifestations (erythema, pruritis, and urticaria)
- Gastrointestinal manifestations (muscle cramping, nausea and vomiting, incontinence)
- Respiratory manifestations (coughing, wheezing, dyspnea, laryngeal edema)
- Cardiovascular manifestations (palpitations, tachycardia, hypotension, unconsciousness, cardiac arrest).

Table 2
Management of local anesthesia–related allergic manifestations

Manifestation	Symptom Occurrence	Signs/Symptoms	Management
Localized Skin Reaction	Usually	Erythema, edema, pruritus	Monitor patient without intervention, or oral antihistamine (Benadryl 25–50 mg)
Generalized Skin Reaction	Often	Pruritus, urticaria, macular rash	Oral antihistamine (Benadryl 25–50 mg), or IM antihistamine (diphenhydramine 25–50 mg)
Respiratory Implication	Occasionally	Bronchoconstriction, laryngeal edema, dyspnea	Epinephrine IM or SC (0.3 mg); oxygen, maintain airway, EMS activation. Supplemental Therapy: IM diphenhydramine (50 mg); IM or IV glucocorticoids
Anaphylactic Shock	Rarely	Skin reactions, bronchoconstriction, edema, dyspnea, marked hypotension, cardiovascular collapse	EMS activation, epinephrine IM or SC (0.3 mg); oxygen, BLS/CPR as indicated. Supplemental Therapy: IM diphenhydramine (50 mg); IM or IV glucocorticoids

Abbreviations: BLS, basic life support; CPR, cardiopulmonary resuscitation; EMS, emergency medical services; IM, intramuscular; IV, intravenous; SC, subcutaneous.

Prompt detection and response to emergent allergic reactions will alter the extent of the reaction. It is important to note that, when applicable, the removal of any remaining traces of a possible allergen should always be the initial treatment step. The management of allergic reactions will also follow a progressive pattern of treatment depending on the severity of the patient's response. **Table 2** outlines the management of allergic responses to local anesthetics.

SUMMARY

True allergic reactions to local anesthetics are rare adverse reactions. At the most, they represent less than 1% of all adverse local anesthetic reactions.[25,40,41] When true allergic reactions have been confirmed, the reactions are most commonly the type I anaphylactic and type IV delayed hypersensitivity responses. The type I immediate hypersensitivity reactions are the most severe and may be life-threatening.[24,41]

In the event a potential allergic reaction occurs in a dental office, the dentist needs to properly evaluate the events leading up to the reaction and provide a differential diagnosis. Patients presenting with hives, wheezing, angioedema, bronchospasm, hypotension, unconsciousness, and cardiovascular collapse may have a true allergic reaction. The dentist needs to catalog all drugs and materials that came in contact with the patient to assist in definitive diagnosis. A referral should be given to any patient when an allergic reaction cannot be ruled out as an intravascular injection, toxic overdose, psychogenic reaction, or an idiosyncratic event.

REFERENCES

1. Milam SB, Giovannitti JA. Local anesthetics in dental practice. Dent Clin North Am 1984;28:493–508.
2. Gouda M, Dabarakis KP. Is allergy to local anesthetics in dentistry possible? Res J Biol Sci 2009;4:899–904.
3. Miller RD, Stoelting RK. Basics of anesthesia. 5th edition. Philadelphia (PA): Churchill Livingstone; 2007. p.124–6.
4. Giovannitti JA, Bennett CR. Assessment of allergy to local anesthetics. J Am Dent Assoc 1979;98:701–9.
5. Ball IA. Allergic reactions to lignocaine. Braz Dent J 2003;186:224–6.
6. Lukawska J, Caballero RM, Tsabour S, et al. Hypersensitivity to local anaesthetics—6 facts and 7 myths. Curr Allergy Clin Immunol 2009;22(3): 117–20.
7. Daublander M, Muller R, Lipp MD. The incidence of complications associated with local anesthesia in dentistry. Anesth Prog 1997;44:132–41.
8. Moore PA. Adverse drug reactions to local anesthesia. Dent Clin North Am 2002; 46:747–57.
9. Scott DS, Hirschman R. Psychologic aspects of dental anxiety in adults. J Am Dent Assoc 1982;10:27–31.
10. Haas DA. An update on local anesthetics in dentistry. J Can Dent Assoc 2002; 68(9):546–51.
11. Grimes E. The syncopal patient in the dental office. J Practical Hygiene 2001 (Nov/Dec) 39–42.
12. Marieb EN. Human anatomy & physiology. 4th edition. Menlo Park (CA): Benjamin/Cummings Science Publishing; 1998. p. 791–93.
13. Gonzalez-Delgado P, Anton R, Soriano V, et al. Cross-reactivity among amide-type local anesthetics in a case of allergy to mepivacaine. J Investig Allergol Clin Immunol 2006;16(5):311–5.
14. Larson CE. Methylparaben—an overlooked cause of local anesthetic hypersensitivity. Anesth Prog 1977;24:72–4.
15. Schamberg IL. Allergic contact dermatitis to methy and propyl paraben. Arch Dermatol 1967;95:626–8.
16. Noormalin A, Shahnaz M, Rosmilah M, et al. IgE-mediated hypersensitivity reaction to lidocaine—case report. Trop Biomed 2005;22:179–83.
17. Schorr WP, Mohajerin AH. Paraben sensitivity. Arch Dermatol 1966;93:721–3.
18. Stoelting RK. Allergic reactions during anesthesia. Anesth Analg 1983;62: 341–56.
19. Covino BG, Vassallo HH. Local anesthetics: mechanisms of action and clinical use. New York: Grune and Stratton; 1976. p. 9–11.
20. Aldrete JA, Johnson DA. Allergy to local anesthetics. JAMA 1969;207:356–61.
21. De Jong RH. Physiology and pharmacology of local anesthesia. 2nd edition. Springfield (IL): Charles C. Thomas Books; 1970. p. 206.
22. Aldrete JA, Johnson DA. Evaluation of intracutaneous testing for investigation of allergy to local anesthetic agents. Anesth Analg 1970;49:173–81.
23. Gall H, Kaufmann R, Kalveram CM. Adverse reactions to local anesthetics: analysis of 197 cases. J Allergy Clin Immunol 1996;97(4):933–7.
24. Haugen RN, Brown CW. Case reports: type I hypersensitivity to lidocaine. J Drugs in Dermatology 2007;6:1222–3.
25. Fuzier R, Lapeyre-Mstre M, Mertes PM, et al. French association of regional pharmacovigilance centers. Immediate- and delayed-type allergic reactions to amide

local anesthetics: clinical features and skin testing. Pharmacoepidemiol Drug Saf 2009;18:595–601.

26. The Associated Press. FDA plans warning on drugs with sulfites. New York (NY): The New York Times; 1986.
27. Simon RA. Adverse reactions to food and drug additives. Immunology and Asthma Clinics of North America 1996;16(1):228.
28. Koo YH, Dym H. An unusual complication with local anesthetic injection. Columbia Dental Review 2000;5:30–2.
29. Campbell JR, Maestrello CI, Campell RI. Allergic response to metabisulfite in lidocaine anesthetic solution. Anesth Prog 2001;48:21–6.
30. FDA/New York Times. FDA plans warning on drugs with sulfites. AP, 1986.
31. Stevenson D, Simon R. Sensitivity to ingested metabisulfites in asthmatic subjects. J Allergy Clin Immunol 1981;68:26–32.
32. Poley GE, Slater JE. "Latex allergy". J Allergy Clin Immunol 2000;105(6):1054–62.
33. CDC. National Center for Health Statistics. Vital and Health Statistics Series 1996; 13(134).
34. Shojaei AR, Hass DA. Local anesthetic cartridges and latex allergy: a literature review. J Can Dent Assoc 2002;68(10):622–6.
35. Jastak JT, Yagiela JA, Donaldson D. Local anesthesia of the oral cavity. Philadelphia: WB Saunders Co. 1995. p.297–98.
36. Canfield DW, Gage TW. A guideline to local anesthetic allergy testing. Anesth Prog 1987;34:157–63.
37. Malamed SF. Handbook of local anesthesia. 5th edition. St Louis (MO): Elsevier Mosby; 2004.
38. Bassett KB, DiMarco AC, Naughton DK. Local anesthesia for dental professionals. Saddle River (NJ): Pearson Education Inc; 2010. p. 360.
39. Mertes PM, Laxenaire MC. Allergic reactions occurring during anaesthesia. Eur J Anaesthesiol. 2002;19:240–62.
40. Schatz M. Skin testing and incremental challenge in the evaluation of adverse reactions to local anesthetics. J Allergy Clin Immunol 1984;74:606–16.
41. Chih-Yung C, Tzou-Yien L, Shao-Hsusan H, et al. Systemic anaphylaxis following local lidocaine administration during a dental procedure. Pediatr Emerg Care 2004;20:178–80.

Acquired Methemoglobinemia Revisited

Larry Trapp, DDS, MS[a],*, John Will, DDS[a,b]

KEYWORDS

- Acquired methemoglobinemia • Benzocaine
- Prilocaine • Dentistry

Acquired methemoglobinemia remains a source of morbidity and mortality in dental and medical patients despite the fact that it is better understood now than it was even a decade ago. It is in the interest of all dental patients that their treating dentists review this disorder. The safety of dental patients mandates professional awareness.

THE PHYSIOLOGY OF HEMOGLOBIN IN THE RED BLOOD CELL

Hemoglobin is a molecule that constitutes a large fraction of the nonwater content of the red blood cell in humans. The important physiologic role of hemoglobin in humans includes the distribution of oxygen from the lungs to all peripheral tissues and the removal of all metabolically derived carbon dioxide from peripheral tissues by returning it to the lungs for elimination.

Each molecule of hemoglobin contains 4 iron atoms. All 4 of the iron atoms normally have an atomic valence of +2 (each is referred to as a ferric ion).[1] As blood passes through the lungs, molecules of oxygen are exposed to the hemoglobin in the red blood cells. The oxygen molecules are bound by the ferrous ions in hemoglobin and transported to the peripheral tissues. In the periphery, the oxygen gradient reverses and the acidic environment (lower pH) reduces the affinity of hemoglobin for oxygen and the oxygen is released into the surrounding peripheral tissues. The affinity of hemoglobin for carbon dioxide increases once the oxygen has been released. The carbon dioxide is bound by the deoxygenated hemoglobin and it is transported back to the lungs where the affinity for carbon dioxide is decreased and it moves into the alveoli and is subsequently exhaled. The cycle of oxygen and carbon dioxide transport then repeats itself.

[a] Department of Dental Anesthesiology, Loma Linda University School of Dentistry, 11092 Anderson Street, Loma Linda, CA 92350, USA
[b] 135 Tyler Ct, Leoma, TN 38468, USA
* Corresponding author.
E-mail address: ltrapp@llu.edu

Dent Clin N Am 54 (2010) 665–675
doi:10.1016/j.cden.2010.06.007
0011-8532/10/$ – see front matter © 2010 Elsevier Inc. All rights reserved.

How is Methemoglobin Created?

If hemoglobin is exposed to an agent or chemical that is able to extract an electron from 1 or more of the 4 ferrous ions in hemoglobin, the iron atom(s) adopt a +3 atomic valence (known as a ferric ion).[1] The molecule of hemoglobin now has at least 1 iron atom in the ferric state. A molecule of hemoglobin with 1 or more of its iron atoms in the ferric ion status is referred to as *methemoglobin*. Inorganic chemistry teaches that the process whereby an iron atom's valence is increased from +2 to +3 is referred to as oxidation. The agent or chemical causing the increased valence is called an oxidant.[1,2]

As soon as even one of hemoglobin's 4 iron atoms has been oxidized to the ferric state, the methemoglobin molecule then has an *increased* affinity for its bound oxygen and a *decreased* affinity for any unbound oxygen. Thus, less oxygen is transported by methemoglobin and the smaller amount of oxygen that is transported is not readily released in the peripheral tissues (ie, the oxyhemoglobin dissociation curve is shifted to the left). With less oxygen being transported to the periphery and less oxygen being released by methemoglobin in the periphery, the affinity of methemoglobin for carbon dioxide is decreased and less carbon dioxide is removed from the peripheral tissues. It is thought that the transition from hemoglobin to methemoglobin alters the molecule's shape (ie, molecular conformation) and that this alteration of molecular shape is sustained by the presence of one or more ferric ions. The fraction of hemoglobin oxidized dictates the extent of compromise in oxygen delivery and carbon dioxide removal (ie, toxicity) and it is directly related to the efficacy of exposure to the oxidizing agent. If the exposure to an oxidant is great enough, cyanosis or color change in the blood and skin becomes apparent followed by progressively more serious signs and symptoms of methemoglobinemia (**Table 1**).[3]

Reducing Methemoglobin is a Physiologic Process

A blood level of methemoglobin between 0% and 2% is detectable in the human population at all times. This level is thought to exist because the body uses and is dependent on a prototypical oxidant, oxygen. Blood is continuously exposed to this oxidant because it must necessarily and continually transport oxygen. The human body has more than one compensatory physiologic mechanism to reduce ferric iron to ferrous iron. These systems continually reduce methemoglobin to hemoglobin and thereby maintain homeostasis of the oxygen delivery system in the body. The predominant enzyme system for the physiologic reduction of methemoglobin to hemoglobin is cytochrome b5 methemoglobin reductase. An alternate enzyme system that normally reduces only a small fraction of methemoglobin is referred to as nicotinamide adenine dinucleotide phosphate ($NADPH_3$).[1,2]

Table 1	
Symptoms and signs of methemoglobinemia	
Methemoglobin Level %	**Symptoms and Signs[1,2]**
≤ 2	None (physiologic)
2–15	None
15–20	Cyanosis
20–30	Mental changes (headache, fatigue, dizziness), exercise intolerance, syncope, tachycardia
30–50	Fatigue, confusion, tachypnea, tachycardia
50–70	Dysrhythmias, seizures, coma, acidosis
>70	Death

How Methemoglobin Levels Increase

When the body encounters an exogenous oxidant exposure of sufficient dosage and potency, the physiologic capacity for methemoglobin reduction is overwhelmed and increasing methemoglobin levels ensue. As methemoglobin levels increase, the reading on a conventional pulse oximeter falls to between 85% and 90%, and remains in that range.[4] The pulse oximeter reading is unresponsive to the administration of supplemental oxygen. Methemoglobin concentrations approaching 10% to 15% may be associated with cyanosis in light-skinned individuals. Methemoglobin blood levels of 20% to 45% produce additional symptoms, which include nausea, lethargy, tachycardia, headache, and dizziness. Consciousness deteriorates as methemoglobin levels reach the range of 50% to 55%, and levels of 70% are usually fatal (see **Table 1**).[1]

Measuring Methemoglobin Blood Levels

Before 2005, a laboratory test was required to identify the blood level of methemoglobin. This test was named oximetry analysis (commonly referred to as a co-oximetry test) and required that a blood specimen be drawn.[1] The methemoglobin level was generally measured and reported as a percent of hemoglobin present in the blood. A noninvasive device that looks like a pulse oximeter was marketed in 2005 (Masimo, Inc, Irvine, CA, USA) that could reliably identify blood levels of methemoglobin and carboxyhemoglobin as well as the hemoglobin saturation of oxygen. The new monitor uses additional light transmission technology. It is of interest that this new device correctly reads elevated methemoglobin levels, whereas the pulse oximeter component may erroneously read, as previously described.[5]

Potential Etiologies of Methemoglobinemia

Oxidation of hemoglobin to methemoglobin occurs continuously in the absence of any exogenous toxin or oxidizing medication and levels of 1% to 2% are the result of a physiologic process. As stated previously, this low methemoglobin level may be caused by the transport of oxygen and its inherent ability to act as an oxidant. In this discussion of etiologies of methemoglobinemia, only causes of methemoglobin levels that are more than those described as physiologic will be considered.

Congenital methemoglobinemia is a rare metabolic disorder of the newborn and is difficult to diagnose. The metabolic ability to reduce methemoglobin to hemoglobin is either absent or diminished.[6] The diagnosis and treatment of this perinatal disease is important but it does not require the attention of the dental profession.

The most common etiology of methemoglobinemia is referred to as *acquired* methemoglobinemia. The first clinical descriptions of acquired or toxic methemoglobinemia date back to 1886.[7] Many cases of acquired methemoglobinemia have as their etiology an oxidizing substance that may be one of a large number of medications or other exogenous toxins.[5,8,9] Oxidizing medications that are used in dentistry include the topical anesthetic benzocaine (eg, Hurricaine) and the injected local anesthetic prilocaine (Citanest), or more accurately the two metabolites of prilocaine: o-toluidine and nitrosotoluidine.[10] There are many other oxidants, including aniline (used in the manufacture of polyurethane), nitrites (used to treat angina, cyanide toxicity), nitrobenzene (a precursor of aniline), dapsone (Aczone, an antibiotic for acne), and phenazopyridine (Pyridium, a urologic antibiotic). The rate of increase and the peak levels of methemoglobin are a function of dose and route of absorption. Nitrous oxide has been implicated as an oxidant of hemoglobin by a few publications and is discussed later in detail.

In some cases of methemoglobinemia an etiology is never identified. In this situation, the diagnosis becomes idiopathic methemoglobinemia.

Interactions Between Oxidizing Agents and Diseases

Patients that are diagnosed with diseases that may compromise oxygen delivery to the peripheral tissues need to be assessed for the potential negative interaction with any oxidizing agents administered during dental or other treatments. This task is sometimes difficult because diseases vary as to their mechanism for decreasing oxygen delivery to peripheral tissues. Examples include patients with chronic kidney failure who commonly manifest a low hemoglobin value, patients diagnosed with sickle cell anemia and who are beginning a sickle cell crisis, and patients with pulmonary fibrosis who have hypoxemia caused by an oxygen-diffusion barrier in their lungs. Patients with any of these diagnoses may experience a life-threatening reduction in oxygen delivery to their peripheral tissues if they receive a modest dose of an agent or medication that oxidizes hemoglobin to methemoglobin.[3]

Medications Used in Dentistry That Induce Methemoglobinemia

As previously mentioned, the dental profession in the United States commonly administers two medications that are well recognized as oxidants of hemoglobin. The two medications are discussed sequentially starting with prilocaine. Two other medications used in dentistry, lidocaine and nitrous oxide, have been held responsible for being oxidants of hemoglobin. However, after extensive review, they have not been clearly demonstrated to cause methemoglobinemia.

Prilocaine

The evidence supporting the oxidation of hemoglobin to methemoglobin subsequent to the clinical use of prilocaine has been clearly demonstrated for many decades. Investigations into the mechanism of oxidation clarified that prilocaine itself did not oxidize hemoglobin in vitro; however, oxidation did occur in vivo. Subsequently, it was discovered that two metabolites of prilocaine are responsible for the oxidation of hemoglobin. These metabolites have been identified as o-toluidine and nitrosotoluidine.[10]

Parenteral local anesthetics are packaged in 1.8 mL cartridges for dental administration in the United States. The medications in cartridges include lidocaine, mepivacaine, prilocaine, articaine, and bupivacaine. These local anesthetics are packaged with and without vasoconstricting agents that enhance the duration and intensity of local anesthetic action and decrease the central nervous system toxicity. Prilocaine is packaged as a 4% solution without an agent for vasoconstriction and a 4% solution with an added agent for vasoconstriction (one 4% dental cartridge of 1.8 mL volume contains 72 mg of prilocaine). Of the listed local anesthetics packaged for parenteral use in the United States, only prilocaine is well documented to cause the oxidation of hemoglobin to methemoglobin (see later discussion).

Other injectable local anesthetics and methemoglobinemia

The only injectable local anesthetics cited in the literature as oxidizers of hemoglobin are prilocaine, lidocaine, tetracaine, and cocaine.[7] Lidocaine has not been shown to be an oxidizer of hemoglobin after extensive review (see later discussion).[7] Tetracaine is a local anesthetic with an ester structure that is used exclusively in medical anesthesiology for spinal anesthesia and is not available in dental cartridges in the United States. There is inadequate evidence to label tetracaine as an oxidizer of hemoglobin.[7] Cocaine has not been used as an injectable local anesthetic in more than 100 years.

There is no suggestion or evidence in the literature that mepivacaine, bupivacaine, or septocaine oxidizes hemoglobin and thereby causes methemoglobinemia.

Benzocaine

Benzocaine is commonly used by the dental profession as a topical anesthetic on oral mucosa before administering a local anesthetic injection and as a topical anesthetic on oral mucosa and gingiva before having the teeth cleaned. Less frequently, benzocaine is used to minimize pain from radiographic film when taking intraoral radiographs. Benzocaine spray is infrequently used by dental and medical anesthesiologists during laryngoscopy for endotracheal intubation under special circumstances. Benzocaine is marketed as an aerosol, gel, cream, liquid, and oral spray in concentrations ranging from 7.5% to 20.0%. It is marketed for all oral pain, including teething pain in infants. It is available in many over-the-counter products. Benzocaine is a well-documented but poorly understood cause of methemoglobinemia.[7]

EUTECTIC MIXTURE OF LOCAL ANESTHETIC

A topical anesthetic product containing prilocaine and lidocaine is commercially available as EMLA (eutectic mixture of local anesthetic) cream. Prilocaine and lidocaine are placed in an oil base and, upon mixing, the physical properties of both local anesthetics change to that of a eutectic mixture. A eutectic mixture is created when two or more substances are mixed and their respective melting points decrease below that for each of the individual constituents. Hence, the local anesthetics change from a mixture of anesthetic crystals to local anesthetics in a liquid state. The manufacturer (AstraZeneca) then emulsifies the oil into a cream and the product is ready to apply to the skin. The final product contains prilocaine 2.5% and lidocaine 2.5%.[11]

The product was designed for application onto intact skin. However, application to oral mucous membranes has been evaluated in the last decade and a product has been marketed (Oraqix).[11] Topical skin application requires placing a specified amount of the product as a thin layer over a given area of skin. Both the amount of the product and the area covered are based on age and weight (eg, 2 g over 20 cm^2 if body weight is >5 kg). An occlusive dressing, such as Tegaderm, is then placed over the area for 1 hour after which time topical anesthesia is obtained. Pediatric applications include use as an adjunct to circumcision. Placing too large an amount over too large an area may place the younger pediatric patient at risk for methemoglobinemia. Oral mucosal application is limited to deep periodontal pockets to facilitate mechanical removal of debris from the pocket. The product is marketed as a gel with the same concentrations of lidocaine and prilocaine (2.5% for both). The gel is applied by means of a blunt-tipped applicator device. Each applicator contains 1.7 g (1.7 mL). The maximum to be applied is 5 applicators or 212 mg of prilocaine.[11] Any use of prilocaine by injection at the same appointment would be additive if given in the same time frame.

Does Lidocaine Oxidize Hemoglobin to Methemoglobin?

Although lidocaine has been listed as an oxidizer of hemoglobin to methemoglobin in a few medical references,[3,5] a recent and thorough review of methemoglobinemia as it relates to local anesthetics resulted in the author concluding that the capability of lidocaine to induce methemoglobin formation and methemoglobinemia is *not well demonstrated.*[7] Neither does the dental literature (and vast clinical experience with lidocaine in dentistry) support lidocaine as an oxidant of hemoglobin and a cause of methemoglobinemia.[8] For this reason, lidocaine is not considered as an oxidizing agent in this review.

Does Nitrous Oxide Induce Methemoglobin Formation?

One published paper surmised that a pediatric dental patient receiving nitrous oxide/oxygen for sedation and prilocaine for local anesthesia experienced severe cyanosis, methemoglobinemia, seizures, and a stuporous mental status.[12] The Ludwig article correctly attributes the methemoglobinemia to prilocaine. However, a subsequent publication[3] incorrectly referenced the Ludwig article and one other article[13] as having provided evidence that nitrous oxide is an oxidant of hemoglobin and a potential cause of methemoglobinemia. Authors have continued to cite and reproduce the table in the Ash-Bernal article and have thereby supported the spurious role of nitrous oxide as a oxidant of hemoglobin.[5] Nitrous oxide administered with at least 50% oxygen is a venerable anxiolytic in dentistry, and nitrous oxide is a supplement to inhalation general anesthesia, which has been in clinical use for more than 150 years. Thus, any author that incriminates nitrous oxide in the oxidation of hemoglobin must have compelling evidence and, if it is true, will require a paradigm shift in dental anxiolysis, dental anesthesia, and medical anesthesia. The ramifications of these statements require that the cited articles be reviewed to assess if, indeed, the evidence for nitrous oxide as an oxidant of hemoglobin is compelling.

Dr Scott Ludwig authored the first case–report article. A 5-year-old Caucasian boy, previously in good health, was brought by paramedics to an emergency room in Springfield, Missouri from a dental office where the patient had exhibited severe cyanosis and generalized tonic-clonic seizures. Before arriving at the hospital, the paramedics administered oxygen at a rate of 8 L per minute and, after starting an intravenous line, administered 5 mg of diazepam intravenously. Upon arrival at the emergency room, the patient was not exhibiting seizure activity but remained severely cyanotic and was described as stuporous. The medical history proved unremarkable and the patient was taking no medications. A tentative diagnosis of methemoglobinemia was made within 15 minutes of arrival at the emergency room and the patient was given methylene blue (2 mg/kg) by slow intravenous injection. Within 15 minutes of administration, the cyanosis disappeared. The hospital course was one of progressive improvement with posttreatment methemoglobin levels of 10% at 4 hours and 0.7% at 24 hours. The methemoglobin level at admission proved to be 32.5%. No further treatment was necessary. Tests for abnormal hemoglobin and glucose-6-phosphate dehydrogenase (G6PD) were negative. The parents were advised at discharge to avoid prilocaine and other oxidants in the future. Dr Ludwig correctly attributed the cause of methemoglobinemia to the administration of prilocaine 52 mg (1.3 mL of 4% prilocaine; the patient's weight was not specified and, therefore, the dose per kilogram of body weight is unknown). Dr Ludwig did not make any mention of an etiologic role for nitrous oxide nor did he provide any evidence for the role of nitrous oxide in the oxidation of hemoglobin to methemoglobin. This article provided no evidence for the inclusion of nitrous oxide as an oxidant of hemoglobin as it appears in the Ash-Bernal article.[3] Thus, the article by Dr Ludwig lacks *any* compelling evidence.[12]

The second of two references that appeared in Dr Ash-Bernal's article,[3] which *should* provide evidence for the role of nitrous oxide as an oxidant of hemoglobin, was authored by Drs Malatinsky, Kadic, and Kovacik. Dr Malatinsky's article did not attribute any oxidizing ability to nitrous oxide in the article. In fact, the first line of the article states "Pure nitrous oxide (N_2O) is an *inert gas* with anesthetic characteristics." The authors then continue to discuss the contaminants found in tanks of nitrous oxide in small amounts that are referred to as higher nitrogen oxides (eg, NO and NO_2). Thus, the article by Malatinsky and colleagues[13] offered no compelling evidence that nitrous oxide oxidizes hemoglobin or causes methemoglobinemia.

In summary, one can characterize the content of these two articles as lacking any discussion of or compelling evidence for the role of nitrous oxide as an oxidant of hemoglobin. In the absence of evidence in these two articles as well as in the extensive literature on nitrous oxide in medicine and dentistry,[14] the characterization of nitrous oxide as an oxidant of hemoglobin and a possible etiology for methemoglobinemia must be considered erroneous and discarded.

The Diagnosis of Methemoglobinemia

When patients present with cyanosis and an absence of pathology in the respiratory or cardiovascular systems, toxic methemoglobinemia should be considered in the differential diagnosis. To confirm a diagnosis of methemoglobinemia, a specimen of the patients' blood is sent to a hospital laboratory for a co-oximetry test. Multiple wavelengths of light are passed through a sample of the patient's blood. The result specifies the methemoglobin level, which represents the percent of total hemoglobin in the oxidized state.[1] This is a test that has been available for several decades, but does not provide any proactive monitoring capabilities.

In the late 1980s, noninvasive pulse oximetry became an affordable technology and the measurement of the oxygen saturation of hemoglobin rapidly became a widespread, essential, point-of-care test and monitor. This device has significantly and dramatically lowered the morbidity and mortality in dental and medical anesthesia. However, it soon became evident that the much-desired pulse oximeter readings were unexpectedly and erroneously altered to approximately 85% in the presence of increasing methemoglobin levels and these depressed readings were unresponsive to supplemental oxygen administration.[4] Thus, one loses the benefit of knowing the hemoglobin saturation with oxygen in the presence of an unknown level of methemoglobin. In the scenario of office-based treatment, co-oximetry testing is not available. Hence, the treating practitioner is aware that there may be a methemoglobin accumulation developing in patients but they are unaware of the extent of the problem.

In approximately 2005, a device was introduced that, although being a conventional pulse oximeter, also possesses the ability to measure methemoglobin levels and carboxyhemoglobin levels in the blood in a noninvasive fashion similar to pulse oximetry (The Rainbow Rad 57 by the Massimo Corp, Irvine, CA, USA). Peer-reviewed studies of this device have proved it to be reliable and accurate in the methemoglobin range of 0% to 12%.[5] Precision and accuracy outside of the range of 0% to 12% of methemoglobin remains to be determined and published. The small, handheld size of this monitor, along with its noninvasive application, translates to a significant improvement in the ability to diagnose, monitor, and implement the early treatment of methemoglobinemia. The availability of this device obviates the need for drawing blood and using laboratory services and facilitates monitoring for methemoglobinemia in the office-treatment venue.[15] This monitoring system allows a safety net for those practitioners who feel the use of prilocaine or benzocaine is imperative.

The Treatment of Acquired or Toxic Methemoglobinemia

The following discussion of the treatment of methemoglobinemia is limited to acquired or toxic methemoglobinemia. Congenital methemoglobinemia is associated with genetic alterations of metabolism and requires a totally different approach to treatment.[6]

Methylene blue

The first line of treatment for symptomatic, acquired methemoglobinemia is an intravenous infusion of methylene blue (1 to 2 mg/kg). Methylene blue is an intense dye that causes the urine to become green. Treatment with methylene blue is generally reserved for those patients who are symptomatic. Methylene blue may also interfere with pulse oximeter readings. Methylene blue is not the agent that directly reduces methemoglobin. Methylene blue is reduced by an enzyme known as NADPH methemoglobin reductase to leukomethylene blue. Leukomethylene blue then donates an electron (ie, reduces) methemoglobin to hemoglobin. NADPH methemoglobin reductase is not the same enzyme involved in the physiologic reduction of methemoglobin (NADH-cytochrome b5 reductase). In the absence of methylene blue, NADPH methemoglobin reductase is responsible for less than 6% of the restoration of hemoglobin from methemoglobin.[2]

Individuals with glucose-6-phosphate dehydrogenase deficiency lack the ability to produce NADPH. Because the methylene blue treatment requires NADPH as the reductase, methylene blue will be ineffective in individuals with G6PD deficiency and may worsen the methemoglobinemia.[2]

Prognosis

Methemoglobinemia is a potentially life-threatening disorder. In the absence of glucose-6-phosphate dehydrogenase deficiency, individuals experiencing symptomatic acquired methemoglobinemia should be treated with methylene blue to reduce the acute methemoglobin levels in the blood and thereafter allow further metabolic reduction of methemoglobin to physiologic levels, usually over 24 to 36 hours. Any residual morbidity or mortality is a function of peak blood methemoglobin levels achieved and the elapsed time before treatment. Individuals demonstrating severe symptoms of methemoglobinemia have experienced a full recovery when treatment is prompt.[12]

Implications for dentistry

Dentists may now be, or may become in the future, a major contributor to cases of methemoglobinemia. Benzocaine and prilocaine are recognized dental treatments and dentists and dental hygienists are administering these hemoglobin oxidants.[11] However, prilocaine is only one of several local anesthetics that are available for dental use and the opportunity for the development of methemoglobinemia[7] must not be overestimated.

Benzocaine

Benzocaine has been used widely in both dentistry and in operating rooms for many decades (eg, Hurricane [20%] and Cetacaine [14%]). Benzocaine is in many over-the-counter products, such as teething gels for use in infants and children and products for tooth pain in adults. Benzocaine represents a unique problem for individuals promoting medication safety because it has been marketed in such high concentrations. It is currently marketed in concentrations between 7.5% and 20%. These high concentrations increase the likelihood of toxicity because such a small amount of the product may represent an overdose. As an example, one manufacturer of a benzocaine 14% spray (Citanest) recommends that no more than 1 second of spray should be used on the oral mucous membranes of patients. One author that has published recommendations regarding the use of local anesthetics that are associated with methemoglobinemia has concluded that benzocaine should cease to be used at all.[7] Certainly, infant pediatric dental patients are at risk when uninformed and distraught parents provide a teething gel to their sleepless child that contains high concentrations of benzocaine. Children younger than 6 months of age appear to be at an increased risk for methemoglobinemia.

Prilocaine

Prilocaine is marketed and sold to dentistry primarily as a parenteral local anesthetic in a 1.8 mL cartridge containing a 4% of prilocaine without a vasoconstrictor (ie, 72 mg of prilocaine in each cartridge) and a 1.8 mL cartridge containing 4% prilocaine with 1:200,000 epinephrine added as a vasoconstrictor (ie, 9 mcg of epinephrine added to each cartridge). One author has stated that the vasoconstrictor delays the onset but not the magnitude of the response.[7] Another author found that the methemoglobin levels were higher when the prilocaine was given as a higher concentration, irrespective of the total dose.[10]

The ability of prilocaine to induce methemoglobinemia at varying doses per kilogram in patients without comorbidities suggests that the current maximum recommended dose, 8 mg/kg, should be lowered. One author that has evaluated the relationship of prilocaine to methemoglobinemia has suggested that the maximum dose should be 2.5 mg/kg (**Table 2**).[7]

Patients that arrive for routine care in the dental office appear to be increasingly medically complex because more major disorders are managed on an outpatient basis. Examples include congestive heart failure, chronic renal failure, and ischemic heart disease manifesting as stable angina. Medication lists seem to be growing for these individuals. Patients with these disorders may require a lower maximum dose of prilocaine.

Dentists do have local anesthetics that may be substituted for prilocaine, such as lidocaine or mepivacaine. However, some dentists feel that prilocaine offers them clinical advantages in local anesthesia for dentistry and they may choose to continue to use prilocaine despite its unique disadvantage among the injectable local anesthetics for dentistry. It would appear to be an obligation of any dentist making such a decision to become familiar with methemoglobinemia and the predisposing factors that can lower the threshold for the onset of this potentially life-threatening disorder.

Table 2
Lowered maximum dose recommendations for prilocaine

Body Weight (kg)	MRD (mg)[a]	MRV in Cartridges[b]
10	25	0.35
20	50	0.7
30	75	1.0
40	100	1.4
50	125	1.7
60	150	2.1
70	175	2.4
80	200	2.8

Maximum recommended dose with corresponding maximum recommended volume.
Abbreviations: MRD, maximum recommended dose; MRV, maximum recommended volume.
[a] MRD in milligrams based on 2.5 mg/kg body weight.
[b] MRV of 4% prilocaine (1 cartridge = 1.8 mL).
Data from Guay J. Methemoglobinemia related to local anesthetics: a summary of 242 episodes. Anesth Analg 2009;108(3):837–45.

SUMMARY

Dentistry has two medications in its pain management armamentarium that may cause the potentially life-threatening disorder methemoglobinemia. The first medications are the topical local anesthetics benzocaine and prilocaine. The second medication is the injectable local anesthetic prilocaine. The mechanism of action is well understood in that both of these medications oxidize hemoglobin to methemoglobin. Hemoglobin normally carries oxygen from the lungs to the peripheral tissues and removes carbon dioxide from the peripheral tissues and returns it to the lungs in its role as the major constituent of red blood cells. In the oxidized state referred to as methemoglobin, oxygen and carbon dioxide transport is reduced. As the level of methemoglobin continues to increase in the blood, cyanosis develops and additional symptoms appear with the potential for progression to unconsciousness and death. Fortunately, treatment is effective and the prognosis is good if the methemoglobin levels are not too high and if treatment is prompt. Certain conditions and diseases predispose to methemoglobinemia. It is incumbent on the dental profession to take steps to minimize the risk for this preventable disorder. There are 3 actionable items for the dental profession to consider: (1) follow conservative (and in some cases new) guidelines regarding the use of both of these medications, (2) learn patients' diseases and medical conditions as well as the treatment of those diseases and conditions that predispose dental patients to methemoglobinemia, and (3) advise parents of infants regarding the potential toxicity of over-the-counter teething gels that contain benzocaine. Some dental professionals may choose to minimize patient risk by simply not using these medications and substituting other topical or injectable local anesthetics for use in the oral cavity. The author of a recent publication on this subject emphasized the importance of the issues when she said, "Local anesthetic-related methemoglobinemia is an important clinical problem. 40%.... of these episodes have been published in 2000 or after."[7] This fact suggests that dental and medical professionals using oxidizing local anesthetics have become more cognizant and watchful for the toxic side effects of these agents. If an increased awareness of toxic side effects among professionals is a reality, an elevated incidence of reporting of toxic side effects will continue into the next decade.

REFERENCES

1. Wright RO, Lewander WJ, Woolf AD. Methemoglobinemia: etiology, pharmacology, and clinical management. Ann Emerg Med 1999;34(5):646–56.
2. Umbreit J. Methemoglobin - it's not just blue: a concise review. Am J Hematol 2007;82:134–44.
3. Ash-Bernal R, Wise R, Wright SM. Acquired methemoglobinemia: a retrospective series of 138 cases at 2 teaching hospitals. Medicine 2004;83(5):265–73.
4. Barker S, Tremper K, Hyatt J. Effects of methemoglobin on pulse oximetry and mixed venous oximetry. Anesthesiology 1989;70:112–7.
5. Barker S, Curry J, Redford D, et al. Measurement of carboxyhemoglobin and methemoglobin by pulse oximetry. Anesthesiology 2006;105(5):892–7.
6. Da-Silva SS, Sajan I, III Underwood JP. Congenital methemoglobinemia: a rare cause of cyanosis in the newborn-a case report. Pediatrics 2003;112(2):158–61.
7. Guay J. Methemoglobinemia related to local anesthetics: a summary of 242 episodes. Anesth Analg 2009;108(3):837–45.
8. Wilburn-Goo D, Lloyd LM. When patients become cyanotic: acquired methemoglobinemia. J Am Dent Assoc 1999;130(6):826–31.

9. Bradberry S, Gazzard B, Vale J. Methemoglobinemia caused by the accidental contamination of drinking water with sodium nitrite. J Toxicol Clin Toxicol 1994; 32(2):173–8.
10. Vasters FG, Eberhart LH, Koch T, et al. Risk factors for prilocaine-induced meth-aemoglobinaemia following peripheral regional anaesthesia. Eur J Anaesthesiol 2006;23:760–5.
11. Wynn R, Meiller T, Crossley H, editors. Drug information handbook for dentistry. 12th edition. Hudson (OH): Lexi-Comp; 2006.
12. Ludwig S. Acute toxic methemoglobinemia following dental analgesia. Ann Emerg Med 1981;10(5):265–6.
13. Malatinsky J, Kadlic T, Kovacik V. Acute poisoning by higher nitrogen oxides. Anesth Analg 1973;52(1):94–9.
14. Eger EI. Nitrous oxide N O. 1st edition. New York: Elsevier; 1985. p. 357.
15. Annabi EH, Barker SJ. Severe methemoglobinemia detected by pulse oximetry. Anesth Analg 2009;108(3):898–9.

Ocular Complications Associated with Local Anesthesia Administration in Dentistry

Sean G. Boynes, DMD, MS[a],[*], Zydnia Echeverria, DMD[a],[b],
Mohammad Abdulwahab, DMD, MPH[a]

KEYWORDS

• Amaurosis • Mydriasis • Ptosis • Diplopia

The most widely used method for controlling pain during dental procedures is the intraoral administration of local anesthetics. The anesthetic solution is deposited in close proximity to a specific nerve or fiber to obtund nerve conduction. The most commonly anesthetized nerves in dentistry are branches or nerve trunks associated with the maxillary and mandibular divisions of the trigeminal nerve (cranial nerve V). However, other nerves may be inadvertently affected by intraoral local anesthesia injections, resulting in anesthetic complications of structures far from the oral cavity.[1–3]

One such distant complication is of the eye. Symptoms of this unexpected complication have been described as blurring of vision and amaurosis (temporary blindness).[1,3] In addition, anesthesia of motor neurons can result in mydriasis (pupillary dilation), ptosis (droopy eyelid), and diplopia (double vision). Horner-like manifestations involving ptosis, enophthalmos (recession of the eyeball within the orbit), and miosis (papillary restriction) have also been reported.[1] Generally, symptoms develop immediately after injection of the anesthetic solution and last for several hours. These symptoms are attributed to the anesthetic solution reaching the orbit or cavernous sinus.[4]

When these complications occur, they can be distressing to both the patient and the dentist. Although permanent damage to tissues, nerves, and eyes is rare, the

[a] Department of Anesthesiology, University of Pittsburgh, School of Dental Medicine, 3501 Terrace Street, 622 Salk Hall, Pittsburgh, PA 15261, USA
[b] University of Pittsburgh Graduate Dental Anesthesiology Program, University of Pittsburgh, School of Dental Medicine, 3501 Terrace Street, 622 Salk Hall, Pittsburgh, PA 15261, USA
* Corresponding author.
E-mail address: seangboynes@hotmail.com

Dent Clin N Am 54 (2010) 677–686
doi:10.1016/j.cden.2010.06.008
0011-8532/10/$ – see front matter © 2010 Elsevier Inc. All rights reserved.

practitioner should be able to detect and effectively treat the complication to avoid the development of permanent sequellae.

CLINICAL REPORTS AND IMPLICATIONS

In 1962, Cooper[5] presented one of the most cited ocular complication cases in the dental literature. The case describes a 46-year-old woman who was given a right mandibular block with 2% mepivacaine with vasoconstrictor. She immediately experienced transitory blindness followed by diplopia, which continued for 5 hours. The ophthalmologists who examined her 15 minutes after local anesthetic administration discovered a total paralysis of the right lateral rectus muscle. The patient was without ocular signs and symptoms when she was evaluated the following day.

Blaxter and Britten[6] similarly reported several cases involving transient loss of vision, diplopia, and amaurosis. They postulated that an intra-arterial injection of the inferior alveolar artery occurred, with a retrograde flow pattern carrying the anesthetic to the area of the eye. In all of their reported cases, the patients recovered completely. Goldenberg[7] reported a similar case following a mandibular injection, in which the patient developed dizziness, diplopia, and blanching of the ipsilateral upper eyelid. The proposed cause was traced to the lacrimal artery, which affected the innervation to the lateral rectus muscle. Dryden[8] reported a case following a Gow-Gates injection, in which the patient complained of a burning sensation around the infraorbital region after the second injection. Diplopia of the right eye developed, as well as blanching of the skin coinciding with the infraorbital artery.

The most calamitous ocular outcome of a local anesthetic injection was reported in 1957 by Walsh.[9] In his report, the patient experienced permanent blindness immediately after an intraoral injection of 2% procaine-adrenaline (1:50,000) solution. The patient stated a sensation of blue color for a moment followed by a reduced perception of light. Examination 4 days after the injection revealed areas of early retinal damage and lack of visual acuity.

A review of literature since 1957 revealed a total of 48 cases (including the new report presented later in the article) involving ophthalmic complications. Twenty-seven reports occurred after maxillary injection (posterior superior alveolar nerve block or middle superior alveolar field block) and 21 reports were related to mandibular injections (inferior alveolar nerve block). The symptoms associated with the maxillary and mandibular injections are listed in **Table 1**. The demographic data overall were somewhat inconclusive; however, a predilection was observed with 72.9% of cases (n = 48) involving women.

As shown in **Fig. 1**, the onset times of symptomatic response are not always reported. For the cases in which onset was documented, most symptoms were seen within the first 5 minutes following the injection. It should be noted that comparisons between onset times and location of injection revealed no statistically significant difference between maxillary or mandibular injection techniques.

The duration of symptoms was examined for these reports from literature (see **Fig. 1**). Forty reports (83.3%) have described transient manifestations that disappeared within 6 hours of anesthetic administration. However, because of the usually benign and transient nature of the manifestations, most patients never received detailed examinations by an ophthalmologist and specifics of the ocular deficits are not well documented.

As shown in **Table 1**, the most common symptom identified by the investigators of the 48 case reports was diplopia (17 manifestations), followed by muscle paralysis (14 manifestations), ptosis (12 manifestations), mydriasis (9 manifestations), and

Table 1
Evaluation of ocular complication symptom reports following intraoral local anesthetic administration in literature[a]

Symptom/Manifestation	Total Reports	Maxillary Injections	Mandibular Injections
Ophthalmoplegia (Paralysis of eye muscles)	14	12	2
Ptosis of the eyelid	12	7	5
Mydriasis	9	6	3
Amaurosis (Blindness/Loss of vision)	9	3	6
Diplopia	7	3	4
Diplopia by lateral rectus palsy	8	3	5
Diplopia by medial rectus palsy	2	1	1
Miosis	3	3	0
Dizziness	6	2	4
Blurred vision	4	1	3
Partial paresis	1	1	0
Blanching	2	0	2
Burning sensation	1	0	1
Horner syndrome	1	0	1
Nausea	1	0	1
Tearing	1	0	1
Totals	81	42	39

[a] Based on 48 case reports (including the case report presented in the article). All manifestations were included, allowing for multiple symptom reports in an individual article.

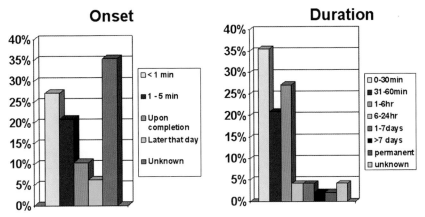

Fig. 1. Onset and duration comparisons of reported symptoms with ocular complications following intraoral anesthetic injections. As shown with the onset evaluation, approximately 47% of symptoms are reported within the first 5 minutes of local anesthetic administration. It should also be noted that 83% of the patients in reports of ocular complications recover from these adverse events within 6 hours of anesthetic administration.

blindness or loss of vision (9 manifestations). In addition, most patients experience approximately 2 symptoms per manifestation. On evaluating these literature reports by injection location, 42 symptoms followed maxillary injections and 39 symptoms followed mandibular injections. Comparisons of symptoms revealed that ophthalmoplegia, mydriasis, and ptosis were more commonly seen with maxillary injections, whereas amaurosis, diplopia, and blurred vision were observed more frequently after mandibular injections.

The authors also completed an evaluation of the types of anesthetic used and their relation to ocular complications (**Table 2**). A particular pattern was discovered as it relates to articaine and maxillary injections. It was noted that in 15 of the 27 (55.6%) case reports relating to ophthalmic complications with maxillary injections, 4% articaine with 1:100,000 epinephrine was used. Conversely, articaine was not involved with any of the mandibular injection complications. Given that the most commonly proposed cause of ocular manifestations with maxillary injections is diffusion, it could be proposed that the diffusion properties of articaine may be more extensive than those of the other local anesthetics evaluated. Given the increased use of articaine in North America in the last few years, this pattern may continue to be seen in the future.

ETIOLOGY OF OCULAR COMPLICATIONS

There is currently no agreement to the exact cause of ocular complications seen following intraoral local anesthesia injections.[10] However, it is generally agreed that (1) the local anesthetic solution reaches the area of the orbit through vascular, neurologic, myofascial, and/or lymphatic networks and (2) the cause is likely to be different for the injections administered in the maxilla or mandible.[4,11]

Proposed Causes of Ocular Complication with Mandibular Nerve Block Injections

Arterial

This theory is supported by the frequent symptoms of temporary dizziness, blanching of the skin, and anesthesia of the eyelids, which are supplied by the lacrimal nerve that

Table 2
Analysis of the type of anesthetic used in 48 case reports of ocular complications with local anesthesia for dentistry

Type of Anesthetic	Total	Maxillary Injections	Mandibular Injections
1% Lidocaine with Adrenaline	1	1	0
2% Lidocaine with 1:80,000 Adrenaline	6	2	4
2% Lidocaine Plain	1	1	0
2% Lidocaine with 1:100,000 Epinephrine	9	2	7
3% Mepivacaine Plain	4	2	2
2% Mepivacaine with Vasoconstrictor	2	0	2
4% Articaine with 1:100,000 Epinephrine	15	15	0
Procaine	1	1	0
Procaine with 1:300,000 Adrenaline	3	0	3
Butethamine hydrochloride with 1:100,000 Adrenaline	1	0	1
Unknown/Not Reported	5	3	2

depends on the lacrimal artery.[12] The inferior alveolar artery runs posterior to the inferior alveolar nerve, and therefore, local anesthetic solution may accidentally be injected into the artery.[10] Given that the solution is injected under pressure, the solution may be forced back into the maxillary artery (via retrograde flow) and gain access to the middle meningeal artery (**Fig. 2**). The ophthalmic branch of the middle meningeal artery may anastomose with the lacrimal artery.[10] The blood supply of the lateral rectus muscle derives from the lacrimal artery and from the lateral muscular trunk of the ophthalmic artery. Therefore, the intra-arterial injection of the local anesthetics may reach and paralyze the lateral rectus muscle and cause diplopia.[12]

Venous
This theory suggests that after inadvertent administration into the inferior alveolar vein following an inferior alveolar nerve block, the pressurized injection and diffusion will allow the flow of anesthetic into the pterygoid venous plexus and consequently into the cavernous sinus through emissary veins that traverse the bony foramina.[10,13] Once the anesthetic is positioned within the cavernous sinus, the abducens nerve would be more vulnerable to the effect of the anesthetic because of its immediacy within the sinus.

Myofascial planes
Often considered a cause of anesthetic failure, myofascial plane orientation may create a path of least resistance where the anesthetic solution flows away from the nerve and toward the orbital area. Studies of radiopaque dyes combined with local anesthetics have demonstrated that an injection can be made within the direct area of a nerve without producing an effect, whereas in supplementary illustrations, the solution was administered more than 2 cm away but still generated excellent

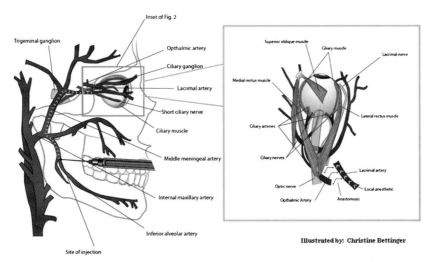

Illustrated by: **Christine Bettinger**

Fig. 2. Anatomic relationships between the mandibular injection site and the orbit. This illustration shows the potential route of local anesthetic following a standard inferior alveolar nerve block injection technique and inadvertent arterial injection with retrograde blood flow. As seen in the detailed illustration (superior view) of the eye (inset), the retrograde flow pattern may allow the local anesthetic to travel through the lacrimal artery and diffuse into the ophthalmic artery via anastomosis, thus affecting the muscles of the eye (such as the ciliary muscles and lacteral rectus muscle) and resulting in some of the symptoms demonstrated in **Table 1**.

anesthesia.[14,15] In the former case, the anesthetic spreads over the path of least resistance away from the nerve; in the latter case, it is directed toward the nerve.[15]

Sympathetic ganglion anesthesia

Campbell and colleagues[16] described a case with a Horner-like syndrome with ptosis, vascular dilatation of the conjunctiva, miosis, hoarseness in vocalization, and widespread rash over the ipsilateral upper body. In their report, it was suggested that the local anesthetic administration resulted in a stellate ganglion block, which may explain the patient's hoarseness of voice.

Proposed Causes of Ocular Complications with Maxillary Injections

Diffusion

As opposed to mandibular injections for which the injection site is further away from the orbit, maxillary injections have an increased opportunity of diffusion carrying the local anesthetic solution into the orbital area. It is proposed that simple diffusion from the pterygomaxillary fossa to the orbit through defects in the bone or via the vascular, lymphatic, and venous networks that link these spaces results in ocular consequences.[4,12,17]

Arterial

Inadvertent intra-arterial injection into the superior alveolar artery, with retrograde flow to the internal maxillary artery and then to the middle meningeal artery, serves as the basis for this theory (see **Fig. 2**). A middle meningeal branch occasionally penetrates the superior orbital fissure and anastomoses with the lacrimal branch of the ophthalmic artery.[6,18] The risk of an ocular complication occurring as proposed by this theory would be increased when the solution is injected rapidly and under pressure.[4]

Venous

This hypothesis proposes an inadvertent venous injection into the pterygoid venous plexus to explain a possible cause of ocular complication.[11,12] The theory proposes that the anesthetic solution would reach the orbit through the cavernous sinus, which receives drainage from the pterygoid venous plexus via the inferior and superior ophthalmic veins, which could communicate with the various musculature associated with the eye.[19]

Orbital injection

Himmelfarb[20,21] reported a case of diplopia after inadvertent injection into the orbit through the inferior orbital fissure. After the injection of the maxillary molar region, in which the needle was suggestively inserted to 2.5 cm, the patient presented with ipsilateral diplopia. The condition resolved after a short period, and no long-term issues were reported by the patient.

When evaluating the reports of ocular complications occurring with local anesthesia injections, the proposed causes of the event are highly variable. Although a true consensus is not supported in literature, similarities in theory should be noted. Because it relates to ocular complications with maxillary injections, the theory of diffusion causing the orbital effects seems to be the most cited explanation in reviewed articles. The theory of simple diffusion seems more acceptable overall because the process has already been recognized via pharmacodynamic and pharmacokinetic studies.[4,17,20,22]

On the other hand, the explanations of cause with mandibular injections prove more difficult to discern. However, a general similarity observed in literature with mandibular nerve block injections focus on retrograde arterial flow and anastomoses (see **Fig. 2**). In reporting several cases involving transient amaurosis and diplopia, Blaxter and Britten[6] suggest that an intra-arterial injection of the inferior alveolar artery had transpired, with the anesthetic agent peripatetic to the internal maxillary artery, the middle meningeal artery, and ultimately to the lacrimal and ophthalmic arteries.[1] Goldenberg[12,22] reported an analogous case following a mandibular injection and traced the anesthetic to the lacrimal artery. Rood[23] also illustrated a likely arterial route for diffusion of a vasoconstrictive agent from the alveolar artery to the internal maxillary and middle meningeal arteries and from the lacrimal to the ophthalmic artery by way of an anastomotic relationship.

The maxillary artery has variable anatomic locations as it relates to the branches of the mandibular neurovascular bundle as well as individual disparity in its topography, diameter, size of the downward loop, and location relative to the mandibular foramen.[24,25] The middle meningeal artery can arise as the second major branch of the maxillary artery.[1] Furthermore, in 4% of patients, the ophthalmic artery is established not from the internal carotid but from the middle meningeal artery, which follows uninterrupted flow from the external carotid artery.[18] These variations have been proposed as possible factors in ocular complications that follow intraoral local anesthetic injections. In addition, other investigators have postulated the existence of vascular anomalies that may generate the retrograde anesthetic diffusion phenomemon.[26,27]

PREVENTION AND TREATMENT

To prevent ocular complications, all local anesthetic injections should be accompanied by aspiration before actual injection. If a significant amount of anesthetic is to be injected, it should be administered slowly and with frequent aspirations.[28] Although ocular complications are rare, they can be severe and will create an anxiety reaction from the patient. Therefore, it is imperative that a practitioner understands the proper management of these cases.

Lee[10] and van der Bijl[11] suggest the following management guidelines:

- Reassure the patient as to the usually transient nature of these complications
- Continue to monitor the patient's vital signs
- Cover the affected eye with gauze dressing to protect the cornea for the duration of anesthesia
- Functional monocular vision will be restored by covering the affected eye. The patient should be escorted home by a responsible adult, because monocular vision is devoid of distance-judging capability
- Should the ocular complications last longer than 6 hours, refer patients to an ophthalmologist for evaluation
- Continue regular follow-up procedures.

A NEW CASE REPORT

A healthy 27-year-old woman presents to the emergency clinic of the University of Pittsburgh School of Dental Medicine complaining of extraoral tenderness in the left mandibular region. After a complete intra- and extraoral evaluation, the patient was diagnosed with an acute apical periodontitis with partial pulpal necrosis of tooth no. 18, caused by extensive dental decay. Alternative treatment plans were discussed, and a decision to proceed with a palliative treatment was made.

In preparation for dental treatment, the patient was placed in a semisupine position and protective eyewear was provided. As a conventional inferior alveolar nerve block was being administered to the left mandibular quadrant, the patient suddenly felt a "squirt from the inside of her eye." At that time 1.8 mL of 2% lidocaine with 1:100,000 epinephrine had been administered. The patient reported not being able to see through her left eye and started to panic. There was complete loss of vision of the eye ipsilateral to the block. The patient started to panic more, which made it difficult to assess the extraocular movements. About 15 to 20 minutes later, the patient regained complete vision on the affected eye after initial loss of visual acuity (ie, the patient had difficulty with accommodation). After the administration of additional local anesthetic using a mandibular infiltration technique (2% lidocaine with 1:100,000 epinephrine), palliative treatment was resumed without further complications, and follow-up telephone interaction revealed no additional adverse events.

DISCUSSION

The case report described is similar to those cases reported by Blaxter and Britten[6] as well as Ngeow and colleagues.[1] In those cases, the patients developed transient blindness that resolved after initial visual acuity loss. The cause of the ocular manifestations postulated by Blaxter and Britten relates to an inadvertent intra-arterial injection of the inferior alveolar artery that travels to the vasculature of the eye via retrograde flow patterns. Given that the patient reported blindness followed by visual acuity or accommodation loss, it can be postulated that paralysis of the ciliary muscle may have occurred via this same retrograde flow pattern.

Visual acuity directly relates to the power of accommodation of the eye.[1] This action depends on the flexibility of the lens capsule and retrenchment of the ciliary muscle, which is innervated by the short ciliary nerves and thus the ciliary ganglion.[29] As shown in **Fig. 2**, the ganglion is generally positioned in proximity to ophthalmic artery. As previously mentioned, a retrograde flow pattern from the inferior alveolar artery allows for the anesthetic to reach the ophthalmic artery, which via anastomoses affects the muscles of the eye, including the ciliary muscle.[29,30]

The loss of power of accommodation, as the patient experienced, is most likely a consequence of the paralysis of the ciliary muscle caused by injury or anesthesia of all or a branch of the cranial nerve III.[1,29] Given that the patient complained of an unidentified pressure change from inside the eye, it can be postulated that paralysis may have affected only a part of the nerve. Therefore, there would be internal strabismus from spasm of the internal rectus (which would result in an unusual feeling within the eye), accommodation issues from spasm of the ciliary muscle, and/or miosis.[1] Unfortunately, the patient was uncooperative for a detailed evaluation because of the understandable anxiety reaction. Therefore, confirmation of specific signs of ciliary muscle paralysis is incomplete.

SUMMARY

Practitioners should be aware of potential ocular complications following intraoral injections in dentistry. These complications include oculomotor paralysis and vision loss. The knowledge of these conditions and their potential cause should alert the dentist to the importance of appropriate injection techniques and an understanding of management protocol.

REFERENCES

1. Ngeow WC, Shim CK, Chai WL. Transient loss of power of accommodation in one eye following inferior alveolar nerve block: report of two cases. J Can Dent Assoc 2006;72:927–31.
2. Brodsky CD, Dower JS. Middle ear problems after a Gow-Gates injection. J Am Dent Assoc 2001;132:1420–4.
3. Penarrocha-Diago M, Sanchis-Bielsa JM. Opthalmologic complications after intraoral local anesthesia with articaine. Oral Surg Oral Med Oral Pathol Oral Radiol Endod 2000;90:21–4.
4. Horowitz J, Almog Y, Wolf A, et al. Ophthalmic complications of dental anesthesia: three new cases. J Neuroophthalmol 2005;25:95–100.
5. Cooper JC. Deviation of eye and transient blurring of vision after mandibular nerve anesthesia. J Oral Surg Anesth Hosp Dent Serv 1962;20:151–5.
6. Blaxter P, Britten M. Transient amaurosis after mandibular nerve block. Br Med J 1967;1:681–4.
7. Goldenberg A. Diplopia resulting from a mandibular injection. J Endod 1983;9:261–2.
8. Dryden J. An unusual complication resulting from a Gow-Gates mandibular block. Compendium 1993;14:94–8.
9. Walsh FB. Clinical neuro-opthlmology. 2nd edition. Baltimore (MD): Williams and Wilkins Company; 1957.
10. Lee C. Ocular complications after inferior alveolar nerve block. Hong Kong Med Diary 2006;11:4–5.
11. van der Bijil P, Meyer D. Ocular complications of dental local anesthesia. SADJ 1998;53:235–8.
12. Goldenberg AS. Transient diplopia as a result of block injections. Mandibular and posterior superior alveolar. N Y State Dent J 1997;63:29–31.
13. Walker M, Drangsholt M, Czartoski TJ, et al. Dental diplopia with transient abducens palsy. Neurology 2004;63:2449–50.
14. Galbreath JC, Eklund MK. Tracing the course of the mandibular block injection. Oral Surg Oral Med Oral Pathol 1970;30:571–82.
15. Jastak JT, Yagiela JA, Donaldson D. Local anesthesia of the oral cavity. Philadelphia: WB Saunders Company; 1995. p. 278–9.
16. Campbell RL, Mercuri LG, Van Sickels J. Cervical sympathetic block following intraoral local anesthesia. Oral Surg Oral Med Oral pathol 1979;47:223–6.
17. Petrelli EA, Steller RE. Medial rectus muscle palsy after dental anesthesia. Am J Ophthalmol 1980;90:422–4.
18. Singh S, Dass R. The central artery of the retina. I. Origin and course. Br J Ophthalmol 1960;44:193–212.
19. Marinho RO. Abducent nerve palsy following dental local analgesia. Br Dent J 1995;179:69–70.
20. Himmelfarb R. Interpreting the cause of diplopia after dental injection. Arch Ophthalmol 1980;98:575.
21. Monheim LM. Local anesthesia and pain control in dental practice. St Louis (MO): CV Mosby Company; 1957. p. 140–2.
22. Goldenberg AS. Transient dipolplia from a posterior alveolar injection. J Endod 1990;16:550–1.
23. Rood J. Ocular complication of inferior dental nerve block: a case report. Br Dent J 1972;132:23–4.

24. Pretterklieber ML, Skopakoff C, Mayr R. The human maxillary artery reinvestigated: I. Topographical relations in the infratemporal fossa. Acta Anat (Basel) 1991;142:281–7.
25. Roda RS, Blanton PL. The anatomy of local anesthesia. Quintessence Int 1994; 25:27–38.
26. Hyams SW. Oculomotor palsy following dental anesthesia. Arch Ophthalmol 1976;94:1281–2.
27. Bandres A, Penarocha M, Sanchis JM. Complicaciones de la anesthesia dental. An Esp Odontoestomatol 1997;3:87–95 [in Spanish].
28. Cooley RL, Cottingham AJ. Ocular complications from local anesthetic injections. Gen Dent 1979;27:40–3.
29. Pickering T, Howden R. Gray's anatomy, descriptive and surgical. 15th edition. London: Chancellor Press; 1985. p. 703–9.
30. Snell RS. Clinical anatomy for medical students. 3rd edition. Boston: Little Brown & Company; 1986. p. 825–7.

Beta-adrenergic Blocking Agents and Dental Vasoconstrictors

Elliot V. Hersh, DMD, MS, PhD[a,b,]*, Helen Giannakopoulos, DDS, MD[a]

KEYWORDS

- Epinephrine • Levonordefrin • Dental vasoconstrictors
- Beta-adrenergic blocking agents • Propranolol • Metoprolol

Adverse drug interactions involving dental vasoconstrictors have been the focus of several reviews and commentaries within the dental literature.[1–8] Considering the many millions of dental local anesthetic cartridges containing epinephrine administered to patients in any given year, reports of serious drug interactions with these agents in the outpatient dental setting have been exceedingly rare. However, based on a case series describing severe hypertensive events in plastic surgery patients who were on chronic propranolol for the treatment of hypertension or migraine headaches and received what was typically high therapeutic dosages of lidocaine with epinephrine,[9] and because this pressor effect has been reproduced in the clinical research setting in patients taking propranolol and other nonselective beta-adrenergic blocking agents when administered epinephrine infusions[10–13] or submucosal dental injections,[14,15] the potential exists for a similar adverse drug interaction in dental patients.

EPINEPHRINE PHARMACOLOGY AND SAFETY

One reason for the relative safety of vasoconstrictors in the current practice of dentistry is that epinephrine is by far the most widely used vasoconstrictive agent. Although epinephrine has α_1 adrenergic effects on some vascular beds, most notably under the skin and mucous membranes leading to vasoconstriction, it also has vasodilatory effects on other vascular beds that contain predominantly β_2 adrenergic receptors, such as those in skeletal muscle resulting in vasodilation (**Table 1**).[1,5]

[a] Department of Oral Surgery and Pharmacology, University of Pennsylvania School of Dental Medicine, 240 South 40th Street, Philadelphia, PA 19104-6030, USA
[b] Office of Regulatory Affairs, University of Pennsylvania, 240 South 40th Street, Philadelphia, PA 19104-6030, USA
* Corresponding author. Department of Oral Surgery and Pharmacology, University of Pennsylvania School of Dental Medicine, 240 South 40th Street, Philadelphia, PA 19104-6030.
E-mail address: evhersh@pobox.upenn.edu

Dent Clin N Am 54 (2010) 687–696
doi:10.1016/j.cden.2010.06.009
0011-8532/10/$ – see front matter © 2010 Elsevier Inc. All rights reserved.

dental.theclinics.com

Table 1	
Some physiologic actions of epinephrine at various receptors	
Receptor	**Response**
α_1 adrenergic	Constriction of blood vessels in skin and mucous membranes
β_1 adrenergic	Increased heart rate Increased contraction force
β_2 adrenergic	Dilation of bronchial smooth muscle Dilation of blood vessels in skeletal muscle and certain internal organs (brain)

This opposing vasodilatory property of epinephrine limits the potential pressor effects of the drug compared with levonordefrin and norepinephrine, which in the case of levonordefrin has approximately 50% less, and in the case of norepinephrine almost no β_2 adrenergic activity.[1,6,16,17] Norepinephrine is no longer available in dental cartridges because clinical research and case reports revealed a significant pressor effect following dental injections with even low therapeutic doses of the drug.[16–18] Levonordefrin is found only in the 2% mepivacaine formulation whose current use dwarfs that of lidocaine, articaine, bupivacaine, and prilocaine formulations, which contain various concentrations of epinephrine.

Typically most systemic effects of epinephrine, whether they involve myocardial stimulation caused by β_1 adrenergic receptor activation or changes in vascular tone, are short-lived, usually of only 10 to 20 minutes duration, because of the drug's short half-life in the blood stream.[19] For example, in a recent study in normal healthy volunteers, the intraoral injection of 7 cartridges (11.9 mL) of 4% articaine with 1:100,000 epinephrine (0.119 mg epinephrine total), which represented the maximum recommended dose of articaine in individuals weighing 68 kg or more, produced only small but significant ($P<.05$) increases in heart rate (9 beats per minute) and systolic blood pressure (6 mm Hg) that completely dissipated within 13 minutes of the final injection.[20] In addition, the β_2 adrenergic effects of epinephrine were demonstrated in this study by small decreases in diastolic blood pressure and total peripheral resistance.

Another factor adding to the safety of epinephrine in dental practice is that for most dental procedures, adequate pain control and/or hemostasis usually requires far less local anesthetic and vasoconstrictor than used in the study by Hersh and colleagues.[20] The few deaths attributed to vasoconstrictor use in the dental office have involved excessive doses of epinephrine, typically in patients with significant cardiovascular disease. A case report describing a fatality in a 58-year-old dental patient with symptomatic angina, 2 previous myocardial infarctions, type 2 diabetes, and a continuing smoking history after the injection of 5 cartridges of 2% lidocaine plus 1:50,000 epinephrine (0.18 mg epinephrine total), clearly supports this assumption.[21] In contrast to this tragic outcome, geriatric patients with a mean age of 70 years on various cardiovascular medications and cardiac arrhythmias confirmed by electrocardiography experienced no adverse sequelae during minor oral surgical procedures when the mean dose of epinephrine was limited to only 0.04 mg.[22] So in reality most serious adverse events reported with epinephrine administration probably involve excessive dosing and/or poor aspirating technique in cardiovascularly compromised individuals, not adverse drug interactions.

CLINICAL PHARMACOLOGY OF BETA-ADRENERGIC BLOCKING AGENTS

Beta-adrenergic blocking agents are classified as either being nonselective, meaning they block both β_1 receptors on the heart and β_2 receptors on the bronchial and the vasculature smooth muscle almost equally well; or they are cardioselective, that is they preferentially block β_1 receptors.[23] **Table 2** classifies some of the more commonly prescribed β-blockers into these categories. Both classes of beta-adrenergic blocking agents are commonly used in the treatment of hypertension, angina, and cardiac arrhythmias, although the cardioselective β-blockers have become more popular in these patient populations because β_2 blockade produced by drugs such as propranolol can lead to bronchoconstriction in sensitive individuals, a potentially lethal event in asthmatic patients and in those with other bronchospastic disorders.[23] However, in individuals who have migraine headache the older nonselective β-blockers are frequently used as prophylactic agents for this condition, because of their ability to block β_2 receptors on the cerebral vasculature, possibly limiting vasospasm, which is associated with some migraine headaches.[23]

THEORETIC BASIS FOR THE INTERACTION

As previously discussed, when epinephrine is absorbed systemically it is not a pure vasoconstrictor because it activates both α_1 and β_2 adrenergic receptors (see **Table 1**). However, if a nonselective β-blocker such as propranolol is used and significant systemic absorption of epinephrine occurs, the β_2 vasodilatory effects (and the β_1 cardiac stimulatory effects) of epinephrine will be blocked, allowing the α vasoconstrictive effects to function unopposed. The actions of epinephrine throughout the body would now resemble that of an almost pure vasoconstrictor like norepinephrine, theoretically resulting in an increase in systolic and diastolic blood pressure, and a compensatory reflex bradycardia.[1,3,19] These types of events in a patient with significant cardiovascular disease could increase the risk of myocardial ischemia and stroke.[11]

CASE REPORTS SUPPORTING THE INTERACTION

Dramatic increases in systolic and diastolic blood pressures have been reported in plastic surgery patients on propranolol for hypertension or migraine prophylaxis who received facial injections of lidocaine with epinephrine.[9] **Table 3** summarizes this case series. All patients were middle aged, were taking chronic propranolol, and had normal blood pressures after preoperative sedation and pain control regimens that included opioids, benzodiazepines (in all cases intravenous diazepam was titrated to effect), and in some cases barbiturates, neuroleptics, and the antihistamine hydroxyzine. Cases 1 and 2 showed significant hypertensive responses with a severe reflex bradycardia after the lidocaine with epinephrine injections. They had received the equivalent epinephrine dose of 5.5 to 6.5 dental cartridges of 2% lidocaine with 1:100,000 epinephrine. Blood pressures returned to normal in these patients within 15 to 60 minutes with no intervention. Case 3, for which preoperative

Table 2 Classification of some beta-adrenergic blocking drugs with common trade names in parentheses	
Nonselective Beta-adrenergic Blockers	**Cardioselective Beta-adrenergic Blockers**
Propranolol (Inderal)	Acebutolol (Sectral)
Nadolol (Corgard)	Atenolol (Tenormin)
Timolol (Blocadren)	Metoprolol (Lopressor)
Sotalol (Betapace)	Bextalol (Kerlone)
Pindolol (Visken)	Bisprolol (Zebeta)

Table 3
Summary of adverse case reports in patients taking therapeutic doses of propranolol and receiving lidocaine with epinephrine

	Case 1	Case 2	Case 3	Case 4	Case 5	Case 6
Sex/Age (y)	F/55	F/61	F/52	F/66	F/52	M/58
Propranolol dose/ indication	40 mg BID/migraines	40 mg BID/ hypertension	40 mg BID/ hypertension	10 mg BID/ hypertension	20 mg TID/ hypertension	20 mg TID/ hypertension
Postsedation blood pressure (mm Hg), pulse (beats/min)	110/70, 72	120/80, 70	Unknown	120/80, 75	120/80, 62	120/80, 60
Volume of lidocaine (%) with epinephrine administered	12 mL 1% with 1:100,000	10 mL 1% with 1:100,000	13 mL 0.5% with 1:200,000	40 mL 0.5% with 1:200,000	40 mL 0.5% with 1:200,000	8 mL 0.5% with 1:200,000
Epinephrine dose (mg)	0.12	0.10	0.065	0.20	0.20	0.04
Equivalent no. of 1:100,000 cartridges	6.5	5.5	3.5	11	11	2
Postinjection blood pressure (mm Hg), pulse (beats/min)	190/110, 38	200/100, 32	200/110, cardiac arrest	210/110, 100	245/145, 58	260/150, 52

Data from Foster CA, Aston SJ. Propranolol-epinephrine interaction: a potential disaster. Plast Reconstr Surg 1983;72(1):74–8.

blood pressure and pulse were unknown, experienced a severe hypertensive response and cardiac arrest that was successfully defibrillated when the amount of epinephrine contained in 3.5 dental cartridges was administered. Cases 4 and 5 were administered amounts of epinephrine that would be considered absolute maximum recommended dosages in healthy adult dental patients and certainly not in dental patients with significant cardiovascular disease.[5,19,24] The patient described in case 4 was also taking a thiazide/potassium–sparing diuretic combination (Dyazide) as well as propranolol. Both patients exhibited dramatic increases in blood pressure. The pulse rate, instead of decreasing, significantly increased in case 4, probably the result of that patient being pretreated with atropine before the procedure, which blocked the compensatory reflex vagal effect of the hypertensive response. In case 5, hydralazine (a vasodilator) was administered intravenously to reduce the severe increase in blood pressure. Case 6 received a relatively small amount of epinephrine approximately equal to the amount found in 2 dental cartridges containing a 1:100,000 solution. As in case 4, a combination thiazides/potassium–sparing diuretic was also being used to control blood pressure. After the injection, blood pressure rose to 260/150 and intravenous hydralazine was used to normalize the blood pressure. Although these cases tend to implicate the presence of the nonselective beta-adrenergic blocking agent propranolol as the culprit in these hypertensive events, as pointed out by other investigators, these patients were taking multiple preoperative drugs and 2 were also taking diuretics, both of which may have played some role in the ultimate course of the adverse interactions.[7]

There is only 1 well documented dental case, described by Mito and Yagiela,[25] in which a 32-year-old female dental patient with a history of mitral valve prolapse who was also taking 60 mg of propranolol per day for dysrhythmias and hypertension, had increases of 40 mm Hg and 15 mm Hg in systolic and diastolic blood pressure, respectively, after the administration of 1.5 cartridges of 2% mepivacaine plus 1:20,000 levonordefrin while under deep sedation. This particular local anesthetic formulation was chosen instead of one that contained epinephrine because it was felt that epinephrine would have a higher chance of promoting dysrhythmias in this particular patient. A second dose of 0.5 cartridge of the same anesthetic given 75 minutes later produced a similar response. These increases in blood pressure were relatively transient, lasting only 15 minutes and the restorative procedures were completed uneventfully. When this same patient was treated with 2 cartridges of 3% mepivacaine plain on a subsequent appointment, no change in any cardiovascular parameter was observed. However, when maxillary anesthesia diminished and 0.5 cartridge of 2% mepivacaine plus 1:20,000 levonordefrin was administered, increases in systolic and diastolic blood pressure of approximately 15 mm Hg and 10 mm Hg, respectively, occurred within several minutes of the injection. As before, these blood pressure increases were transient and did not interfere with the completion of the restorative procedures.

CLINICAL RESEARCH REGARDING THE INTERACTION

One of the most compelling studies supporting the adverse interaction between nonselective beta-adrenergic blocking agents and epinephrine is illustrated in **Figs. 1** and **2**.[10] Five patients were all being treated for long-standing severe hypertension with either the nonselective beta-adrenergic blocking agent propranolol (mean dose 208 mg/d) or the cardioselective beta-adrenergic blocking agent metoprolol (mean dose 260 mg/d) in 2 or 3 divided dosages. They took their usual morning dose of their respective beta-adrenergic blocking agent 2 hours before they

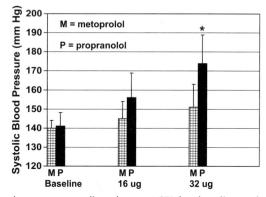

Fig. 1. Systolic blood pressure recordings (mean ± SEM) at baseline and at the end of 16 μg and 32 μg epinephrine infusions in 5 hypertensive patients on long-term metoprolol or propranolol therapy. The study was a crossover design. Three patients were on chronic metoprolol therapy and 2 were taking propranolol before the first set of epinephrine infusions. After crossing over to the alternative beta-adrenergic blocking agent, patients remained on that drug for at least 4 weeks before the second set of epinephrine infusions. Significant increases in systolic blood pressure recordings were observed in patients pretreated with propranolol compared with patients pretreated with metoprolol administered a total epinephrine dose of 32 μg. *$P<.05$ versus metoprolol pretreatment. (*Data from* Houben H, Thien T, van't Laar A. Effect of low-dose epinephrine infusion on hemodynamics after selective and nonselective beta-blockade in hypertension. Clin Pharmacol Ther 1982;31(6):685–90.)

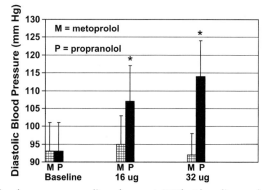

Fig. 2. Diastolic blood pressure recordings (mean ± SEM) at baseline and at the end of 16 μg and 32 μg epinephrine infusions in 5 hypertensive patients on long-term metoprolol or propranolol therapy. The study was a crossover design. Three patients were on chronic metoprolol therapy and 2 were taking propranolol before the first set of epinephrine infusions. After crossing over to the alternative beta-adrenergic blocking agent, patients remained on that drug for at least 4 weeks before the second set of epinephrine infusions. Significant increases in diastolic blood pressure recordings were observed in patients pretreated with propranolol compared with patients pretreated with metoprolol administered total epinephrine doses of 16 μg and 32 μg. *$P<.05$ versus metoprolol pretreatment. (*Data from* Houben H, Thien T, van't Laar A. Effect of low-dose epinephrine infusion on hemodynamics after selective and nonselective beta-blockade in hypertension. Clin Pharmacol Ther 1982;31(6):685–90.)

underwent slow epinephrine infusions of various doses (0.5 μg/min–4 μg/min) over 8 minutes. After the completion of the first session they were crossed-over to the alternative treatment for at least 4 weeks (80 mg of propranolol was considered equipotent to 100 mg of metoprolol) and the infusions took place again. Similar to many hypertensive patients, blood pressure was not being optimally controlled by either regimen with mean systolic/diastolic blood pressures in both groups before the infusions (baseline) of approximately 140/93 (see **Figs. 1** and **2**). As shown in **Fig. 1** following the slow infusion of 16 μg (2 μg/min) of epinephrine, which is slightly less than that found in a single 1.8 mL 1:100,000 epinephrine dental cartridge (18 μg or 0.018 mg), the mean increase in systolic blood pressure was about 15 mm Hg in the propranolol group and only 5 mm Hg in the metoprolol group. As shown in **Fig. 2** the differences in diastolic blood pressure following the 16 μg epinephrine infusion was even more pronounced increasing only 2 mm Hg in the metoprolol group but 14 mm Hg in the propranolol group. This difference reached the level of statistical significance ($P<.05$). When 32 μg of epinephrine was slowly infused (an amount slightly <2 1.8-mL cartridges of a 1:100,000 solution) the metoprolol group exhibited a 10 mm Hg increase in mean systolic blood pressure, whereas the propranolol group exhibited a mean systolic blood pressure increase of 33 mm Hg ($P<.05$). Diastolic blood pressure remained unchanged in the metoprolol group but increased 21 mm Hg in the propranolol group ($P<.05$). Not shown in the figure is that even smaller total infusion doses of epinephrine (4–8 μg) in patients taking propranolol produced small (5 mm Hg–9 mm Hg) but significant ($P<.05$) increases in diastolic blood pressure compared with patients taking metoprolol, in whom diastolic blood pressure remained essentially unchanged. Although one can argue that intravenous infusions do not resemble typical submucosal dental injections, inadvertent intravascular injections do occur in dental practice with injection speeds at least 8 times more rapid (1 cartridge per minute) than the infusion study discussed here.

Other epinephrine infusion studies have reported similar effects in research participants taking nonselective beta-adrenergic blocking agents. In 1 study of 6 normotensive men aged 38 to 46 years who were pretreated with propranolol, intravenous epinephrine infusions of 15 μg (0.015 mg) produced increases in mean arterial blood pressure recordings of 12 mm Hg with a reflex bradycardia (37% mean decrease in heart rate).[11] One individual experienced severe bradycardia with a heart rate of only 28 beats per/minute. In the same study, epinephrine infusions alone only raised mean blood pressure by 5 mm Hg and increased heart rate (because of its β_1 stimulatory effect) by 20%. Cardiovascular changes in both groups were short-lived, only lasting for 5 minutes. Two other studies in normotensive individuals also documented the ability of propranolol and pindolol to eliminate the β_2 vasodilatory effect of infused epinephrine. A decrease in diastolic blood pressure of about 20 mm Hg and a decrease in total peripheral resistance were observed with epinephrine infusions alone; diastolic blood pressure rose by about 20 mm Hg, and total peripheral resistance also significantly increased ($P<.05$) when patients were coadministered or immediately pretreated with intravenous propranolol or pindolol. When the same patients were coadministered or immediately pretreated with the cardioselective beta-adrenergic blocking agents metoprolol or atenolol, significant increases in diastolic blood pressure and peripheral vascular resistance did not occur.[12,13] The lack of significant diastolic blood pressure and total peripheral resistance increases with the cardioselective beta-adrenergic blocking agents during epinephrine infusions is explained by their inability to block the β_2 vasodilatory properties of epinephrine.

There are 2 studies in the literature where individuals on nonselective beta-adrenergic blocking agents received dental injections of lidocaine with epinephrine.

In 1 study, when normal volunteers were pretreated with a single oral dose of the nonselective beta-adrenergic blocking agent pindolol, small (8–9 mm Hg) but significant (P<.05) increases in systolic and diastolic blood pressure and peripheral vascular resistance, with corresponding decreases in heart rate and stroke volume, were observed after the administration of 2 intraoral injections of 2% lidocaine plus 1:80,000 epinephrine (0.045 mg epinephrine total). When these same individuals were not pretreated with pindolol, the administration of the same dose of local anesthetic solution induced small decreases in systolic and diastolic blood pressure, and peripheral vascular resistance.[14] In another study, patients with various cardiovascular diseases in need of dental treatment were administered a single cartridge of 2% lidocaine with 1:80,000 epinephrine (0.0225 mg epinephrine).[15] In 15 patients not receiving beta-adrenergic blocking therapy and in 9 patients receiving chronic cardioselective beta-adrenergic blocking therapy, mean arterial pressure was unchanged following the local anesthetic injection with a corresponding decrease in total peripheral resistance. In the 3 patients on nonselective beta-adrenergic blocking therapy, mean arterial pressure increased by approximately 15 mm Hg 2 minutes after the injection with a corresponding increase in total peripheral resistance. These increases dissipated within 5 to 10 minutes of the injection.

RECOMMENDATIONS

Although there is a dearth of documented case reports of severe hypertensive reactions in patients on nonselective beta-adrenergic blocking agents who subsequently receive local anesthetic injections containing epinephrine in both the dental and medical literature, the magnitude of the blood pressure increases in the plastic surgery case series was alarming and potentially life threatening.[9] Intravenous infusion studies of epinephrine in the presence of the nonselective beta-adrenergic blocking agents propranolol and pindolol clearly support the potential interaction.[10–13] There seems to be a positive dose-response between the amount of epinephrine administered and the magnitude of the pressor response seen in hypertensive patients taking nonselective beta-adrenergic blocking agents.[10] Two studies using submucosal dental injections equivalent to slightly more than 1 to 2 cartridges of a 1:100,000 epinephrine solution in patients on nonselective beta-adrenergic blocking agents were also able to demonstrate the pressor response but at smaller magnitude than the infusion studies.[14,15] However, as shown by the case report of Mito and Yagiela,[25] there can be individual hyper-responders.

Based on the results of these studies and case reports, the following recommendations can be made. In patients on nonselective beta-adrenergic blocking agents requiring simple restorative procedures, complete avoidance of epinephrine or levonordefrin seems rational. For more complex procedures for which hemostasis or a more prolonged duration of local anesthesia is required, keeping initial vasoconstrictor doses to an absolute minimum (a 0.5 cartridge test dose) and injecting carefully to avoid inadvertent intravascular injection seems prudent.[6] Frequent monitoring (every 5 minutes) of blood pressure and heart rate should be performed before giving additional doses,[6] and an absolute maximum dose of 0.036 mg epinephrine (2 cartridges of a 1:100,000 solution) of epinephrine or 0.18 mg of levonordefrin (2 cartridges of a 1:20,000 solution) is advised assuming the absence of a hypertensive response. Using local anesthetic solutions containing 1:200,000 epinephrine including 0.5% bupivacaine for surgical procedures likely to result in significant postoperative pain, and 4% articaine and prilocaine solutions for other procedures for which some degree of localized hemostasis would be beneficial will increase the maximum recommended number of cartridges to 4. The use of 1:50,000 epinephrine and the use of epinephrine impregnated gingival retraction cord, which contain 0.5 to 1 mg of racemic epinephrine per 2.5 cm,[24,26] should be avoided in patients on nonselective beta-adrenergic blocking agents.

SUMMARY

A clinically significant interaction between epinephrine or levonordefrin with nonselective beta-adrenergic blocking agents, although apparently rare in the dental setting, is potentially serious and can lead to significant hypertension with a concomitant reflex bradycardia. Based on the results of epinephrine infusion studies, the severity of the interaction seems dose related; small epinephrine doses cause less of a pressor response than larger doses. The interaction can be seen after intraoral submucosal injections but is generally of a smaller magnitude, at least with only 1 or 2 cartridges of lidocaine plus 1:100,000 epinephrine. However as demonstrated by 1 case report, some individuals are hypersensitive to this interaction. Inadvertent intravascular injections of local anesthetic plus vasoconstrictor and the use of high doses of vasoconstrictor are likely to result in a more pronounced response. Patients with significant cardiovascular disease may be especially vulnerable to the most serious sequelae resulting from the pressor reactions of the drug combination.

REFERENCES

1. Jastak JT, Yagiela JA. Vasoconstrictors and local anesthesia: a review and rationale for use. J Am Dent Assoc 1983;107(4):623–9.
2. Cassidy JP, Phero JC, Grau WH. Epinephrine: systemic effects and varying concentrations of local anesthesia. Anesth Prog 1986;33(6):289–97.
3. Goulet JP, Pérusse R, Turcotte JY. Contraindications to vasoconstrictors in dentistry: part III. Pharmacologic interactions. Oral Surg Oral Med Oral Pathol 1992;74(5):692–7.
4. Hersh EV. Local anesthetics in dentistry: clinical considerations, drug interactions, and novel formulations. Compend Contin Educ Dent 1993;14(8):1020–8.
5. Yagiela JA. Vasoconstrictors agents for local anesthesia. Anesth Prog 1995; 42(3–4):116–20.
6. Yagiela JA. Adverse drug interactions in dental practice: interactions associated with vasoconstrictors. J Am Dent Assoc 1999;130(5):701–9.
7. Brown RS, Rhodus NL. Epinephrine and local anesthesia revisited. Oral Surg Oral Med Oral Pathol Oral Radiol Endod 2005;100(4):401–8.
8. Hersh EV, Moore PA. Adverse drug interactions in dentistry. Periodontol 2000 2008;46:109–42.
9. Foster CA, Aston SJ. Propranolol-epinephrine interaction: a potential disaster. Plast Reconstr Surg 1983;72(1):74–8.
10. Houben H, Thien T, van't Laar A. Effect of low-dose epinephrine infusion on hemodynamics after selective and nonselective beta-blockade in hypertension. Clin Pharmacol Ther 1982;31(6):685–90.
11. Mackie K, Lam A. Epinephrine-containing test dose during beta-blockade. J Clin Monit 1991;7(3):213–6.
12. Hjemdahl P, Akerstedt T, Pollare T, et al. Influence of beta-adrenoceptor blockade by metoprolol and propranolol on plasma concentrations and effects of noradrenaline and adrenaline during i.v. infusion. Acta Physiol Scand Suppl 1983;515:45–53.

13. Rehling M, Svendsen TL, Maltbaek N, et al. Haemodynamic effects of atenolol, pindolol and propranolol during adrenaline infusion in man. Eur J Clin Pharmacol 1986;30(6):659–63.
14. Sugimura M, Hirota Y, Shibutani T, et al. An echocardiographic study of interactions between pindolol and epinephrine contained in a local anesthetic solution. Anesth Prog 1995;42(2):29–35.
15. Niwa H, Sugimura M, Satoh Y, et al. Cardiovascular response to epinephrine-containing local anesthesia in patients with cardiovascular disease. Oral Surg Oral Med Oral Pathol Oral Radiol Endod 2001;92(6):610–6.
16. Boakes AJ, Laurence DR, Lovel KW, et al. Adverse reactions to local anesthetic/vasoconstrictor preparations. A study of the cardiovascular responses to xylestesin and hostacain-with-noradrenaline. Br Dent J 1972;133(4):137–40.
17. van der Bijl P, Victor AM. Adverse reactions associated with norepinephrine in dental local anesthesia. Anesth Prog 1992;39(3):87–9.
18. Barnard DP, Joubert PH, Venter CP. Noradrenaline and local anaesthesia: a review of the literature and a clinical evaluation. J Dent Assoc S Afr 1987; 42(4):185–91.
19. Jastak JT, Yagiela JA, Donaldson D. Pharmacology of vasoconstrictors. In: Local anesthesia of the oral cavity. Philadelphia: WB Saunders; 1995. p. 61–85.
20. Hersh EV, Giannakopoulos H, Levin LM, et al. The pharmacokinetics and cardiovascular effects of high-dose articaine with 1:100,000 and 1:200,000 epinephrine. J Am Dent Assoc 2006;137(11):1562–71.
21. Yagiela JA. Death in a cardiac patient after local anesthesia with epinephrine. Orofac Pain Manage 1991;1:6.
22. Campbell JH, Huizinga PJ, Das SK, et al. Incidence and significance of cardiac arrhythmia in geriatric oral surgery patients. Oral Surg Oral Med Oral Pathol Oral Radiol Endod 1996;82(1):42–6.
23. Piacik MT, Abel PW. Adrenergic blocking drugs. In: Yagiela JA, Dowd FJ, Neidle EA, editors. Pharmacology and therapeutics for dentistry. 5th edition. St Louis (MO): Elsevier Mosby; 2004. p. 113–24.
24. Naftalin LW, Yagiela JA. Vasoconstrictors: indications and precautions. Dent Clin North Am 2002;46(4):733–46.
25. Mito RS, Yagiela JA. Hypertensive response to levonordefrin in a patient receiving propranolol: report of case. J Am Dent Assoc 1988;116(1):55–7.
26. Kellam SA, Smit JR, Scheffel SJ. Epinephrine absorption from commercial gingival retraction cords in clinical patients. J Prosthet Dent 1992;68(5):761–5.

Local Anesthetic Use in the Pregnant and Postpartum Patient

Edgar P. Fayans, DDS*, Hunter R. Stuart, DDS, MS,
David Carsten, DDS, Quen Ly, DDS, DMD, Hanna Kim, DDS

KEYWORDS

• Local anesthesia • Pregnant • Postpartum • Fetus

The use of systemically absorbed drugs in the gravid and in the lactating patient is of concern to the dentist. The need for interventional dental treatment occurs in virtually all stages of life, and during pregnancy is no exception. This article reviews concerns for the health and safety of the mother, developing fetus, and neonate involving local anesthetics. The effects of medications on successful pre- and postpartum human development and maternal health became evident in the 1960s when the drug thalidomide altered our awareness of maternal and fetal drug complications. This article reviews available literature on the use of local anesthetics for dentistry in the pregnant and postpartum patient. In addition, the physiology of the pregnant and postpartum woman is reviewed because this is essential to understanding potential interplay with local anesthesia and the stress of a dental appointment.

FIRST TRIMESTER

Any discussion of the use of local anesthetics both during pregnancy and the postpartum period requires a brief explanation of teratogenicity (the capability of an agent to initiate fetal malformation) and mutagenicity. The specific definition of a mutagen involves an agent that can alter genetic material and increase the incidence of mutations compared with background levels. A teratogen is an agent that initiates abnormalities of fetal development. The primary focus here is teratogenicity of local anesthetics.

Birth defects occur in about 3% of live births each year in the United States, and have been the leading cause of infant mortality.[1] Drug and chemical exposure is believed to be responsible for about 1% of these occurrences.[2] Birth defects account for 20% of all infant deaths and are consequently the leading cause of infant mortality in the United States. Extensive diagnoses or treatments of birth defects are required

---

Dental Anesthesiology Residency, Lutheran Medical Center, 150-55th Street, Brooklyn, NY 11220, USA
* Corresponding author.
E-mail address: efayans@hotmail.com

Dent Clin N Am 54 (2010) 697–713
doi:10.1016/j.cden.2010.06.010
0011-8532/10/$ – see front matter © 2010 Published by Elsevier Inc.

dental.theclinics.com

for 7% to 10% of all children,[3] and approximately 65% of birth defects have no identifiable cause.[4] Intrauterine vulnerability of the embryo led to the development and refinement of The Six Principles of Teratology, as found in Jim Wilson's 1959 monograph Environment and Birth Defects. For our purposes, the principles that apply to teratogenic effects are genotype, developmental stage, agent-specific actions, and fetal absorption.[5–7]

Early investigations were centered on gross deformities in animal models, but, for human studies, pregnancy registries serve as large prospective studies that record outcomes and provide information about possible risks of medications or exposures in pregnancies. Exposure to teratogens can result in a wide range of structural abnormalities such as cleft lip, cleft palate, dysmelia, anencephaly, or ventricular septal defect. In most cases, specific agents produce a specific teratogenic response. There is a long list of agents and environmental factors that has been discovered to be teratogenic, and commonly used local anesthetics have not been included. Teratogenic agents are categorized as radiation, infections, metabolic imbalances, drugs, or environmental chemicals.

By the end of the first month of development following fertilization, the fetus has a closed neural tube, hematopoesis has begun, and a primitive heart is present.[8] The embryonic period reaches from conception to the 10th gestational week, with the embryo then becoming a fetus and the first trimester culminating at the end of the 13th week. Organogenesis has occurred, the heart is beating, there is fetal movement, limb buds are developing and the fetus can already make a fist. All major structures are formed by this point and continue to develop throughout the gestational period. Once the embryo has become a fetus, the risk of environmental damage is reduced, but still present to a degree.[9]

During this early stage of pregnancy, it is crucial to be aware that a pregnancy may exist. Because the possibility of embryonic or fetal damage is a concern, a missed menstrual period may be the first sign; however, a urine pregnancy test may be suggested when there is doubt. Human chorionic gonadotropin (hCG), a glycoprotein secreted by the placenta shortly after implantation, is measured in urine in milliinternational units (mIU). Urine tests reacting to a level of 20 mIU/mL hCG are more sensitive and can detect a pregnancy earlier (at approximately 8 days) than those requiring a higher level.[10] Blood tests can confirm a positive urine test. Over-the-counter testing products are required to list their sensitivity level in their packaging, aiding choice in home product use. On average, a pregnant woman's level of hCG is approximately 25 mIU/mL at 10 days after ovulation and 100 mIU/mL at about 14 days. Home pregnancy test kits used by experienced technicians are almost as accurate as professional laboratory testing (97.4%), but, when used by consumers, the accuracy can be reduced to 75%. Improper usage may cause both false negatives and false positives.[11] If your patient is at risk for pregnancy, careful consideration must be given to the possible negative outcomes before initiating treatment. Consultation with the patient's obstetrician is the customary practice.

Most drugs cross the placenta by simple diffusion; hence our concern for the possibility of their teratogenic effects.[12] Although the embryo is within the predifferentiation period from 2 to 4 weeks it is resistant to teratogenic effects.[13] The most risk occurs following this period, when organogenesis takes place, during the 4 to 10 weeks following the last menstrual period.[13] Because of the level of sensitivity of the embryo and fetus, it is generally recommended that any dental treatment be deferred until the first trimester is complete.[14]

If emergent care is required in the first trimester, the negative consequences of allowing an active infection to progress untreated in a pregnant patient outweigh the risks of providing care.[15] Radiographs may be taken as necessary, with appropriate precautions being taken to protect the fetus and the patient, such as a lead apron, a tightly collimated beam, and high-speed film.[16] In choosing the local anesthetic for care in this situation, both the maternal and fetal effects are considered. The local anesthetic with the longest record of use is lidocaine. Because lidocaine is not available in a dental cartridge without epinephrine, the effects of this second drug become an issue. The use of 1:100,000 epinephrine as the vasoconstrictor in accidental intravascular injection can deliver 10 μg/mL of epinephrine. Clinically significant intravascular doses of α-adrenergic agents are to be avoided to maintain appropriate placental perfusion and fetal viability.[17–19] Normally used dental dosages of local anesthetic with vasoconstrictors, without inadvertent intravascular injection, do not expose the fetus or uterus to significant levels of epinephrine. The possibility of the formation of methemoglobinemia in the fetus with the use of prilocaine, the reduced level of fetal protein binding, as well as reduced liver metabolism, give lidocaine the least risk.[2]

SECOND TRIMESTER

The second trimester is weeks 14 to 27 of gestation. Teratogenicity risk in the second trimester is a diminishing concern. After 8 weeks, major organogenesis has occurred. In order to avoid labor, supine hypotensive syndrome, and general discomfort it is often suggested that elective dental care should be done during the second trimester. Many obstetricians believe that dentists are overly cautious about providing dental care.[20] Pregnancy loss is the primary concern, mainly occurring between the 14th and 23rd week of gestation, during which time 1% to 2% of all pregnancies are lost.[21] The main reasons for fetal loss during the second trimester include inflammation of fetal membranes, umbilical cord inflammation, and the placental viral infection.[21] A fetus with a major chromosome abnormality usually does not survive to the 14th week of gestation. A maturing fetus reaches 50% survivability if born prematurely, at approximately 22 to 25 weeks.[22]

Dentists should perform a risk assessment that should include past medical history, reproductive history, and physical examination including blood pressure and heart rate. Because dentists do not commonly assess reproductive history, this article includes a review of the tool that obstetricians use. The term, prematurity, abortion, living (TPAL) system is a 4-digit numerical system to summarize reproductive history. The first digit is the number of times the woman has come to term (T). The second digit is the number of premature infants (P). The third digit is the number of abortions, miscarriages, or ectopic pregnancies (A). The fourth digit is the number of living children (L). Therefore, P1001 is a woman who has given birth once and has 1 living child. Women who have a series of bad pregnancy outcomes are at high risk, and a thorough consultation with the obstetrician should be obtained.[23] Gravidity is the number of times a woman has been pregnant, including the present pregnancy. Parity is the number of times a woman has come to term and delivered a baby.

There are many conditions that heighten pregnancy risk. Hypertensive disorders occur in approximately 8% of all pregnancies.[24] Hypertensive disorders include preeclampsia, chronic hypertension, gestational hypertension, and eclampsia. Preeclampsia usually occurs after the 20th week and shows blood pressures of approximately 140/90 and protein in the urine. If seizures occur, it is then considered eclampsia. In the pathogenesis of eclampsia, the first stage of the disease occurs when the spiral arteries fail to become dilated, resulting in reduced placental perfusion. The second stage includes an increased maternal sensitivity to vasopressors, activation of the coagulation cascade with concomitant microthrombi, and decreased intravascular volume. Inadvertent intravenous (IV) vasopressor injection may result in a more profound response in the pregnant patient.[24]

Gestational diabetes mellitus may occur in a seemingly healthy woman with no prior history. It is defined as glucose intolerance diagnosed during pregnancy.[24] The average incidence is 4%.[25] Because this hyperglycemia causes premature placental aging, uteroplacental deficiencies, delayed fetal lung maturation, and birth defects (example cardiac abnormalities), it is often aggressively treated. The primary risks are an increase in miscarriages, congenital malformations, preterm birth, pyelonephritis, preeclampsia, in utero meconium, fetal heart rate abnormalities, cesarean deliveries, and stillbirths. The risk of recurrence in future pregnancies is about 60%.[25] After pregnancy there is a 40% to 60% likelihood of developing diabetes later in life.[24]

Fetal toxicity from local anesthesia depends on the amount of free drug that reaches the fetus. Factors that influence the fetal exposure are total dose, route of administration, presence of vasoconstrictive agents, rate of maternal metabolism and excretion, maternal and fetal pH, pKa of the drug, and degree of maternal and fetal protein binding.[26] Because of higher vascularity, head and neck administration of local anesthesia carries a risk of higher plasma levels, and therefore a higher drug concentration to the fetus.

Lidocaine, the agent most commonly used, has a maximum recommended dose of 5 mg/kg without vasoconstrictor and 7 mg/kg with vasoconstrictor. Diluted blood volume and decreased protein binding may reduce the maximum safe dosage. Intravascular injection combined with decreased protein binding may allow a reduced dose to precipitate seizures, particularly in the patient with preeclampsia or eclampsia. Because of decreased protein binding, the medical provider may reduce seizure medications during pregnancy. The maximum recommended local anesthetic doses are too small to reach significant fetal levels in most circumstances.[26]

Dental anesthetic cartridges with vasoconstrictors such as epinephrine or levonordephrin contain either sodium bisulfite or metabisulfite as an antioxidant.[27] Although true anesthetic allergies are uncommon, allergies to the preservative or antioxidant in the anesthetic are not.[28] If bisulfite allergy is suspected, referral for evaluation or skin testing may be indicated. If the local anesthetic is preservative and antioxidant free, this evaluation and skin testing may be avoided.

Local anesthetics (without vasoconstrictors) can exert direct effects on uterine smooth muscle. High concentrations of lidocaine or procaine in vitro can cause contraction. Direct injection of myometrium with 1% procaine results in uterine hyperstimulation and fetal distress. There is no evidence that IV infusion of clinically relevant concentrations has a measurable effect.[29] Bupivacaine may be considered for use in the pregnant patient to reduce the exposure to postoperative analgesics. Bupivacaine 0.75% for spinal and epidural anesthesia is no longer used because of cardiac arrests as a result of blocking cardiac conduction.[30] Bupivacaine in the 0.75% concentration is not used in dental delivery systems. Toxic side effects associated with excessive doses of local anesthetics include methemoglobinemia, seizures, coma, respiratory arrest, and cardiac depression.

Fetal uptake and distribution of local anesthetics are strongly influenced by high maternal protein binding (as high as 95% for bupivicaine) that limits placental transfer. Fetal/maternal ratios of local anesthetics seem to be inversely related to the degree of plasma protein binding because only the free unbound drug is available for placental transfer. Bupivacaine has a low fetal/maternal ratio (0.2:0.4). In animal studies, fetal bradycardia can result from high concentrations of lidocaine, bupivacaine, or mepivacaine injected in the vicinity of the umbilical artery.[29]

Fetal plasma has a significantly lower capacity to bind drugs, but experimental data has not shown this to be significant with regard to toxicity.[26] Drugs that compete for maternal plasma protein binding could increase drug availability. If the fetus were to become acidotic (ie, fetal distress), this could make more anesthetic available. Rapid maternal metabolism limits the amount of local anesthetic available to the fetus, reducing this as a factor.[23] Though local anesthetics can freely cross the placental barrier, direct effects on the fetus are minimal, even at near–maximum recommended doses.[31]

Prilocaine and benzocaine are causes of iatrogenic methemoglobinemia in clinical use. In methemoglobinemia, hemoglobin iron atoms are oxidized to a ferric state and cannot carry oxygen to the same degree as normal. If severe, maternal anoxia is potentially lethal to the fetus as well as the mother. A large dose of local anesthetic in a susceptible patient could theoretically cause a crisis. In patients who have no other toxic exposure or genetic defect, the dose of prilocaine must far exceed the maximum recommended dose for significant oxidation of hemoglobin iron to occur.[25] There are no reports in the literature of any added hazard to mother or fetus compared with other anesthetics.[32]

Allergic reactions can be life threatening to mother and fetus. Ester anesthetics carry the highest allergic potential. The amide anesthetic itself is rarely antigenic. Allergic reactions to the esters are almost entirely caused by sensitivity to their metabolite, para-aminobenzoic acid (PABA), and does not result in cross-allergy to amides. Articaine, although it has an ester link, rapidly breaks down to the inactive metabolite articainic acid, which is quickly excreted.[33] Sensitivity to the preservatives was discussed earlier.

Vasoconstrictors decrease the toxicity of local anesthetics by decreasing absorption. There are no significant contraindications for the use of epinephrine in the recommended dosages, provided intravascular injection does not occur.[31] Epinephrine improves local anesthesia, reducing peak blood levels of local anesthetics, and it intensifies and prolongs neural blockade. Epinephrine in the spinal column has been shown to mediate antinociception through the α_2 receptor.[34] Epinephrine in the blood has dose-related effects on uterine blood flow and contractility, causing both a decrease in blood flow and a decrease in uterine activity.[17] Agents that decrease uterine activity are called tocolytics. Epinephrine can also cause constriction of the umbilical artery but it has proved to be of possible significance only when there is fetal compromise.[29]

A major multicenter study that examined the safety of anesthetics was the Collaorative Perinatal Project. It was conducted from 1959 to 1965, prospectively reviewing 60,000 pregnancies. The data did not show that the administration of benzocaine, procaine, tetracaine and lidocaine resulted in any increased rate of fetal complications.[35]

THIRD TRIMESTER

During the third trimester, there are many physiologic changes that make dental treatment more challenging. As physiologic stress increases and childbirth begins, it is essential for the dentist to understand these changes.

The cardiac output of the gravid patient increases 30% to 50%, secondary to a 20% to 30% increase in heart rate as well as a 20% to 50% increase in stroke volume.[36,37] Most of this cardiovascular increase occurs by the 10th week, with a gradual increase up to 24 weeks, when the output plateaus.[38] During the second and third trimesters, a dramatic decrease in blood pressure and cardiac output can occur while the patient is in a supine position. This has been attributed to decreased venous return to the heart as a result of compression of the inferior vena cava by the gravid uterus. This compression can result in a 14% reduction in the cardiac output.[39,40] Decreased blood flow to the common iliac arteries can also occur with compression of the descending aorta.[41] This condition is known as supine hypotensive syndrome and is characterized by lightheadedness, hypotension, tachycardia, and syncope.[42] About 30% of pregnant women will demonstrate aortocaval compression when supine.[43] This usually occurs in the third trimester. The treatment is to place the patient in a 5 to 15 degree left lateral position to reduce the uterine pressure on the vena cava, and administer 100% oxygen.[14] If the hypotension is still not relieved, a full left lateral position may be needed.[44]

The pulmonary system of the gravid patient begins to change in the first trimester with hyperventilation. This may increase up to 42% in late pregnancy.[45] The hyperventilation results from the decreased resting arterial carbon dioxide tension (<30 mm Hg) and the increased renal bicarbonate excretion.[45] Hyperventilation is also caused by the respiratory stimulant effects of progesterone.[46] If patients are allowed to significantly hyperventilate (such as in a stressful situation), it may be extrapolated from studies that this could decrease uterine artery flow and could cause a decrease in fetal oxygenation.[47,48] Two factors significantly decrease oxygen reserve of the gravid patient.[39] (1) The diaphragm of a gravid patient is displaced upward approximately 4 cm, which is compensated by an increase in the transverse diameter of the thorax and the chest circumference. This diaphragmatic displacement results in a 40% increase in the vital capacity,[49] but it still leads to a 15% to 20% reduction in functional residual capacity.[50] (2) There is a 15% baseline increase in oxygen consumption by the gravid uterus. It is recommended that the inspired oxygen concentration should be increased before any anticipated period of apnea.[51]

Braxton Hicks contractions, also known as false labor or practice contractions, can begin as early as the second trimester; however, they are most common in the third trimester. The muscles of the uterus tighten for approximately 30 to 60 seconds, but can contract for as long as 2 minutes. Braxton Hicks contractions are described as irregular in intensity, infrequent, unpredictable, nonrhythmical, and more uncomfortable than painful. They do not increase in intensity or frequency, and taper off and disappear altogether. Possible triggers of Braxton Hicks contractions are increased activity of mother or fetus, abdominal contact, full bladder, or dehydration. These contractions may be alleviated by changing position, rhythmical breathing, hydration, or urination. If doing any of these does not alleviate contractions, the patient's obstetrician should be contacted as labor may have started.

Opioid analgesics should be used cautiously and only when indicated. A common postsurgical analgesic is codeine; however, it is a US Food and Drug Administration (FDA) category C drug that has been associated with fetal toxicity at less than the maternal toxic dose levels in mice and hamster models, resulting in decreased fetal body weight. Studies have found that codeine did not induce any increase in structural malformations in mice.[52] A prospective study of the use of codeine and propoxyphene during human pregnancy suggested that both drugs are associated with multiple congenital defects, including heart defects and cleft lip or palate.[53]

Aspirin and nonsteroidal antiinflammatory drugs (NSAIDs) have the common mechanism of inhibiting prostaglandin synthesis. Prostaglandin is one of the hormones involved in induction of labor. NSAIDs may also prolong pregnancy. In addition, prostaglandin inhibitors raise concerns about premature fetal ductus arteriosus constricture, resulting in pulmonary hypertension in the fetus. These concerns were derived from studies of patients taking large doses of aspirin and extrapolated to apply to other NSAIDs.[54] Ingest by mothers of 5 to 10 g of aspirin 5 days before delivery resulted in infant bleeding tendencies, specifically intracranial hemorrhage. No bleeding tendencies were found if aspirin was taken at least 6 days before delivery.[55] Ibuprofen has had no published reports linking its use with congenital defects.[56] Aspirin and other NSAIDs should be avoided, especially during the third trimester of pregnancy.[56] The alternative to aspirin and other NSAIDs is acetaminophen, which causes less gastric irritation and does not cause bleeding tendencies. The dosage of acetaminophen should be closely monitored to preclude hepatic effects.

Local anesthesia may affect nerve impulse transmission differently between pregnant and nonpregnant patients. The time required for 50% depression of the action potential of A, B, and C fibers from pregnant and nonpregnant animal models was determined after the application of bupivacaine. Conduction blockade occurred more rapidly in each type of nerve fiber in the pregnant as opposed to nonpregnant animal (differences were shown to be highly significant).[57] Preliminary findings suggest a slowing of nerve conduction velocity in humans with the progression of pregnancy.[58] The study may imply that the pregnant patient may be easier to anesthetize using local anesthetics.

Most local anesthetics used in dentistry are commonly dispensed with a 1:100,000 or 10 μg/mL epinephrine concentration for vasoconstriction. The concern with epinephrine-containing local anesthetics is accidental intravascular injection, which results in uterine artery vasoconstriction and decreased uterine blood flow. In animal models, blood levels of 15 μg/mL of epinephrine have shown a decrease in uterine blood flow. The magnitude and duration of this decrease is equivalent to the decrease in uterine blood flow caused by a single uterine contraction.[17] Clinically large doses of α-adrenergic agents (ie, phenylephrine) should be avoided to preserve placental perfusion. In general, there does not seem to be any significant contraindication to the careful use of lidocaine with epinephrine in pregnant patients.

Levonordefrin, another vasoconstrictor used in local anesthetic solutions, has pharmacologic activity similar to epinephrine. In equal concentrations, levonordefrin is less potent than epinephrine in raising blood pressure or as a vasoconstrictor. In dental carpules, the concentration of levonordefrin (1:20,000) is 5 times the normally employed concentrations of epinephrine (1:100,000). The high concentration of levonordefrin is a more potent vasoconstrictor, and therefore carries a higher risk to the fetus. This makes this vasoconstrictor a poorer choice in the pregnant patient.

In 1979, the FDA established a drug classification system based on the risks to pregnant women and their fetuses.[59] The classification consists of 5 categories: A, B, C, D, and X. Categories A and B are considered safe for use and show no evidence of risk in humans. The difference between categories A and B is that category A studies were performed on humans and category B studies were limited to animal subjects. In category C are drugs in which teratogenic risk cannot be ruled out. Category D includes drugs that have demonstrated risks in humans, and category X drugs clearly should be avoided because they have been shown to be harmful to pregnant women and their fetuses (**Table 1**). The dentist may treat pregnant patients on multiple medications and, if needed, prescribe additional ones. Attention must be given to their effect on maternal and fetal health (**Table 2**).[60]

THE POSTPARTUM PERIOD

The postpartum period can be an overwhelming experience for the mother. Patients may have delayed their dental care and actively sought treatment soon after delivery. Drug excretion into breast milk, along with the potential risks to the breast fed infant, is a common concern. Most drugs given to the mother are excreted into breast milk to

Table 1
FDA pregnancy risk factor definitions

Category	Definitions
A	Controlled studies in pregnant women fail to demonstrate a risk to the fetus in the first trimester with no evidence of risk in later trimesters. The possibility of fetal harm is unlikely
B	Either animal-reproduction studies have not demonstrated a fetal risk, but there are no controlled studies in pregnant women, OR animal-reproduction studies have shown an adverse effect (other than a decrease in fertility) that was not confirmed in controlled studies in women in the first trimester and there is no evidence of a risk in later trimesters
C	Either studies in animals have revealed adverse effects on the fetus (teratogenic or embryocidal effects or other) and there are no controlled studies in women, OR studies in women and animals are not available. Drugs should be given only if the potential benefits justify the potential risk to the fetus
D	There is positive evidence of human fetal risk, but the benefits from use in pregnant women may be acceptable despite the risk (eg, if the drug is needed in a life-threatening situation or for a serious disease for which safer drugs cannot be used or are ineffective)
X	Studies in animals or humans have demonstrated fetal abnormalities or there is evidence of fetal risk based on human experience, or both, and the risk of the use of the drug in pregnant women clearly outweighs any possible benefit. The drug is contraindicated in women who are, or may become, pregnant

some degree. If a drug needs to be used that has significant effects on the newborn, an alteration of the mechanics of breastfeeding (stored breast milk) or formula may be substituted.

During lactation, the infant may consume approximately 1% of the entire maternal drug dose.[61] Factors affecting the excretion of drugs can vary with blood flow in the breast, plasma concentration, the speed of breast milk production, and, specifically, the pharmacodynamics of the drug.[61] Lipid solubility, molecular mass, ionization, and protein binding are important variables in determining the drug's potential to be excreted. In order to maximize benefits to the mother and minimize adverse affects to the infant, necessary maternal drugs should have a short half-life to decrease the frequency of the infant's exposure. Timing the medication directly after the last feeding can decrease drug levels in breast milk. The advantages to the mother should exceed any potential disadvantages to the infant to justify the use of a drug.

The American Academy of Pediatrics considers lidocaine to be safe and compatible for use in the breastfeeding mother.[62] Both the infant and fetus are able to metabolize lidocaine.[63,64] Levels of lidocaine and its metabolite monoethylglycinexylidide (MEGX) in breast milk were examined in a prospective study following local anesthesia for dental procedures. The nursing mothers received 3.6 to 7.2 mL of 2% lidocaine without epinephrine and were instructed to dispose of their breast milk for 36 hours following the local anesthesia injection. Presuming the infant had 90 mL of breast milk every 3 hours, the daily dosage for lidocaine was determined to be 73.4 µg/L/d and 66.1 µg/L/d for MEGX. It was concluded that a mother undergoing dental treatment after local anesthesia using lidocaine without epinephrine can continue breastfeeding safely.[65] In different articles, reported idiosyncratic reactions from other components of the local anesthetic (methylparaben or sulfite) suggested the use of local anesthetics without epinephrine to avoid these additional components.[66–68]

After giving birth, the patient may require specific considerations relating to coagulapathy. Hematologic regulation and return to balance continue for weeks after pregnancy.[69] In general, there is a progressive increase in coagulation factors (fibrinogen, V, VII, VIII, IX, X, XII, and von Willebrand factor) during pregnancy, most significant in the third trimester.[70–72] Decreased levels of fibrinolytic protein C during all trimesters of pregnancy can exaggerate this hypercoagulable state.[72,73] Nevertheless, this may be considered an evolutionary advantage to offset blood loss related to placental delivery and postpartum hemorrhage (PPH).[74]

The immediate postpartum period is associated with a higher risk of thrombosis than during pregnancy.[75,76] Specifically, the first few weeks after labor have the highest risk.[77] Boer and colleagues[78] hypothesized that increased tissue factor (TF) levels activate coagulation, which explains why the thrombotic risk is highest in the postpartum period. In particular, the physical removal of the placenta leads to the release of TF into the maternal circulation. This released TF quickly forms a complex, causing magnification of coagulation: a thrombin burst.[79–81] A prospective study concluded that a period of high-risk thrombosis exists until day 25 after delivery.[69] A patient remains in this hypercoagulable state for a minimum of 2 to 3 weeks, if not more.[74] Prophylactic medication for hypercoagulable states may be recommended by the obstetrician for up to 25 days after delivery.[82] Hydration, speedy ambulation, compression stockings, and, occasionally, low molecular weight heparin should be considered for use in conjunction with therapy.[83] There are no routinely used blood tests that quantify effectiveness of the low molecular weight heparins.

PPH is categorized as primary and secondary. Primary PPH is classified as blood loss more than 500 mL in the first 24 hours after delivery. Secondary PPH is described as excessive bleeding that occurs between 24 hours and 6 weeks after delivery. Because of this consumption of clotting factors, replacement therapy may be used to prevent hemorrhage for a minimum of 3 days following vaginal delivery and 5 days after cesarean section.

It is important for the dentist to be aware of how local anesthesia could affect coagulation. Epinephrine may increase levels of thrombin and clotting factor VIII[84]; this would initiate the coagulation cascade and potentially worsen the hypercoagulable state. Although vasoconstrictor would expose the patient to an extremely low dose of exogenous epinephrine, the possible effect on a hypercoagulable patient should be considered. However, if the mother is on anticoagulant therapy, a hematoma-related complication during a dental injection is of concern. Consultation and evaluation by a hematologist or obstetrician may be necessary before the start of dental treatment.

In the infant, the presence of natal teeth may be a cause for early dental intervention. Laceration to the mother's breasts, discomfort during suckling, sublingual ulceration (Riga-Fede disease) with feeding refusal, and swallowing or aspiration are common issues related to requesting removal.[84,85] Despite these potential problems, natal teeth are generally benign and extraction is generally not needed unless it is a supernumary or it is an aspiration hazard.[85–87] The prevalence of natal and neonatal teeth ranges from 1:1000 to 1:30,000.[88] It is slightly more common in girls, uncommon in extremely preterm infants, and has a stronger predilection for infants of some American Indian tribes.[85,89,90] Although the exact cause is unknown, natal teeth affect 2% of infants with unilateral cleft lip and palate and 10% of infants with bilateral cleft lip and palate.[91] Infants may have a lower seizure threshold and a lessened ability to metabolize the drug so, although the maximum dosage of lidocaine for a 3-kg infant

Table 2
Drugs commonly used in dentistry

Drugs	FDA Category	Use in Pregnancy	Use in Nursing	Possible Side Effects
Analgesics				
Acetaminophen	B	Yes	Yes	Not reported
Aspirin	C	Not in third trimester	No	Postpartum hemorrhage
Ibuprofen	B	Not in third trimester	Yes	Delayed labor
Naproxen	B/D	Not in second half of pregnancy	Yes	Delayed labor
Codeine	C	With caution	Yes	Multiple birth defects
Oxycodone	B	With caution	With caution	NRD
Hydrocodone	C/D[a]	With caution	With caution	NRD
Morphine	B	Yes	Yes	Respiratory depression
Propoxyphene	C	With caution	Yes	Not reported
Meperidine	B	Yes	Yes	Not reported
Pentazocine	C	With caution	With caution	Not reported
Antibiotics, Antimicrobials				
Amoxicillin	B	Yes	Yes	Not reported
Metronidazole	B	Yes	Yes	Not reported
Erythromycin	B	Yes	Yes	Not reported
Penicillin V	B	Yes	Yes	Not reported
Cephalosporins	B	Yes	Yes	Not reported
Gentamicin	C	Yes	Yes	Fetal ototoxicity
Clindamycin	B	Yes	Yes	Not Reported
Tetracycline	D	No	No	Discoloration teeth
Chloramphenicol	C	No	No	Maternal toxicity/fetal death
Chlorhexidine	B	No data	No data	Not reported

Local Anesthetics				
Lidocaine	B	Yes	Yes	Not reported
Articaine	C	With caution	With caution	Not reported
Mepivacaine	C	With caution	Yes	Fetal bradycardia
Prilocaine	B	Yes	Yes	Not reported
Bupivacaine	C	With caution	Yes	Fetal bradycardia
Corticosteroids				
Prednisolone	B	Yes	Yes	Not reported
Sedative/Hypnotics				
Nitrous oxide	Not assigned	Avoid in first trimester	Yes	Spontaneous abortions
Barbiturate	D	Avoid	No	NRD
Benzodiazepines	D or X[b]	No	No	Cleft lip/palate

Abbreviation: NRD, neonatal respiratory distress.

[a] D indicates caution if used for prolonged periods of time, or in high doses.

[b] Category X benzodiazepines include flurazepam, estazolam, temazepam, quazepam, and triazolam.

Data from Suresh L, Radfar L. Pregnancy and lactation. Oral Surg Oral Med Oral Pathol Oral Radiol Endod 2004;97:672–82.

may be calculated to be 15 to 21 mg, a reduction in the calculated dose is advised. Neonatal blood volume is 85 mL/kg. This correlates to a low tolerance for blood loss and low circulation of coagulation factors; therefore, the use of epinephrine may be wise, coupled with zealous postextraction pressure. Consultation with a neonatologist is recommended.

SUMMARY AND RECOMMENDATIONS

Local anesthetics may be safely used when treating pregnant and postpartum patients if careful guidelines are followed. Because teratogenic risks are highest in the first trimester, the second trimester is usually the period chosen for nonemergent and routine dental care. Dental care is generally deferred during the late third trimester and immediately after giving birth. Awareness of the potential maternal and fetal effects of any drug used during dental care is of prime importance.

Anesthetic and treatment precautions during pregnancy include:

- Avoidance of treatment in the first 10 weeks of pregnancy because teratogenic risk is highest. Keep in mind that an active infection may have a higher risk of adverse outcome than necessary treatment. Ideally, defer routine care between weeks 14 and 27.
- Sulfonamides, nitrofurantoins, tetracyclines and quinolones seem to be associated with birth defects and should be avoided.
- Radiographs may be taken as necessary, with appropriate precautions being taken to protect the fetus and the patient, such as a lead apron, a tightly collimated beam, and high-speed film.
- All pregnant women requiring care need a thorough risk assessment including TPAL and medical history, with particular attention given to blood pressure (preeclampsia) and blood sugar (gestational diabetes).
- Strict adherence to good local anesthetic technique is required. Aspiration to avoid intravascular injection, needle placement accuracy, and limiting to safe dosages is advised.
- Vasoconstrictors decrease toxicity of anesthetics and can be used safely if intravascular injection is avoided.
- Ester anesthetics should be avoided because of allergenicity. History of sulfite allergies should be considered.
- Lidocaine is the local anesthetic most studied and least associated with medical complications. Other amide or hybrid anesthetics can also be used safely, albeit with slightly higher risk of adverse outcome.
- In second and third trimesters, blood pressure should be monitored and the patient placed in left lateral position to avoid or relieve supine hypotensive syndrome. The angle of positioning can be determined empirically. Supplemental oxygen should be considered if hypotension occurs.
- NSAIDs and aspirin should be avoided, especially in the last trimester and just after delivery. Acetaminophen can be used safely if dosages avoid hepatotoxicity.

A summary of the anesthetic and treatment considerations for patients who are breastfeeding include:

- The American Academy of Pediatrics considers lidocaine to be safe for the breastfeeding mother. Vasoconstrictors necessitate the use of preservatives in local anesthetics. During lactation, the neonate can have idiosyncratic reactions to these preservatives, thus local anesthetics without vasoconstrictors may be associated with a lower incidence of adverse side effects.

- Drugs administered to the mother may be passed on to the breast-fed infant. If the drugs have significant levels to the fetus, stored milk or formula should be substituted. To minimize, advise effects of breast milk–containing drugs; this should have a short half-life, and be given immediately after feeding.
- A hypercoaguable state often exists for a minimum of 2 to 3 weeks after giving birth unless the patient had significant blood loss related to delivery. Epinephrine carries a risk of increasing coagulability.
- Natal teeth are generally benign unless aspiration is a concern. The use of local anesthetics with epinephrine for the neonate may be wise because toxicity of the anesthetic is decreased.

REFERENCES

1. Wang Y, Hu J, Druschel CM. A retrospective cohort study on mortality among children with birth defects in New York State 1983 to 2006. Birth Defects Res A Clin Mol Teratol 2010. [Epub ahead of print].
2. Rood JP. Local analgesia during pregnancy. Dent Update 1981;8(7):483–5 Update Publications, Guilford Press.
3. Dicke JM. Teratology: principles and practice. Med Clin North Am 1989;73(3): 567–82.
4. Rang HP. Pharmacology. 3rd edition. New York: Churchill Livingstone; 1995.
5. Wilson JG. Environment and birth defects (environmental science series). London: Academic Press; 1973.
6. Bracken MB, Holford TR. Exposure to prescribed drugs in pregnancy and association with congenital malformations. Obstet Gynecol 1981;58(3):336–44.
7. O'Rahilly R, Müller F. Human embryology & teratology. New York: Wiley-Liss; 2001.
8. O'Rahilly R, Müller F. Developmental stages in human embryos. Washington, DC: Carnegie Institution of Washington; 1987.
9. Moore KL. The developing human. 3rd edition. Philadelphia: WB Saunders; 1982.
10. Waddell RS. Home pregnancy test hCG levels and FAQ. 2006. Available at: http://www.fertilityplus.org/faq/hpt.html. Accessed June 17, 2006.
11. Bastian LA, Nanda K, Hasselblad V, et al. Diagnostic efficiency of home pregnancy test kits. A meta-analysis. Arch Fam Med 1998;7(5):465–9.
12. Stacey TE. Placental transfer. In: Hytten F, Chamberlain G, editors. Clinical physiology in obstetrics. 2nd edition. Oxford (UK): Blackwell Scientific; 1991.
13. Simpson JL, Globus MS, Martian AO, et al. Genetics in obstetrics and gynecology. New York: Grune and Stratton; 1982. p. 203–10.
14. Mishkin DJ, Johnson KE, Javed T. Dental diseases. In: Gleicher N, editor. Principles and practice of medical therapy in pregnancy. Stamford (CT): Appleton and Lange; 1998. p. 1093–5.
15. Moore PA. Selecting drugs for the pregnant patient. J Am Dent Assoc 1998;129: 1281–6.
16. Little JW, Falace DA. Dental management of the medically compromised patient. 4th edition. St Louis (MO): CV Mosby Co; 1993. p. 383–9.
17. Hood DD, Dewan DM, James FM III. Maternal and fetal effects of epinephrine in gravid ewes. Anesthesiology 1986;64:610–3.
18. Turner M, Aziz SR. Management of the pregnant oral and maxillofacial surgery patient. J Oral Maxillofac Surg 2002;60:1479–88.

19. Cenzig SB. The pregnant patient: considerations for dental treatment and drug use. Quintessence Int 2007;38:133–42, 171.e.

20. Michalowicz, DiAngelis AJ, Novak MJ, et al. Examining the safety of dental treatment in pregnant women. J Am Dent Assoc 2008;139(6):685–95.

21. Srinivas SK, Ernst LM, Edlow AG, et al. Can placental pathology explain second-trimester pregnancy loss and subsequent pregnancy outcomes? Am J Obstet Gynecol 2008;199(4):402, e1–5.

22. MacDonald H, American Academy of Pediatrics, Committee on Fetus and Newborn. Perinatal care at the threshold of viability. Pediatrics 2002;110(5): 1024–7.

23. Lipsky M, King M. Blueprints in family medicine. Malden (MA): Wiley-Blackwell; 2003.

24. Duke J. Anesthesia secrets. 3rd edition. Philadelphia (PA): Mosby; 2006. p. 403–7.

25. Spong CY, Guillermo L, Kuboshige J, et al. Recurrence of gestational diabetes mellitus: identification of risk factors. Am J Perinatol 1998;(1):23–33.

26. Mattison GD. Obstetric and fetal pharmacology. Global Library of Women's Medicine, 2008; January 2009.

27. Campbell JR, Maestrello CL, Campbell RL. Allergic response to metabisulfite in lidocaine anesthetic solution. Anesth Prog 2001;48:21–6.

28. Eggleston ST, Luch LW. Understanding allergic reactions to local anesthetics. Ann Pharmacother 1996;30:851–6.

29. Chestnut D. Obstetric anesthesia: principles and practice. 3rd edition. Philadelphia (PA): Mosby; 2004. p. 198–9.

30. Albright G. Cardiac arrest following regional anesthesia with etidocaine or bupivicaine. Anesthesiology 1979;51:285–7.

31. Turner M, Singh F, Glickman R. Dental management of the gravid patient. N Y State Dent J 2006;72:22–7.

32. Watson AK. Local anaesthetics in pregnancy [letter]. Br Dent J 1988;165:278–9.

33. Oertel R, Ebert U, Rahn R, et al. Clinical pharmacokinetics of articaine. Clin Pharmacokinet 1997;33(6):420.

34. Collins JG, Kitahata LM, Matsumoto M, et al. Spinally administered epinephrine suppresses noxiously evoked activity of WDR neurons in the dorsal horn of the spinal cord. Anesthesiology 1984;60:269–75.

35. Turner MD, Singh F, Glickman RS. Dental management of the gravid patient. N Y State Dent J 2006;72(6):22–7.

36. Mabie WC, DiSessa TG, Crocker LG, et al. A longitudinal study of cardiac output in normal human pregnancy. Am J Obstet Gynecol 1994;170:849–56.

37. Spatling L, Fallenstein F, Huch A, et al. The variability of cardiopulmonary adaptation to pregnancy at rest and during exercise. Br J Obstet Gynaecol 1992;99 (Suppl):1–40.

38. Adams MD, Keegan KA Jr. Physiologic changes in normal pregnancy. In: Gleicher N, editor. Principles and practice of medical therapy in pregnancy. Stamford (CT): Appleton & Lange; 1998. p. 25–40.

39. Lee W. Cardio respiratory alterations during normal pregnancy. Crit Care Clin 1991;7:763.

40. Vorys N, Ullery JC, Hanusck GE. The cardiac output changes in various positions in pregnancy. Am J Obstet Gynecol 1961;82:1312.

41. Marx GF, Bassel GM. Hazards of the supine position in pregnancy. Clin Obstet Gynecol 1982;9:255.

42. Kinsella SM, Lohmann G. Supine hypotensive syndrome. Obstet Gynecol 1994; 83:774–88.

43. DeCherney A, Nathan L, Murphy Goodwin T, et al. Current diagnosis & treatment obstetrics & gynecology. 10th edition. Lange; 2007. Chapter 8, p. 158.
44. Katz VL. Physiologic changes during normal pregnancy. Curr Opin Obstet Gynecol 1991;3:750.
45. Skartrud JJB, Dempsey JA, Kaiser DG. Ventilatory response to medroxyprogesterone acetate in normal subjects. J Appl Physiol 1978;44:939.
46. O'Day MP. Cardiorespiratory physiological adaptation of pregnancy. Semin Perinatol 1997;21:268.
47. Levinson G, Shnider SM, DeLorimier AA, et al. Effects of maternal hyperventilation on uterine blood flow and fetal oxygenation and acid-base status. Anesthesiology 1974;40(4):340–7.
48. Low JA, Boston RW, Cerveneko FW. Effect of low maternal carbon dioxide tension on placental gas exchange. Am J Obstet Gynecol 1970;106:1032–41.
49. Rosman J. Pulmonary physiology. In: Gleicher N, editor. Principles and practice of medical therapy in pregnancy. 2nd edition. East Norwalk (CT): Appleton & Lange; 1992. p. 733–7.
50. Weinberger SE, Weiss ST, Cohen WR. Pregnancy and the lung. Am Rev Respir Dis 1980;121:559.
51. Awe RJ, Nicotra MB, Newsom TD. Arterial oxygenation and alveolar-arterial gradients in term pregnancy. Obstet Gynecol 1979;53:182.
52. Williams J, Price CJ, Sleet RB. Codeine: developmental toxicity in hamsters and mice. Fundam Appl Toxicol 1991;16:401.
53. Heinonen OP, Slone D, Shapiro S. Birth defects and drugs in pregnancy. Littleton (MA): Publishing Sciences Group; 1997.
54. Schoenfeld A, Bar Y, Merlob P, et al. NSAIDS: maternal and fetal considerations. Am J Reprod Immunol 1992;28:141.
55. Stuart MJ, Gross SJ, Elrad H. Effects of acetylsalicylic acid ingestion on maternal and neonatal hemostasis. N Engl J Med 1981;307:909.
56. Hayes DP. Teratogenesis: a review of the basic principles with a discussion of selected agents. Part 2. Drug Intell Clin Pharm 1981;15:542–65.
57. Datta S, Lambert DH, Gregus J. Differential sensitivities of mammalian nerve fibers during pregnancy. Anesth Analg 1983;62:1070–2.
58. Sevarino FB, Gilbertson LI, Gugino LD. The effect of pregnancy on the nervous system response to sensory stimulation. Anesthesiology 1988;69: A695–6.
59. United States Food and Drug Administration. Labeling and prescription drug advertising: content and format for labeling for human prescription drugs. Federal Register 1980;44:37434–67. Available at: http://www.fda.gov/downloads/Drugs/GuidanceComplianceRegulatoryInformation/Guidances/ucm075082.pdf Accessed June 15, 2010.
60. Suresh L, Radfar L. Pregnancy and lactation. Oral Surg Oral Med Oral Pathol Oral Radiol Endod 2004;97:672–82.
61. Dillon AE, Wagner CL, Wiest D, et al. Drug therapy in the nursing mother. Obstet Gynecol Clin North Am 1997;24:675–96.
62. Committee on Drugs, American Academy of Pediatrics. The transfer of drugs and other chemicals into human milk. Pediatrics 1994;93:137–50.
63. Brown WU Jr, Bell GC, Lurie AO, et al. Newborn blood levels of lidocaine and mepivacaine in the first postnatal day following maternal epidural anesthesia. Anesthesiology 1975;42:698–707.
64. Kuhnert BR, Knapp DR, Kuhnert PM, et al. Maternal, fetal, and neonatal metabolism of lidocaine. Clin Pharmacol Ther 1979;26:213–20.

65. Giuliani M, Grossi G, Pileri M, et al. Could local anesthesia while breast-feeding be harmful to infants? J Pediatr Gastroenterol Nutr 2001;32(2):142–4.

66. Schatz M, Fung DL. Anaphylactic and anaphylactoid reactions due to anaesthetic agents. Clin Rev Allergy Immunol 1986;4:215–27.

67. Sindel LJ, De Shazo RD. Accidents resulting from local anaesthetics. Clin Rev Allergy Immunol 1991;9:379–95.

68. Catz CS, Giacoia GP. Drug and breast milk. Pediatr Clin North Am 1972;19: 151–66.

69. Saha P, Stott D, Atalla R. Haemostatic changes in the puerperium '6 weeks postpartum' (HIP Study) – implications for maternal thromboembolism. BJOG 2009; 116:1602–12.

70. Hellgren M, Blomback M. Studies on blood coagulation and fibrinolysis in pregnancy, during delivery and in the puerperium. I. Normal condition. Gynecol Obstet Invest 1981;12:141–54.

71. Stirling Y, Woolf L, North WR, et al. Haemostasis in normal pregnancy. Thromb Haemost 1984;52:176–82.

72. Clark P, Brennand J, Conkie JA, et al. Activated protein C sensitivity, protein C, protein S and coagulation in normal pregnancy. Thromb Haemost 1998;79: 1166–70.

73. Bremme KA. Haemostatic changes in pregnancy. Best Pract Res Clin Haematol 2003;16:153–68.

74. Hellgren M. Hemostasis during normal pregnancy and puerperium. Semin Thromb Hemost 2003;29:125–30.

75. James AH, Tapson VF, Goldhaber SZ. Thrombosis during pregnancy and the postpartum period. Am J Obstet Gynecol 2005;193:216–9.

76. Heit JA, Kobbervig CE, James AH, et al. Trends in the incidence of venous thromboembolism during pregnancy or postpartum: a 30-year population-based study. Ann Intern Med 2005;143:697–706.

77. Romero A, Alonso C, Rincon M, et al. Risk of venous thromboembolic disease in women. A qualitative systematic review. Eur J Obstet Gynecol Reprod Biol 2005; 121:8–17.

78. Boer K, den Hollander IA, Meijers JCM, et al. Tissue factor-dependent blood coagulation is enhanced following delivery irrespective of the mode of delivery. J Thromb Haemost 2007;5:2415–20.

79. Butenas S, Mann KG. Blood coagulation. Biochemistry (Mosc) 2002;67:5–15.

80. Versteeg HH, Peppelenbosch MP, Spek CA. The pleiotropic effects of tissue factor: a possible role for factor VIIa-induced intracellular signaling? Thromb Haemost 2001;86:592–3.

81. Norris LA. Blood coagulation. Best Pract Res Clin Obstet Gynaecol 2003;17: 369–83.

82. O'Riordan MN, Higgins JR. Haemostasis in normal and abnormal pregnancy. Best Pract Res Clin Obstet Gynaecol 2003;17:385–96.

83. Kadir R, Chi C, Bolton-Maggs P. Pregnancy and rare bleeding disorders. Haemophilia 2009;15:990–1005.

84. Rickles FR, Hoyer LW, Rick ME, et al. The effects of epinephrine infusion in von Willebrand's disease. J Clin Invest 1976;57:1618–25.

85. Leung AK. Natal teeth. Am J Dis Child 1986;140:249–51.

86. Seminario AL, Ivancakova R. Natal and neonatal teeth; a study among Chinese in Hong Kong. Br Dent J 1958;105:163–72.

87. Buchanan S, Jenkins CR. Riga-Fedes syndrome: natal or neonatal teeth associated with tongue ulceration. Case report. Aust Dent J 1997;42:225–7.

88. Cunha R, Carrilho Boer F, Torriani DD, et al. Natal and neonatal teeth: review of literature. Pediatr Dent 2001;23:159–62.
89. Sureshkumar R, McAulay AH. Natal and neonatal teeth. Arch Dis Child Fetal Neonatal Ed 2002;87:F227.
90. Leung AK. Natal teeth in American Indians. Am J Dis Child 1986;140:1214.
91. de Almeida CM, Gomide MR. Prevalence of natal/neonatal teeth in cleft lip and palate infants. Cleft Palate J 1996;33:297–9.

Paresthesias in Dentistry

Paul A. Moore, DMD, PhD, MPH[a,b,c,d,]*, Daniel A. Haas, DDS, PhD[e,f,g,h]

KEYWORDS

- Paresthesia • Articaine • Prilocaine • Lidocaine

Alterations to normal oral sensory function can occur after restorative and surgical dental procedures. These sensory abnormalities, generally described as paresthesias, can range from slight to complete loss of sensation and can be devastating for the patient. This article reviews the extent of this oral complication as it relates to dental and surgical procedures, with specific emphasis on paresthesias associated with local anesthesia administration. This review establishes a working definition for paresthesia as it relates to surgical trauma and local anesthesia administration, describes the potential causes for paresthesia in dentistry, assesses the incidence of paresthesias associated with surgery and local anesthesia administration, addresses the strengths and weaknesses in research findings, and presents recommendations for the use of local anesthetics in clinical practice.

DEFINITION OF PARESTHESIA

What is meant by paresthesia? Stedman's Medical Dictionary[1] defines a paresthesia as an abnormal sensation, such as of burning, pricking, tickling, or tingling. Paresthesias are one of the more general groupings of nerve disorders known as neuropathies. Paresthesias may manifest as total loss of sensation (ie, anesthesia), burning or tingling feelings (ie, dysesthesia), pain in response to a normally nonnoxious stimulus (ie, allodynia), or increased pain in response to all stimuli (ie, hyperesthesia).[2]

---

[a] Department of Dental Anesthesiology, School of Dental Medicine, University of Pittsburgh, Pittsburgh, PA 15261, USA
[b] Pharmacology and Dental Public Health, School of Dental Medicine, University of Pittsburgh, Pittsburgh, PA 15261, USA
[c] School of Pharmacy, University of Pittsburgh, Pittsburgh, PA 15261, USA
[d] School of Public Health, University of Pittsburgh, Pittsburgh, PA 15261, USA
[e] Clinical Sciences, Faculty of Dentistry, University of Toronto, 124 Edward Street Toronto, ON M5G 1G6, Canada
[f] Department of Pharmacology, University of Toronto, ON, Canada
[g] Faculty of Medicine, University of Toronto, ON, Canada
[h] Sunnybrook Health Sciences Centre, ON, Canada
* Corresponding author. Department of Dental Anesthesiology, School of Dental Medicine, University of Pittsburgh, Pittsburgh, PA 15261.
E-mail address: pam7@pitt.edu

Dent Clin N Am 54 (2010) 715–730
doi:10.1016/j.cden.2010.06.016
0011-8532/10/$ – see front matter © 2010 Elsevier Inc. All rights reserved.

dental.theclinics.com

In reviewing the dental anesthesiology literature regarding paresthesias, some confusion exists when describing this as an adverse reaction after the administration of local anesthesia. Depression of nerve function and associated anesthesia are the clinical functions of the local anesthetic agents, and altered sensations, such as dysesthesias, are an expected component of the recovery process following local anesthesia. It is now commonplace to include an element of duration to the definition to permit expected pharmacologic alterations in sensory nerve function to be differentiated from abnormal and potentially permanent adverse reactions. In describing paresthesia as a complication of local anesthesia, the anesthesia or altered sensation is required to "persist beyond the expected duration of action of a local anesthetic injection."[3]

Most cases of paresthesia that are reported after dental treatment are transient and resolve within days, weeks, or months.[4–9] The best data regarding rate of recovery are provided in the article by Queral-Godoy and colleagues,[8] in which survival curves are presented for recovery from surgical paresthesias. These data suggest that complete recovery at 8 weeks had occurred in only 25% to 30% of the patients. When reevaluated at 9 months, complete recovery had occurred in 90% of the patients. The time when a paresthesia should be considered permanent is not absolute and is often not known with certainty. Paresthesias that last beyond 6 to 9 months can be described as persistent and are unlikely to recover fully, although some still can. Reports of recovery of sensory function beyond a year are extremely rare.[5,10]

These persistent neuropathies are the authors' primary concern. Few treatments are available that effectively improve symptoms or completely correct persistent paresthesias after dental procedures.[11] Microsurgical repairs of traumatic nerve damage after oral surgical procedures have reported some success in obtaining useful sensory recovery or complete recovery of nerve function.[12] Scientific analyses that establish risk factors for the development of paresthesias must continue to be performed, and treatment options that may prevent this potentially serious complication should be disseminated to those practicing the profession.

REPORTS OF PARESTHESIA AFTER DENTAL TREATMENT

Persistent paresthesias are most commonly reported after oral surgical procedures in dentistry. Needle trauma, use of local anesthetic solutions, and oral pathologies have been less frequently documented.

Third Molars

It has been estimated that 5 to 10 million impacted third molars are removed every year in the United States.[13,14] Peripheral nerve injuries associated with this common oral surgical procedure may be caused by stretching of the nerve during soft tissue retraction, nerve injury caused by compression, as well as partial and complete resection.[4] During removal of third molars, the inferior alveolar nerve (IAN) and the lingual nerve are most likely injured.[12,15] Bataineh,[15] in reviewing more than 30 reports of nerve impairment immediately after third molar extraction, found that the incidence of lingual nerve paresthesia was 0% to 23% and that of IAN paresthesia was 0.4% to 8.4%. Risk factors for these surgical paresthesias include procedures involving lingual flaps and osteotomies, operator experience, tooth angulations, and vertical tooth sectioning.[16,17] IAN and lingual nerve sensory impairments are transient and usually recover fully. Recovery has been reported to occur more rapidly during the first months.[8] As indicated in **Table 1**, estimates for the prevalence of persistent paresthesias (lasting at least 6–9 months) after third molar extraction range from 0.0% to 0.4%.

Table 1
Paresthesia associated with third molar extractions

Investigators	Total Number of Patients	Initial Paresthesia Number (Rate%)	Persistent Paresthesia Number (Rate%)
Queral-Godoy et al[8]	3513	23 (0.65)	1 (0.02)
Genu and Vasconcelos[70]	50 teeth (25 patients)	4 (8.0)	0 (0)
Valmaseda-Catellion et al[16]	946	15 (1.5)	4 (0.4)
Bataineh[15]	741	48 (6.4)	0 (0)
Alling[6]	367,170	1731 (0.47)	81 (0.02)
Jerjes et al[18]	3236	48 (1.5)	20 (0.6)

A recent study evaluating 3236 patients reported that the prevalence of IAN and lingual nerve injury after third molar extractions was initially 1.5% and 1.8% at 1 month, 1.4% and 1.6% at 6 months, and 0.6% and 1.1% at 18 months.[18] Improved surgical procedures and more accurate imaging is likely to limit the risk of this surgical complication.[19]

Dental Implants

Placement of mandibular dental implants has also been associated with inferior alveolar, lingual, and mental nerve paresthesias. As shown in **Table 2**, alterations in nerve function seen initially after mandibular implant placement have been reported to be as high as 37%.[20] Most of these initial events are related to compression of the IAN by the dental implant and can be resolved by removing or repositioning the implant. Persistent alterations in nerve function may also be caused by nerve damage during preparation for the implant placement. Recent recognition of this potential complication has resulted in an increased awareness among practitioners and an apparent decrease in the incidence of this adverse event. Improvements in patient evaluation, treatment planning, and surgical procedures are likely to significantly decrease the occurrence of this complication in the future.

Oral Pathologies

Paresthesia after dental procedures may in rare instances be caused by oral pathologies. Reactivation of varicella-zoster virus has been reported in 6 patients who exhibited facial palsy after dental or orofacial treatment.[21] The presence of infection or abscesses may increase the likelihood of neurologic complications after third molar

Table 2
Paresthesias associated with mandibular dental implants

Investigators	Total Number of Patients	Initial Paresthesia Number (Rate%)	Persistent Paresthesia Number (Rate%)
Bartling et al[71]	94	8 (8.5)	0 (0)
van Steenberghe et al[72]	93	16 (17.6)	6 (6.5)
Astrand et al[73]	23	9 (39)	4 (19)
Ellies[74]	212	78 (37)	27 (13)
Ellies and Hawker[20]	87	31 (36)	11 (13)

extractions.[22,23] Infection and associated endodontic treatment have also been implicated as causes of oral paresthesia.[24]

Local Anesthesia Administration

Local anesthesia administration has also been associated with paresthesia (**Table 3**). There are several proposed mechanisms for paresthesia after local anesthetic injection. These possible causes include hemorrhage into the neural sheath, direct trauma to the nerve by the needle with scar tissue formation, or possible neurotoxicity associated with certain local anesthetic formulations.[2]

Local anesthetics are generally considered to be safe drugs. Yet, because of the large number of dental local anesthetic injections administered annually, even rarely occurring adverse events, such as persistent paresthesia, can represent significant morbidity. It has been estimated that dentists in the United States administer more than 300 million cartridges every year.[25] Even using the lowest incidence rates delineated in **Table 3**, this could represent nearly 100 patients a year developing this post-anesthetic complication.[26]

Local Anesthetic Agents and Formulations Solutions

To obtain Food and Drug Administration (FDA) approval for the introduction of articaine in the United States, a large multicenter randomized clinical trial (RCT) demonstrating its efficacy and safety was performed. The results of this study were published in 2000 and 2001.[27,28] These reports described the efficacy and safety of articaine in 1325 subjects administered either 4% articaine with 1:100,000 epinephrine or 2% lidocaine with 1:100,000 epinephrine. The study on efficacy showed that articaine was comparable to lidocaine for mandibular blocks and maxillary infiltrations, a finding replicated in the RCTs published since that time.[29–31] Although sensory alterations lasting beyond the expected period of anesthesia were reported, all alterations were found to be transient and complete recovery of sensory function occurred within days to weeks. The published safety data concluded that the adverse event profile of articaine was similar to that found with lidocaine.[28]

A large epidemiologic study has suggested that the 4% solutions used in dentistry, namely prilocaine and articaine, are more likely associated with reports of paresthesias after local anesthesia administration. Articaine has been available in Germany since 1976 and in Canada since 1983. In 1995, Haas and Lennon[32] conducted a retrospective study evaluating the incidence of paresthesia from 1973 to 1993 in Ontario, Canada. The database accessed was from the insurance carrier that administered malpractice insurance to all licensed dentists in that province. At the time of the study, there were approximately 6200 dentists in Ontario. In their data set, it was assumed that these paresthesias were persistent and lasted much longer than 8 weeks. It was concluded that there was an overall incidence of 1 paresthesia out of every 785,000 injections. Compared with the other local anesthetics, a statistically significant higher incidence was noted when either articaine or prilocaine was used. The lingual nerve was involved in 64% of the cases, with the IAN involved in the vast majority of the remainder. There was no apparent association with any other factor, such as needle gauge. A follow-up study was done using the same methodology with data from 1994 to 1998.[33] For this period, the incidence of nonsurgical paresthesia in dentistry was 1 in 765,000, similar to the previous finding. The conclusions were the same in that prilocaine and articaine were more commonly associated with this event than the other local anesthetics. The lingual nerve was involved in 70% of the cases, with the IAN involved in the vast majority of the remainder. The same database was used to assess nonsurgical paresthesia reports from 1999 to

Table 3
Paresthesia associated with local anesthesia

Investigators	Reported Rates[a]	Comments
Haas and Lennon,[32] 1995	1 in 439,897 cartridges of articaine and 1 in 588,154 cartridges of prilocaine	Overall incidence of 1 in 785,000 cartridges
Pogrel and Thamby,[11] 2000	1 per 160,571 IAN blocks (all anesthetics)	Inclusion of additional patients interviewed by telephone but not seen increased this estimate to 1 per 26,762. Most patients reported painful injection experience
Miller and Haas,[33] 2000	1 in 452,000 cartridges of prilocaine, 1 in 550,000 cartridges of articaine, 1 in 2,555,000, for lidocaine, and 1 in 2,620,000 for mepivacaine	Results were consistent with the 1995 Canadian study
Rahn et al,[26] 2000	1 in 3,200,000 cartridges of articaine	Estimated number of exposures to articaine was 775 million. Data obtained from the manufacturer of articaine
CRA Newsletter,[50] 2001	2 per 13,000 injections of articaine	Description of both paresthesias suggested trauma as the probable cause
Malamed et al,[28] 2001	14 in 882 injections of articaine, 3 in 443 injections of lidocaine	Duration of these events was from less than 1 day to 18 days after the procedure. In all cases, the paresthesia ultimately resolved
Dower,[3] 2003	1 in 220,000 cartridges of articaine	Calculated from published data that articaine had a 20-fold increase and prilocaine had a 15-fold increase in paresthesia compared with lidocaine
Legarth,[35] 2005	1 in 140,000 cartridges of articaine	3% prilocaine had no reports of paresthesias
Danish Medicines Agency,[42] 2005	1 in 3,700,000 injections with articaine	Not all were believed to be permanent
Hillerup and Jensen,[10] 2006	1 in 957,000 cartridges of articaine	An overall incidence of 1:22,700,000 for all other anesthetics combined
Moore et al,[39] 2006; Hersh et al,[40] 2006; Moore et al,[41] 2007	1 per 361 subjects (1060 injections) of articaine	Total of 4 clinical trials performed to acquire FDA approval of 4% articaine with 1:200,000 epinephrine. One case of prolonged numbness resolved within 24 hours
Pogrel,[36] 2007	1 in 20,000 mandibular injections	Whereas prilocaine may have a higher incidence of paresthesias, no disproportionate nerve involvement from articaine was seen
Gaffen and Haas,[34] 2009	1 in 410,000 injections of articaine, 1 in 332,000 injections of prilocaine	The incidence estimated for lidocaine was 1 in 2,580,000
Garisto et al,[37] 2010	1 in 2,070,678 injections of prilocaine, 1 in 4,159,848 injections of articaine compared to 1 in 124,286,050 injections of lidocaine	Spikes in reporting of paresthesias were seen after initial marketing of the prilocaine and articaine

[a] For consistency, each reported injection assumes one cartridge of anesthetic.

2008 to see if the findings were consistent with those from 1973 to 1998.[34] Once again, the observed frequencies for reporting paresthesia were greater for both articaine and prilocaine, and the tongue was the most common structure affected, involving 79.1% of the reports, with the lower lip being affected in the majority of the remainder.

These 3 analyses were remarkably consistent in their findings. The estimated incidence of persistent paresthesia from either prilocaine or articaine approximated 1 in 500,000 injections for each drug, which was approximately 5 fold higher than that found with lidocaine or mepivacaine. No reports of paresthesia were associated with bupivacaine.

What articaine and prilocaine have in common is that they are the only 4% solutions used in dentistry. A 4% solution means that the concentration of the drug is 40 mg/mL. The other agents available in dental cartridges in the United States and Canada are all more dilute. Lidocaine is a 2% solution, mepivacaine is either 2% or 3%, and bupivacaine is 0.5%. This information led the authors to consider that it was not the specific drug that was the factor, but maybe the concentration administered.

Articaine was introduced in 2000 in Denmark. A Danish study[35] was conducted, and it used a format similar to the one used by Haas and Lennon[32] in Canada in 1995. Using data from the Danish Dental Association's Patient Insurance Scheme, the investigators reviewed reports of paresthesia from 2002 to 2004 in that country. During this period, 32 lingual nerve injuries were registered. Articaine had been administered in 88% of the cases, even though it constituted only 42% of the market. Mepivacaine, as the 3% formulation, was given in the other 12% of cases, and it constituted 22% of the market. Lidocaine, with 22% of the market, had no reports of paresthesia. Prilocaine had 12% of the market and no reports of paresthesia. In Denmark, prilocaine is formulated as a 3% solution, as opposed to 4% in the United States and Canada. The incidence of paresthesia was reported to be 1 in 140,000 for articaine and 1 in 540,000 for mepivacaine.

Another recent study used standardized tests of neurosensory function to determine the cause of injection injury to the oral branches of the trigeminal nerve.[10] The investigators concluded from the assessment of these 56 consecutive patients that there was neurologic evidence of neurotoxicity, not mechanical injury, which resulted in irreparable damage. Consistent with previous clinical studies, the lingual nerve was the most common nerve involved, accounting for 81% of the cases, with the IAN making up the rest. There was also a significant difference in the drugs associated with this neurologic injury. In these patients, articaine was shown to contribute to more than a 20-fold increase in reported paresthesia compared with all other local anesthetics combined. The investigators noted a substantial increase in the number of injection injuries since articaine was introduced into the Danish market.

In a prospective US study of 83 patients referred to a tertiary care center with the diagnosis of persistent alterations of sensory function after local anesthesia administration, only prilocaine was associated with a higher-than-expected incidence of paresthesia.[11] This report evaluated patients treated before articaine was introduced in the United States. The findings were consistent with those previously reported.[32] The overall rate of local anesthetic–induced paresthesias was estimated at 1 per 160,571 IAN blocks.[11] In a follow-up report of an additional 57 patients with paresthesias, the investigators concluded that although prilocaine may have a higher incidence of paresthesias, the rate of paresthesias associated with articaine did not seem to be grossly disproportionate to its use.[36]

In Germany, more than 80 million injections of local anesthetics are administered each year. Articaine, which represents 90% of the market, was introduced in 1975.

A report of all adverse reactions for articaine collected by the manufacturer during the period 1975 to 1999 found 242 adverse neurologic reactions described as hyperesthesia and paresthesias. The incidence of neurologic adverse effects based on an estimated 775 million injections of articaine given during this period was 1 in 3.2 million.[26]

A recent analysis of voluntarily submitted reports of adverse reactions to dental local anesthetics used the FDA's Adverse Event Reporting System (AERS) computerized information database.[37] Nonsurgical paresthesias reported following local anesthesia administration from November 1997 through August 2008 were evaluated (**Fig. 1**). Of the 248 cases of nonsurgical paresthesia reported during this period, 89% involved the lingual nerve. The statistical analysis indicated a higher rate of paresthesias associated with prilocaine (1 in 2,070,678) and with articaine (1 in 4,159,848) compared to lidocaine (1 in 124,286,050).[37]

PROSPECTIVE CLINICAL TRIALS

A prospective RCT is the most sensitive method to study the efficacy of multiple treatments. However, when comparing infrequent side effects of drugs, RCTs are almost always underpowered. For truly rare events such as paresthesias associated with local anesthetic agents, a properly designed RCT would need to enroll millions of subjects to be able to determine significant differences. Because of the small sample sizes, the RCT reported by Malamed and colleagues[27,28] for 4% articaine with 1:100,000 epinephrine as well as the 4 RCTs required for FDA approval of 4% articaine with 1:200,000 epinephrine are not useful in assessing the incidence rates of paresthesias or the possible differences between treatment groups.[38–41]

On a positive note, prospective clinical trials collect more comprehensive information regarding adverse reactions to treatment. This information can then be investigated, properly diagnosed, and followed until the reactions resolve, which allows one to determine if the adverse reaction is transient or persistent in nature. For example, the 4 FDA-required studies of 4% articaine with 1:200,000 epinephrine

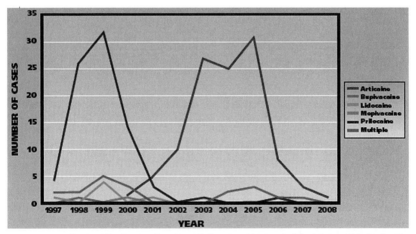

Fig. 1. Reports of paresthesias in dentistry following the use of local anesthetics in the US between 1987 and 2008. (*From* Garisto GA, Gaffen AS, Lawrence HP, et al. Occurrence of paresthesia after dental local anesthetic administration in the United States. J Am Dent Assoc 2010;141:836–44; with permission.)

reported 3 cases of prolonged numbness after administration of articaine.[39–41] All cases reporting this possible adverse reaction returned to the clinic and were examined within 24 hours. Among them, 2 had sensory alterations (discomfort) that were not caused by nerve dysfunctions, but were determined to be caused by soft tissue trauma; all 3 cases had resolved within 24 hours. None of the cases were diagnosed with persistent paresthesias. Yet it should be noted that these studies had a total sample size of 361 subjects receiving only 1060 injections, making conclusions about the incidence of rarely occurring paresthesias difficult, if not impossible.

Similarly, in reporting the safety findings of the clinical trial of 4% articaine with 1:100,000 epinephrine, Malamed and colleagues[28] reported 14 (of 882 injections) paresthesias or hypesthesias after articaine administration and 3 (of 443 injections) after lidocaine administration. All subjects were reevaluated, the nature of the patient report was assessed, a tentative diagnosis and causality assessment was made, and follow-up evaluation was provided. None of the reports were considered persistent, and all cases resolved within 18 days.

RETROSPECTIVE STUDIES

Retrospective data collected from a large population sample provide the best scientific data regarding rare complications. The reports by Haas and Lennon,[32] Rahn and colleagues,[26] and the Danish Medicines Agency[42] are excellent examples of large sample size evaluations. The findings of these studies suggest that the incidences of paresthesias are quite small.

To determine the rate of paresthesias after local anesthesia, one must determine the number of reports of patients having the complication (the numerator) as well as the number of patients exposed to the agent (the denominator). Strategies to determine the denominator have included estimates of the population within the referral base,[11,43] estimates of the population of the country for the national registers,[42] and estimates of the use of the specific agent.[37] One of the approaches to determining the denominator for an epidemiology study was carried out by Haas and Lennon.[32] Having reports of paresthesia from the sole insurance carrier in Ontario, Haas surveyed dentists in Ontario to determine the quantity of each local anesthetic purchased during the same period. The same method was used for the follow-up study by Gaffen and Haas.[34]

Some retrospective studies suggest that the incidence of paresthesia after local anesthesia increased significantly when articaine was first introduced, implying that articaine, because it may be relatively more concentrated than lidocaine, has a greater potential to cause neurotoxicity. However, increased reporting of side effects when a new drug is first marketed is a well-documented phenomenon. This increase in the rate of reporting of adverse events, referred to as the "Weber Effect", was first reported with the introduction of several of the new nonsteroidal antiinflammatory drugs. The Weber Effect increased reporting of side effects by as much as 20 fold during the first few years after a drug is marketed.[42] This finding, first recognized by Weber in Great Britain, has been confirmed for the same agents after their introduction in the United States.[44] The phenomena of a preferential increase in reporting of adverse reactions for a new drug during its first few years of marketing may explain, in part, the peaks in paresthesias seen for prilocaine and articaine (see **Fig. 1**) as recently reported in the US database.[37]

Conversely, on closer examination, the Weber effect may give much more credence to the validity that paresthesia after articaine administration is a real phenomenon reported by the Canadian and Danish investigators.[10,32–35] The Weber Effect states that the number of reported adverse reactions for a drug increases until about the middle to end of the second year of marketing, peaks, and then steadily declines despite steadily increasing prescribing rates. **Fig. 2** shows the reports of paresthesia in Ontario, Canada, from 1973 to 1998.[32,33] The Weber effect would have predicted that the increase in paresthesia reports should have been restricted to 1985 and 1986, after articaine's introduction in Canada in 1983. As can be seen in this figure, the increase in the number of reports lasted much longer than the 2 years predicted by the Weber effect. In fact, the most recent study in 2009 from Ontario shows that the increase in the number of reports for articaine persists for more than 25 years since its introduction in Canada.[34] This finding rules out the hypothesis that the increase in reporting seen in these Canadian data was entirely because of the Weber effect.

An alternative cause for reporting bias is shown in **Fig. 3**, whereby an increased rate of reporting of paresthesias to the Danish Medicines Agency[45] during August and September 2005 was thought to be because of the discussion of paresthesia in the media (stimulated reporting). Increased reporting may also be stimulated by new drug advertising, letters from insurance companies, Internet reports, and editorials published in professional journals.[46–49]

PROPER DEFINITION AND DIAGNOSIS

Reporting of rare clinical events such as paresthesia can be misleading if the event is not accurately evaluated or diagnosed. An example is the Clinical Research Associates (CRA) Newsletter report of 2 paresthesias that occurred after the administration of 13,000 articaine anesthetics.[29] The CRA Newsletter described these paresthesias as follows:

1. One case of paresthesia of the lateral border of the tongue lasting more than 3.6 months resulted after placement of endogenous implants at the site of tooth numbers 29 and 30.
2. A case of paresthesia of the left mandible lasting 36 hours was reported after an articaine block followed by an X-Tip intraosseous injection for the treatment of tooth number 19 with a crown preparation on a patient with a long history of achieving anesthesia.

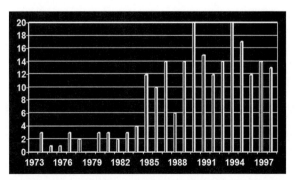

Fig. 2. Reports of nonsurgical paresthesia to the Professional Liability Program of Ontario from 1973 to 1998. (*Data from* Haas DA, Lennon D. A 21 year retrospective study of reports of paresthesia following local anesthetic administration. J Can Dent Assoc 1995;61:319–30, and Miller PA, Haas DA. Incidence of local anesthetic-induced neuropathies in Ontario from 1994–1998 [abstract]. J Dent Res 2000;79:627.)

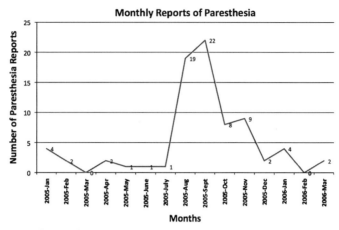

Fig. 3. Reports of paresthesias to the Danish Medicines Agency during January 2005 through March 2006. (*From* Danish Medicines Agency. Adverse reactions from anaesthetics containing articaine (Septanest, Septocaine, Ubistesin, Ubistesin Forte). Reported March 30, 2006. Available at: http://www.dkma.dk/1024/visUKLSArtikel.asp?artikelID=8701. Accessed December 16, 2009; with permission.)

In evaluating these cases, one must wonder if either of these reports represents a paresthesia associated with the use of articaine as anesthetic or were caused by procedural trauma unrelated to the anesthetic agent.

In 2003, Dower published a review of paresthesias associated with administration of local anesthetics.[3] This review analyzed previous studies[27,28,33,50,51] and by making several alternative assumptions estimated the incidence of paresthesia for articaine after mandibular block injections to be 1 in 220,000, higher than that previously reported. Specifically, it was stated that articaine had a 20-fold higher rate of paresthesia than lidocaine and that prilocaine had a 15-fold higher incidence. In addition, using the previously described CRA cases of questionable causation, Dower[3] has suggested articaine's rate of paresthesias after lingual or mandibular blocks to be possibly as high as 1 in 3250, and using FDA data submitted for articaine's new drug application (NDA), has suggested that the possible rate is 1 in 21.[52,53] These unwarranted suggestions have the potential to be misinterpreted and could create inappropriate safety concerns.

UNDERREPORTING AND OVERREPORTING OF RARE ADVERSE EVENTS

Underreporting is a significant problem with any spontaneous reporting system. Because there is no regulated oversight or required reporting, many adverse events are not submitted to government registries and other databases. The extent of underreporting probably relates to the severity of the complication and the availability of multiple sources of input to the registries. Pogrel and Thamby[11] estimated the incidence of paresthesias associated with local anesthesia at 1 in 160,571 based on the number of patients referred and examined at their clinic. In addition, based on logged telephone calls of patients who had contacted them during that period but were never examined or followed up over time, the investigators believed the true incidence was potentially 5 times greater (1 in 26,762).[11]

Conversely, overreporting can also occur when adverse events do not determine the duration of the complication (transient or persistent), include a thorough assessment and diagnosis, and do not have a mechanism for follow-up evaluations. For example, the Danish Medicines Agency notes that some of the 54 patients who reported paresthesias had recovered, suggesting that their incidence rate may have overestimated the true incidence of persistent paresthesias.[46]

PLAUSIBILITY

As early as 1976, it was noted that rats injected with lidocaine at the trigeminal ganglion exhibited inhibition of rapid axonal transport in distal nerve segments in a dose-dependent manner.[54] An investigation of the effects of lidocaine on resting membrane potentials and action potentials of single crayfish giant axons showed a dose-dependent effect resulting in irreversible conduction blockade, with complete loss of resting membrane potential at higher doses.[55] High concentrations of local anesthetics, such as 5% lidocaine, have been shown to result in irreversible conduction block, an effect not found with 1.5% lidocaine.[56] Other studies also support the hypothesis that all local anesthetics have the potential for neurotoxicity, an effect that is dose dependent.[57,58]

Histologic studies have primarily supported the hypothesis that local anesthetics have neurotoxic potential,[59,60] although one study using microinjections into rat sciatic and cat lingual nerves showed no significant effect.[61] This latter study, however, suffered from potential methodological problems of using no control group, using a sample size of 5 for each group, and injecting only 20 μL of local anesthetic into the rat sciatic nerve. The opposite findings to this latter study were shown when a saline control group was used, the sample size was increased to 16, the volume of anesthetic injected in the rat sciatic nerve was increased to 50 μL, and the effects were assessed electrophysiologically.[62]

In a study investigating neuronal cytoplasmic calcium concentrations and neuronal cell death, it was shown that lidocaine in concentrations less than 1% caused minimal changes, whereas 2.5% and, to a greater degree, 5% lidocaine caused much larger changes and cell death.[63] When the concentrations were kept the same, lidocaine and prilocaine had equivalent neurotoxicity in rats.[64] In a study of lidocaine, mepivacaine, bupivacaine, and ropivacaine, all these local anesthetics produced growth cone collapse and neurite degeneration,[65] suggesting that neurotoxicity is not restricted to one agent.

A proposed mechanism for this irreversible nerve injury is membrane disruption, characteristic of a detergent effect,[66] and that local anesthetic neurotoxicity relates to their octanol/buffer coefficients. An assessment of apoptosis induced by different local anesthetics on neuroblastoma cell lines also demonstrates this dose-response relationship of local anesthetics.[67] Their *in vitro* findings indicated that all local anesthetics induced dose-dependent apoptosis. This study also determined that, at the anesthetic concentrations used in dentistry, only prilocaine, but not articaine, was more neurotoxic than lidocaine.[67]

One interesting question is why is the lingual nerve the most common nerve affected? To answer this, a study published in 2003 examined the histologic characteristics of lingual nerves in 12 cadavers.[68] This study showed a range in the number of fascicles present within this nerve, being anywhere from 1 to 8. Of the 12 nerves, 4 (33%) had only 1 fascicle. The investigators speculated that a unifascicular nerve may be injured more easily than a multifascicular one. To date, this seems to be the most plausible explanation for the finding of the predilection of the lingual nerve for permanent paresthesia.

CLINICAL APPLICATION OF THE EVIDENCE

How does the practicing dentist make use of this information? Should a dentist wait for the publication of an RCT proving that articaine and prilocaine are more likely to cause permanent paresthesia than other local anesthetics? Because of the rarity of this event, elucidation of these local anesthetic risk factors is statistically problematic, a finding that has occurred elsewhere in anesthesiology.[69] With published incidence rates estimated to be anywhere from 1 in 160,571,[11] 1 in 140,000,[35] 1 in 785,000,[32] 1 in 3,200,000,[26] 1 in 3,700,000,[50] to 1 in 4,159,848,[37] it would take an unrealistically large RCT to detect a statistically significant difference. The largest RCT on articaine published to date had a sample size of only 1325,[27,28] far too small to be able to detect a statistically significant difference, if one were to exist. The 4 RCTs on the use of articaine with 1:200,000 epinephrine, which when combined included a total of 361 subjects (1060 injections), also have inadequate power to draw conclusions.[39–41] None of the RCTs involving articaine or prilocaine published to date have a sample size large enough to detect this potential difference. No conclusions regarding permanent paresthesia should be made from these particular studies. To quote Hillerup and Jensen,[10] "Since the incidence of injury as such is extremely rare, the finding of nerve injury in a clinical trial is comparable with the finding of a needle in a haystack." Given this reality, they go on to say, "This feature imposes a methodological obstacle to the power of conclusion from prospective clinical studies on injection injuries, and circumstantial evidence, experimental research and retrospective surveys on great number of patients must be taken into account."

SUMMARY

Persistent paresthesias after dental treatment are reported rarely and are most often the result of surgical trauma. The lingual nerve is most often affected, followed by the IAN. The large majority of these complications are transient and result in full recovery within a year. Although a few cases of recovery after several years have been reported, it is generally accepted that paresthesias lasting longer than 6 to 9 months are unlikely to recover fully.

Because the occurrence of local anesthesia–related paresthesias is extremely rare, data from prospective trials having limited sample sizes are not useful. Conversely, data collected retrospectively, suggesting an association with specific anesthetic agents may be incomplete and may have the potential to reflect reporting bias. Thus there is no definitive proof of a cause and effect relationship between 4% solutions and paresthesia. Nevertheless, there exist data that suggest that these solutions are potentially associated with an increased likelihood of paresthesia.

Therefore, having reviewed the literature regarding local anesthesia–induced paresthesias, until future research proves otherwise, the authors agree that a conservative therapeutic strategy is prudent. The authors recommend that the use of 4% articaine or 4% prilocaine for the mandibular nerve block should generally be avoided. This conservative approach is recommended because there is no scientific indication that either agent (articaine or prilocaine) provides greater anesthetic efficacy than the current gold standard in North America, 2% lidocaine with 1:100,000 epinephrine, for the IAN block. As always, dentists should carefully assess the risks and benefits of any drug they prescribe or administer.

REFERENCES

1. Stedman's Online Medical Dictionary. Paresthesia (definition). Available at: www. stedmans.com/section.cfm/45. Accessed April 16, 2007.
2. Haas DA. Articaine and paresthesia: epidemiological studies. J Am Coll Dent 2006;73(3):5–10.
3. Dower JS. A review of paresthesia in association with administration of local anesthesia. Dent Today 2003;22(2):64–9.
4. Girald KR. Considerations in the management of damage to the mandibular nerve. J Am Dent Assoc 1979;98:65–71.
5. Elian N, Mitsias M, Eskow R, et al. Unexpected return of sensation following 4.5 years of paresthesia: case report. Implant Dent 2005;14(4):364–70.
6. Alling CC. Dysesthesia of the lingual and inferior alveolar nerves following third molar surgery. J Oral Maxillofac Surg 1966;44:454–7.
7. Nickel AA. A retrospective study of paresthesia of the dental alveolar nerves. Anesth Prog 1990;37:42–5.
8. Queral-Godoy E, Figueiredo R, Valmaseda-Castellon E, et al. Frequency and evolution of lingual nerve lesions following lower third molar extraction. J Oral Maxillofac Surg 2006;64(3):402–7.
9. Articaine HCL 4% with epinephrine 1:100,000–update '05. CRA Newsletter 2005; 29(6):1–2.
10. Hillerup S, Jensen R. Nerve injury caused by mandibular block analgesia. Int J Oral Maxillofac Surg 2006;35:437–43.
11. Pogrel MA, Thamby S. Permanent nerve involvement resulting from inferior alveolar nerve blocks. J Am Dent Assoc 2000;131:901–7.
12. Bagheri SG, Meyers RA, Khan HA, et al. Retrospective review of microsurgical repair of 222 lingual nerve injuries. J Oral Maxillofac Surg 2010;68:715–23.
13. Friedman JW. The prophylactic extraction of third molars: a public health hazard. Am J Public Health 2007;997(9):1554–9.
14. Moore PA, Nahouraii HS, Zovko J, et al. Dental therapeutic practice patterns in the U.S. Part I: anesthesia and sedation. Gen Dent 2006;54(2):92–8.
15. Bataineh AB. Sensory nerve impairment following mandibular third molar surgery. J Oral Maxillofac Surg 2001;9(9):1012–7.
16. Valmaseda-Castellon E, Berini-Aytes L, Gay-Escoda C. Inferior alveolar nerve damage after third molar surgical extraction: a prospective study of 1117 surgical extractions. Oral Surg Oral Med Oral Pathol Oral Radiol Endod 2001;92:377–83.
17. Wofford DT, Miller RI. Prospective study of dysesthesia following odontectomy of impacted mandibular third molars. J Oral Maxillofac Surg 1987;45(1):15–9.
18. Jerjes W, Talwinder U, Priya S, et al. Risk factors associated with injury to the inferior alveolar and lingual nerves following third molar surgery-revisited. Oral Surg Oral Med Oral Pathol Oral Radiol Endod 2010;109(3):335–45.
19. Park W, Choi J, Kim J, et al. Cortical integrity of the inferior alveolar canal as a predictor of paresthesia after third-molar extraction. J Am Dent Assoc 2010; 141:271–8.
20. Ellies LG, Hawker PB. The prevalence of altered sensation associated with implant surgery. Int J Oral Maxillofac Implants 1993;8:674–9.
21. Furuta Y, Ohtani F, Fukura S, et al. Reactivation of varicella-zoster virus in delayed facial palsy after dental treatment and oro-facial surgery. J Med Virol 2000;62(1): 42–5.
22. Tolstunov L. Lingual nerve vulnerability: risk analysis and case report. Compendium 2007;28(1):28–32.

23. Costantinides F, Biasotto M, Gregori D, et al. "Abscess" as a perioperative risk factor for paresthesia after third molar extraction under general anesthesia. Oral Surg Oral Med Oral Pathol Oral Radiol Endod 2009;107:e8–13.
24. Morse DR. Endodontic-related inferior alveolar nerve and mental foramen paresthesia. Compend Contin Educ Dent 1997;18(10):963–81.
25. Malamed SF. Handbook of local anesthesia. 5th edition. St Louis (MO): Mosby; 2004. p. 285.
26. Rahn R, Jacobs W, Ihl-Beste W, et al. Haufigkeit von Nebenwirkungen bei zahnarztlicher lokalanasthesie: auswertung der nebenwirkungsmeldungen von Ultracain von 1975 bis 1999. ZWR 2000;109(12):678–81 [in German].
27. Malamed SF, Gagnon S, Leblanc D. Efficacy of articaine: a new amide local anesthetic. J Am Dent Assoc 2000;131:635–42.
28. Malamed SF, Gagnon S, Leblanc D. Articaine hydrochloride: a study of the safety of a new amide local anesthetic. J Am Dent Assoc 2001;132:177–85.
29. Claffey E, Reader A, Nusstein J, et al. Anesthetic efficacy of articaine for inferior alveolar nerve blocks in patients with irreversible pulpitis. J Endod 2004;30:568–71.
30. Mikesell P, Nusstein J, Reader A, et al. A comparison of articaine and lidocaine for inferior alveolar nerve blocks. J Endod 2005;31:265–70.
31. Ram D, Amir E. Comparison of articaine 4% and lidocaine 2% in paediatric dental patients. Int J Paediatr Dent 2006;16:252–6.
32. Haas DA, Lennon D. A 21 year retrospective study of reports of paresthesia following local anesthetic administration. J Can Dent Assoc 1995;61:319–30.
33. Miller PA, Haas DA. Incidence of local anesthetic-induced neuropathies in Ontario from 1994–1998 [abstract]. J Dent Res 2000;79:627.
34. Gaffen AS, Haas DA. Retrospective review of voluntary reports of nonsurgical paresthesia in dentistry. J Can Dent Assoc 2009;75(8):579.
35. Legarth J. Lesions to the lingual nerve in connection with mandibular analgesia. Tandlaegebladet 2005;109:10.
36. Pogrel MA. Permanent nerve damage from inferior alveolar nerve blocks- an update to include articaine. J Calif Dent Assoc 2007;35(4):271–3.
37. Garisto GA, Gaffen AS, Lawrence HP, et al. Occurrence of paresthesia after dental local anesthetic administration in the United States. J Am Dent Assoc 2010;141:836–44.
38. Malamed SF, Gagnon S, Leblanc D. A comparison between articaine HCl and lidocaine HCl in pediatric dental patients. Pediatr Dent 2000;22:307–11.
39. Moore PA, Boynes SG, Hersh EV, et al. Dental anesthesia using 4% articaine 1:200,000 epinephrine: two controlled clinical trials. J Am Dent Assoc 2006; 137(11):1572–81.
40. Hersh EV, Giannakopoulos H, Levin LM, et al. Pharmacokinetics and cardiovascular effects of high dose articaine with 1:100,000 and 1:200,000 epinephrine. J Am Dent Assoc 2006;137:1562–71.
41. Moore PA, Delie RA, Doll B, et al. Hemostatic and anesthetic efficacy of 4% articaine HCl with 1:200,000 epinephrine and 4% articaine HCl with 1:100,000 epinephrine when administered intraorally for periodontal surgery. J Periodontol 2007;78(2):247–53.
42. Danish Medicines Agency. Study of adverse reactions from anaesthetics for dental treatment. 2005. Available at: http://www.dkma.dk/1024/visUKLSArtikel.asp?artikelID=6619. Accessed February 11, 2009.
43. Weber JCP. Mathematical models in adverse drug reaction assessment. In: D'Arcy FF, Griffin JP, editors. Iatrogenic diseases. Oxford (UK): Oxford University Press; 1986. p. 102–7.

44. Hartnell NR, Wilson JP. Replication of the Weber effect using postmarketing adverse event reports volunaritly submitted to the United States Food and Drug Administration. Pharmacotherapy 2004;24(6):743–9.
45. Danish Medicines Agency. Adverse reactions from anaesthetics containing articaine (Septanest, Septocaine, Ubistesin, Ubistesin Forte). 2006. Available at: http://www.dkma.dk/1024/visUKLSArtikel.asp?artikelID=8701. Accessed December 16, 2009.
46. Pedlar J. Prolonged paresthesia [letter]. Br Dent J 2003;195:119.
47. Royal College of Dental Surgeons of Ontario. Paraesthesia following local anaesthetic injection. Dispatch Summer 2005;9:26.
48. Randall C. Anaesthetic solutions [letter]. Br Dent J 2003;195:482.
49. van Eeden SP, Patel MF. Letter to the editor: prolonged paraesthesia following inferior alveolar nerve block using articaine. Br J Oral Maxillofac Surg 2002;40: 519–20.
50. Anesthetics, local (articaine HCL 4% with epinephrine 1:100,000). CRA Newsletter 2001;25(6):1–2.
51. FDA Center for Drug Evaluation and Research Approval package for: application number 20–971. Statistical review, 1998. p. 1–19.
52. Peltier B, Dower JS. The ethics of adopting a new drug: articaine as an example. J Am Coll Dent 2006;73(3):11–20.
53. Dower J. Fact sheet. Available at: http://www.nodentalpain.com/ArticaineParesthesia.html. Accessed May 20, 2010.
54. Fink BR, Kish SJ. Reversible inhibition of rapid axonal transport in vivo by lidocaine hydrochloride. Anesthesiology 1976;44(2):139–46.
55. Kanai Y, Katsuki H, Takasaki M. Graded, irreversible changes in crayfish giant axon as manifestations of lidocaine neurotoxicity in vitro. Anesth Analg 1998;86:569–73.
56. Lambert LA, Lambert DH, Strichartz GR. Irreversible conduction block in isolated nerve by high concentrations of local anesthetics. Anesthesiology 1994;80: 1082–93.
57. Selander D. Neurotoxicity of local anesthetics: animal data. Reg Anesth 1993;18: 461–8.
58. Kalichman MW, Moorhouse DF, Powell HC, et al. Relative neural toxicity of local anesthetics. J Neuropathol Exp Neurol 1993;52:234–40.
59. Kalichman MW, Powell HC, Myers RR. Quantitative histologic analysis of local anesthetic-induced injury to rat sciatic nerve. J Pharmacol Exp Ther 1989;250: 406–13.
60. Kalichman MW. Physiologic mechanisms by which local anesthetics may cause injury to nerve and spinal cord. Reg Anesth 1993;18:448–52.
61. Hoffmeister B. Morphologic veranderungen peripherer nerven nach intraneuraler lokalanasthesieinjektion. Dtsch Zahnarztl Z 1991;46:828–30 [in German].
62. Cornelius CP, Roser M, Wietholter H, et al. Nerve injuries due to intrafascicular injection of local anesthetics experimental findings. J Craniomaxillofac Surg 2000;28(Suppl 3):134–5.
63. Johnson ME, Saenz JA, DaSilva AD, et al. Effect of local anesthetic on neuronal cytoplasmic calcium and plasma membrane lysis (necrosis) in a cell culture model. Anesthesiology 2002;97:1466–76.
64. Kishimoto T, Bollen AW, Drasner K. Comparative spinal neurotoxicity of prilocaine and lidocaine. Anesthesiology 2002;97:1250–3.
65. Radwan IA, Saito S, Goto F. The neurotoxicity of local anesthetics on growing neurons: a comparative study of lidocaine, bupivacaine, mepivacaine, and ropivacaine. Anesth Analg 2002;94:319–24.

66. Kitagawa N, Oda M, Totoki T. Possible mechanism of irreversible nerve injury caused by local anesthetics. Anesthesiology 2004;100:962–7.
67. Werdehausen R, Fazeli S, Braun S, et al. Apoptosis induction by different local anesthetics in a neuroblastoma cell line. Br J Anaesth 2009;103(5):711–8.
68. Pogrel MA, Schmidt BL, Sambajon V, et al. Lingual nerve damage due to inferior alveolar nerve blocks a possible explanation. J Am Dent Assoc 2003;134:195–9.
69. Hopwood MB. Statistics: can we prove an association for a rare complication? Reg Anesth 1993;1:428–33.
70. Genu PR, Vasconcelos BC. Influence of the tooth section technique in alveolar nerve damage after surgery of impacted lower third molars. Int J Oral Maxillofac Surg 2008;37(10):923–8.
71. Bartling R, Freeman K, Kraut RA. The incidence of altered sensation of the mental nerve after mandibular implant placement. J Oral Maxillofac Surg 1999;57(12): 1408–12.
72. van Steenberghe D, Lekholm U, Bolender C. Applicability of osteointegrated oral implants in the rehabilitation of partial edentulim: a prospective multicenter study of 558 fixtures. Int J Oral Maxillofac Implants 1990;5:272–9.
73. Astrand P, Borg K, Gunne J, et al. Combination of natural teeth and osteointe-grated implants as prosthesis abutments: a 2-year longitudinal study. Int J Oral Maxillofac Implants 1991;6:305–12.
74. Ellies LG. Altered sensations following mandibular implant surgery: a retrospec-tive study. J Prosthet Dent 1992;68:664.

Needle Phobia: Etiology, Adverse Consequences, and Patient Management

Chester J. Sokolowski, DDS*, Joseph A. Giovannitti Jr, DMD,
Sean G. Boynes, DMD, MS

KEYWORDS

- Needle phobia • Patient management • Avoidance behavior
- Physiologic consequences

Needle phobia is a formal medical condition affecting approximately 10% of the world population and characterized within the American Psychiatric Association Diagnostics and Statistical Manual of Mental Disorders (DSM-IV) by the presence of fear and the occurrence of avoidance behavior.[1] An individual's avoidance of health care to eliminate any preconceived exposure to needles is the central premise to the diagnosis of needle phobia.[1] In conjunction with avoidance behavior, there are also physiologic changes in blood pressure, heart rate, electrocardiogram (ECG), and stress hormone levels.[1] Therefore, needle phobia can be defined as a combination of objective clinical parameters as well as subjective symptoms.

Because much of modern medicine depends on the hypodermic needle for medical testing and/or drug therapies, clinicians should be aware that needle phobia is a common condition that may lead to avoidance of medical treatment, severe health and dental problems, and significant social and legal difficulties. Furthermore, there have been reports in peer-reviewed literature of needle phobia–related syncope/vasovagal/fainting reactions that have led to asystole and death. Clinicians should be aware of the underlying pathophysiology, possible severe sequelae, and the prevention and treatment of the possible adverse events that can occur.

PREVALENCE

In a review of literature, Hamilton[1] states that, because needle phobia has recently been defined, only indirect estimates of its prevalence can be inferred from the literature.

Department of Anesthesiology, University of Pittsburgh School of Dental Medicine, 3501 Terrace Street, Pittsburgh, PA 15261, USA
* Corresponding author. Department of Anesthesiology (G-87 Salk Hall), University of Pittsburgh School of Dental Medicine, 3501 Terrace Street, Pittsburgh, PA 15261.
E-mail address: chs120@pitt.edu

Dent Clin N Am 54 (2010) 731–744
doi:10.1016/j.cden.2010.06.012
0011-8532/10/$ – see front matter © 2010 Elsevier Inc. All rights reserved.

In a Canadian community study completed by Costello,[2] 449 Canadian women were interviewed and administered the Present State Examination (PSE) to allow for a standardized identification of psychiatric classification. The investigators found that 21.2% experienced mild to intense fear, and 4.9% had a phobic level of fear of injections, doctors, dentists, and hospitals. In addition, Agras and colleagues[3] reported findings that estimated that 9% of the population of the United States 10 to 50 years of age have an injection phobia and 5.7% have seen a physician about this phobia. In an English study presented by Keep and Jenkins[4] the dread of a painful injection was present in 11% of 100 British office patients.

Through in-hospital interviews, 22% of 184 teenaged maternity patients in Nashville, Tennessee, were found to have an increased fear of blood drawing that inhibited them from maintaining routine prenatal care within a public clinic.[5] In random questionnaire-based surveys, 23% of 200 Swedish and 27% of 177 American college students reported needle phobia as the main reason for not donating blood.[6,7]

Several studies have also investigated the associated demographics of needle phobia. It seems that the overall population of needle phobics has a slight female preponderance and is of a younger age. Deacon and Abramowitz[8] recruited 3315 venipuncture participants from hospital-based phlebotomy laboratories. The investigators conducted a series of analyses examining differences between individuals with needle phobia symptoms (n = 72) and those who did not present with any symptoms of needle fear (n = 2787). Compared with those with no needle fear, needle phobics were more likely to be women (68.1% vs 48.9%) and of a younger age (43.3 mean years vs 59.0 mean years). Graham[9] also found a significant correlation of age with anxiety as a predictor for syncope in an older study involving 414 blood donors at a hospital blood bank. This evaluation revealed a definite association between age and the occurrence of fainting. As shown in **Table 1**, the younger the blood donor, the more likely he/she was to faint. The pulse rate also proved to be correlated with syncope. Patients with a higher pulse were more likely to have a syncopal episode (**Table 2**). Anxiety was also a significant factor in predicting syncope. Thirty-two percent admitted to being nervous; of these, 28.6% fainted. Of the remaining 68.2% who denied any anxiety, only 12.9% fainted. Therefore, a donor who admitted to being anxious was twice as likely to faint as to one who denied any anxiety (**Table 3**). Racial differences in needle phobia are conflicting in the literature.[10] In Graham's[9] study, 18% of 352 white subjects, but none of the black subjects, fainted while donating blood. There was no obvious explanation for the racial differences. Statistical evaluation showed no significant differences between the means of the 2 groups in age, initial pulse, systolic blood pressure, mean blood pressure, or admission of nervousness. Another study completed by Callahan and colleagues[11] found

Table 1 Frequency of fainting according to age	
Age (y)	**Proportion Fainted (%)**
50–59	0/21 (0)
40–49	8/79 (10)
30–39	24/125 (19)
20–29	28/117 (24)
10–19	3/10 (30)

Data from Graham DT. Prediction of fainting in blood donors. Circulation 1961;23:903.

Table 2
Frequency of fainting according to initial pulse rate

Pulse Rate (bpm)	Proportion Fainted (%)
>100	15/35 (43)
90–99	15/73 (21)
80–89	21/155 (14)
70–79	8/72 (11)
60–69	4/17 (24)

Abbreviation: bpm, beats per minute.
Data from Graham DT. Prediction of fainting in blood donors. Circulation 1961;23:903.

no racial differences. Further study evaluating the possibility of racial or ethnic genetic characteristics that could predispose one to needle phobia and syncope may be warranted.

A familial predilection for needle phobia has been shown in various research. Hamilton[1] reports that approximately 80% of patients who have needle phobia report strong needle fear in a first-degree relative (ie, a parent, child, or sibling). Numerous other studies have shown that patients with needle phobia have family members with similar traits.[12] A Swedish study showed that 68% of patients with needle phobia had biologic relatives who were needle phobic, a rate that was 3 to 6 times higher than the frequency of corresponding phobias among the relatives of patients treated for agoraphobia, social phobia, dental phobia, or animal phobia.[13] In an American study,[12] 27% of patients with needle phobia had a family history of needle fear. By means of a comparative twin study (monozygotic and dizygotic twins), Torgersen[14] investigated the etiology and nosology of phobic fears. The study established that, apart from separation fears, genetic factors have a consistent role in the strength as well as content of phobic fears.

ETIOLOGY
Evolution of the Needle Phobic Trait

Hamilton[1] postulates the presence of a genetic trait that probably evolved among the human species in response to piercing, stabbing, and cutting injuries. He speculates that most violent deaths in our species' evolutionary history have been caused by penetrations from teeth, claws, fangs, and tusks, and from sticks, stone axes, knives, spears, swords, and arrows.[15] He surmises that a deep-rooted, evolutionarily developed psychological reflex resulted in a strong fear of skin puncture and provided selective values in teaching humans to avoid such injuries.[1] He concludes that, in the past 4 million years or more of human evolution, genes controlling blood pressure,

Table 3
Combination of pulse, age, and anxiety

Age (y)	Pulse Rate (bpm)	Anxiety Level	Proportion Fainted (%)
<30	≥90<100	Not nervous	16/46 (35)
<30	≥90<100	Nervous	11/23 (48)
<30	≥100	Not nervous	6/12 (50)
<30	≥100	Nervous	5/7 (71)

Data from Graham DT. Prediction of fainting in blood donors. Circulation 1961;23:904.

heart rate, cardiac rhythm, and stress hormone release developed to maintain the survival of the human species.

However, not all humans suffer an extreme response to needles. Hamilton[1] concludes his hypothesis of etiology by likening it to other human traits such as weight, height, and intelligence, which vary with each individual human. Therefore, he suggests that the gene for needle phobia is distributed in a normal bell-shaped distribution curve that affects individuals to varying degrees.

Inherited or Learned

There is clear evidence that supports the hypothesis of a hereditary component to needle phobia.[1] Both the vasovagal reflex and needle phobia tend to run strongly in families.[15-18] The heritability of blood-injury phobias that include fear of injections, wounds, blood, and pain have been estimated at 48% in twin studies.[14] The heritability in electrocardiographic variations such as PR, QRS, and QT intervals, as well as heart rate, is at 30% to 60%, respectively.[19] The autonomic control of the cardiovascular system in general, based on these twin comparisons, can be considered genetically influenced.[20] Therefore, during a needle phobic response, a correlation may exist between abrupt decreases in blood pressure, heart rate and ECG changes, and genetic influences.[1]

In addition to genetic factors, there is a learned component to needle phobia.[1] There are several publications that discuss the needle fear that arises after a negative experience at a physician's or dentist's office.[17,21,22] A study completed by Ost[18] of 56 subjects who had injection phobia showed that 56% could trace their fear back to negative conditioning from a health care experience. The mean onset of age was 8.06 years and often correlated with a first-time health care–related appointment. This study also determined that 24% of the subjects could trace their phobias to having seen another child, often a sibling, have a negative experience to needles. It has been surmised that over time, with more needle exposures, this learned fear tends to organize itself and form into a conscious phobia that leads to an anticipatory anxiety before various medical procedures involving needles. This fear then becomes generalized toward objects that are frequently associated with needles, such as syringes, doctors, white laboratory coats, examination rooms, nurses, and even the antiseptic smells of offices and hospitals.[2,10,14]

Based on these studies, it can be hypothesized that the trait of needle phobia is both inherited and learned. A vasovagal reflex is seen in all patients with needle phobia who have been tested, and medical histories show that most have had learning experiences that triggered the needle fear.[23] A reasonable theoretic model might propose that needle phobia depends on both an inherited reflex that is hardwired in neurovascular and neuroendocrine pathways and on the learning of a conscious fear.

Other investigators have reached similar conclusions. Marks[10,24] reports that emotional fainting in response to a needle stimulus may have evolved from the tonic immobility reaction (ie, playing dead) that is seen in many species. In a recent animal study completed by Gabrielsen and colleagues,[25] grouse were found to have an emotional bradycardia when they freeze on being approached. Predators tend to attack prey that is moving, and tend to lose interest when the prey becomes still. Marks[10,24] continues by saying that emotional faints in humans, and tonic immobility in animals, may be mediated by a depressor pathway related to survival that has been found in cats and monkeys.[26] Pool and Ransohoff[27] reviewed the physiology of a tonic immobility reaction in which the rostral cingulated gyrus in the brain serves as the primary action sector. He found that stimulation of that area led to autonomic responses, motor effects, and a suppressor action. In the same report, the autonomic responses were evaluated and there was a marked respiratory slowing and arrest up to 25 seconds. Marked cardiovascular effects were also observed, consisting of vagal slowing of the heart, cardiac arrest, and a marked decrease in blood pressure.[27] Kremer[28] suggested the existence of different functional areas in the cingulated gyrus that were related not only to autonomic responses but emotional responses.

CLINICAL FINDINGS/PHYSIOLOGY

The physical symptoms of needle phobia include syncope, near syncope, light-headedness, or vertigo on needle exposure, along with other autonomic symptoms such as pallor, diaphoresis, and nausea.[1]

The Vasovagal Response

The neurophysiology of the vasovagal reflex is both a vagal bradycardia and a vasodilation from withdrawal of α-sympathetic arteriolar tone, which together cause hypotension.[16] Some studies have shown that the vasovagal reflex is a biphasic response in which there is an anticipatory reaction of increased heart rate and blood pressure before needle puncture followed by a sudden decrease in both heart rate and blood pressure after a needle puncture.[10,15,29,30] However, Hamilton[1] has observed that some patients with needle phobia do not show this initial cardiovascular increase.

The onset of the vasovagal response can be immediate, within 2 to 3 seconds, and is usually brief. However, not all cases of syncope are short lived. Hamilton[1] presented a prospective study demonstrating that of 84 blood donors that fainted, 16.7% experienced syncope from 5 to 30 minutes.[31] Another series of 64 blood donors who fainted found that 14% fainted after leaving the phlebotomy site, sometimes several hours later. Furthermore, although those who faint only do so for several seconds, a survey of 298 fainting patients showed that several had lost consciousness for 10 to 30 minutes, and a few from 1 to 2 hours.[32] These studies show that blood pressure returns to normal after 2 hours and most patients feel well enough to return to their normal activity after several hours. However, some have reported anxiety, malaise, and weakness for 1 to 2 days after the syncopal episode.[31,32]

Cardiovascular Implications

There are several reports of ECG changes during the vasovagal reflex. They include sinus arrhythmias; premature atrial contractions; premature junctional contractions; unifocal and multifocal premature ventricular contractions; bigeminy; first- and second-degree heart block; changes in P waves, ST waves, and T waves; sinus bradycardia; sinus tachycardia; ventricular tachycardia; ventricular fibrillation; and asystole.[15,16,29,30,33–35] Some experts presume that these ECG changes are secondary to vagal influence on the sinoatrial and atrioventricular nodes, and that they also relate to the antagonism between the activated sympathetic and parasympathetic systems on the heart.[29] Such evidence should indicate to the clinician that patients who have needle phobia require cautionary management. Although the condition is rare, any prolonged syncopal event indicates prolonged bradycardia and hypotension, and is thus associated with hypoperfusion of cardiac and brain tissue. Such events always expose the patient to a greater incidence of cardiac or cerebral ischemia.

Hormonal Relationships

Epinephrine and norepinephrine levels do not always become increased during episodes of needle phobia.[15] They have been observed to decrease in 8 patients who fainted after venipuncture. This is presumably related to the withdrawal of sympathetic vascular tone.[36] In another study, 21 young women receiving dental treatment had increased levels of epinephrine, but not norepinephrine.[23] This was likely the result of a severe situational stress response in which epinephrine is secreted by adrenal medullary cells in the manner of a fight-or-flight response. Sympathetic activity can be decreased before or during syncope, which may decrease norepinephrine outflow.[37–39] As the shutdown of norepinephrine reduces vascular tone, epinephrine selectively produces vasodilation in skeletal muscle, which causes pooling of blood in the periphery, reduces venous return, and results in profound sudden hypotension.

Vasopressin or antidiuretic hormone (ADH) has been shown to increase in response to the vasovagal reflex associated with venipuncture.[15,16] This may be caused by a reduction in intravascular volume by the pituitary gland during vasovagal shock.[15,16] Renin also increased by 200% in one patient with needle phobia, which could be an attempt by the body to compensate for syncope by increasing the circulating blood volume.[40] ADH, a potent vasoconstrictor, is responsible for the pallor seen during the vasovagal reflex and also contributes to a nausea effect. The ADH hormone acts during the vasovagal response by sharply decreasing cutaneous blood flow, and its increase may be considerable, reaching 46 times normal levels.[15,41] This extensive increase may be responsible, along with the cathecholamine increase, for the intense fear that victims of needle phobia learn in response to their vasovagal reflex.

Bispectral Index

There were also reports of cases in which there was a decrease in bispectral index (BIS) as an indicator of syncope.[42] BIS provides a numerical value that has been correlated with the patient's hypnotic state and is related to the patient's electroencephalogram (EEG). The EEG is a recording of electrical potentials generated by cells in the cerebral cortex of the brain. Data measured by the EEG are taken through a computer-generated algorithm that results in a numerical readout that correlates with the depth of hypnosis. BIS values of 65 to 85 have been related to varying levels of sedation, whereas patients are considered to be unconscious with BIS values ranging from 40 to 65. The BIS monitoring device is a tool used extensively in anesthesiology to aid the anesthesiologist in gauging a patient's depth of anesthesia.

Win and colleagues[42] reported 2 patients with decreased BIS indexes that were associated with syncope during venipuncture. One patient had a reduced BIS score that occurred during the development of hypotension and bradycardia, and the other patient lost consciousness with decreasing BIS scores before hypotension and bradycardia could occur. Using these case studies as means of analysis, it seems that the cortical processing of emotional fear, stress, and pain may be conveyed to the medullary cardiovascular center through the limbic system. The limbic system regulates emotions, and stimulation of the limbic sympathoinhibitory center can cause hypotension and bradycardia.

ADVERSE EVENTS

Needle phobia can manifest as a powerful and incapacitating mental disorder. Those with needle phobia are often terrified of routine needle procedures. Some patients with needle phobia are so frightened that that they state they would rather die than have a needle procedure.[1] This heightened fear places them at risk for health, social, and legal liabilities. The vasovagal response itself has led to fatalities. Syncope has been reported as the cause of more than half of dental office emergencies.[43] Although syncope occurs most commonly with the patients in a standing position, it can also occur when the patients are supine.[44] Although most venipunctures and dental local anesthetic injections are performed with patients in a supine or semireclining position as a precaution against syncope, syncope may still occur because of the overwhelming effect that fear and anxiety may have on central cardiovascular control. The depression of cardiac function causes a reduced stroke volume, cardiac output, myocardial contractility, and brady-cardia.[37,39,45] Severe vasovagal syncope caused by emotional stress could interact with preexisting cardiovascular disease and lead to death.[29,37,39,46]

Morbidity/Mortality

There have been at least 23 reported deaths attributed solely to needle phobia and its vasovagal reaction during needle procedures such as venipuncture, blood donation, arterial puncture, pleural tap, and intramuscular and subcutaneous injections.[47,48] Other reports and indirect evidence further suggest that needle procedures can result in sudden death.[29,34,35] When morbidity and/or mortality from needle phobia occurs, it is usually related to 2 mechanisms. First, an abrupt drop in heart rate and blood pressure leads to a sudden and severe decrease in systemic and cerebral perfusion. This sudden decrease, especially in a patient with a compromised cardiac condition or in a patient with cerebrovascular disease, could lead to myocardial or cerebral infarction.[48] Second, the vasovagal reflex may increase vagal tone to the extent that it could impair the sinoatrial node or atrioventricular node enough to cause ventricular fibrillation or asystole.[29,37]

The role of stress and syncope in the patient with needle phobia should not be taken lightly. There is considerable documentation to show the relationship of stress to heart rhythm.[49] Cardiac arrhythmias can occur in persons without cardiac disease when they are exposed to routine stress.[49] In his research on emotional causes of sudden death, Dimsdale[49] cited animal studies that support the idea of sudden death under extreme stress. In 2 reviewed studies, spontaneous myocardial necrosis was noted after extreme conditions of stress were imposed in captive and wild squirrels.[50] Dimsdale[49] also cited research by Selye,[51] and Keegan[52] who suggest that emotional stress leads to an increase in cathecholamines and glucocorticoids, which can cause cardiac ischemia and disturbed cardiac conduction. He cited another study that showed that continued electrical stimulation of the right vagus nerve in monkeys resulted in myocardial necrosis.[53,54]

Convulsions during syncope are more frequent than is commonly realized. They are a response of the central nervous system to cerebral hypoxia associated with vasovagal shock. Hamilton[1] cites a study of 84 blood donors who fainted. Fourteen percent had prominent tonic-clonic episodes, and another 27 percent had tonic muscular rigidity.[31] Marks[10] reports that bradycardia in response to needle phobic cues can create asystole lasting as long as 25 seconds, during which convulsions may occur.[9,10]

Avoidance

Patients with needle phobias simply avoid health care; sometimes for many years.[15,17] Several studies have made it a common understanding that patients with needle phobias avoid treatment even when the need for it is compelling.[8,10,15,17,21] Approximately 5% to 15% of the population decline necessary dental treatment primarily for fear of oral injections.[22] As stated earlier, with an incidence of needle phobia of at least 10%, a large hidden population goes without regular health care because of this condition.

Social/Legal

Needle phobia can also cause major social and legal problems. A fear of blood testing or immunization can interfere with or destroy plans for marriage, travel, education, immigration, or employment.[1] Students can be discouraged from biologic, nursing, or medical careers because of their fear of needles, and women wishing to have children may decide against conceiving because of needle fear.[1,10,17]

Legal problems can arise when blood tests are ordered by a court and some victims have been charged by police for failing to agree to blood testing.[10] In the book, *The Blooding*,[54] there are details of the extensive resistance that police faced against mass blood testing to eliminate suspects in a murder case. In the United States, 4 cases of accused drunk drivers, required to take involuntary blood tests, have been appealed to the Supreme Court.[34,55–58]

PATIENT MANAGEMENT
Nonpharmacologic

Dentists and physicians must be knowledgeable about the management of needle fear to treat their patients appropriately. Communicating empathy and respect is paramount; advising patients that they are not alone and that there are many others who share a similar fear. Education and reassurance are the mainstays of a doctor's armamentarium. Patients should be informed that there is an inherited, involuntary nature to needle phobia and that there are various methods to counter it.

Desensitization

The most commonly employed technique, desensitization therapy, requires a motivated patient. The therapy may decondition the autonomic symptoms and fear experienced by patients with mild needle phobia and can extinguish associated needle fears. Marks[10] stresses that treatment of needle phobia is mandatory when it endangers the patient's life through avoidance of life-saving medical procedures such as urgent surgery, blood transfusions, or insulin injection for diabetes. The clinician elicits details of all situations that induce fear and/or faintness and then arranges prolonged exposure to each of those situations. The patient is asked to carry out exposure homework to those situations between sessions and to record details of exposure homework tasks and reactions to them in a daily diary. These tasks are monitored at each session and fresh exposure homework is added as needed. The patients can do most treatment alone as self-exposure homework. The clinician's role is that of a monitor.

Pharmacologic desensitization

Another method of desensitization is through pharmacologic means. Moore and colleagues[59] observed that, through a conscious sedation approach, a desensitization phenomenon can occur. Regardless of the specific method used, the overall strategy requires that fearful patients develop a trusting relationship with their dentist. Conscious sedation enables the patient to be presented with a series of positive experiences from which the fearful patient can develop more realistic expectations for future dental treatments. Moore and colleagues[59] showed that patients were able to be weaned through a series of subsequent visits as the patients developed greater trust with their dentist. Through a careful titration of pharmacologic agents, the presentation of perceived aversive stimuli is controlled and decreasing depths of sedation are needed during subsequent appointments.[59]

Habituation

Habituation is considered the most rapid treatment. Exposure to the offending agent is prolonged for an hour or more at a time and the phobic cues are real or filmed rather than imagined. Marks[10] applies these principles by having patients look at a vial of blood and lurid pictures of surgery and disease, read gory descriptions of disease, and handle needles and syringes of increasing size. The success rate with this treatment regimen seems limited, and only a small number of patients respond favorably.

Perceptive Preparation

Perceptive preparation is a common technique used in dental phobic centers. The process involves several preoperative appointments. Applying several of the techniques used with desensitization, the goal of this treatment is for the patient to undergo a series of practice appointments in which they are slowly introduced to the protocol of treatment as well as the equipment that will be used before any procedure is performed. However, time limitations within most practices create an environment in which this lengthy training cannot be used.

Hypnosis

The use of hypnosis for dental anxiety and fear has recently seen a mild resurgence since its use peaked in the 1960s and 1970s. Dentists have used several methods in the management of needle phobia through hypnosis.[60–62] Dental professionals have treated the phobia diametrically and symptomatically, relying essentially on the relaxation techniques associated with hypnotherapy.[60]

Frankel[63] reported that 58% of a group of 24 patients with phobia were highly responsive to hypnosis when evaluated on a group scale of hypnotic susceptibility. Moore and colleagues[64] evaluated the outcomes of hypnotherapy in adults aged 19 to 65 years. The investigators examined regular attendance behaviors, changes in dental anxiety, and changes in beliefs about dentists and treatment after 3 years. After the 3-year period, 54.5% of patients having hypnotherapy were maintaining regular dental care habits, compared with 46.1% of the reference group who reported going regularly to the dentist. It was concluded that many patients can successfully start and maintain regular dental treatment habits with dentists despite years of avoidance associated with phobic or extreme anxiety. It seems that patients with phobia have success in reducing dental anxiety and improving beliefs about dentists in the long-term when treated with hypnotherapy.

Topical Anesthetics

Topical anesthesia at the needle site can provide some relief (ice, ethyl chloride spray, or topical anesthetics). Ethyl chloride spray can freeze the skin temporarily. This effect lasts for only a few seconds and affects only the superficial layers of the skin before a venipuncture. Topical application of cream-based local anesthetic mixtures (EMLA cream; lidocaine 2.5% and prilocaine 2.5%; Astra Zeneca) have been shown to be efficacious.[65] However, the use of these preparations can be inefficient because it can take up to 1 hour for the preparation to induce enough dermal anesthesia to achieve a comfortable venipuncture.

Iontophoresis enables topical anesthetics to penetrate the skin much faster and more deeply. Lidocaine is a small molecular weight amide local anesthetic with poor bioavailability when applied to intact skin, such as in the EMLA preparations. Iontophoresis allows for the transdermal delivery of small molecular weight, charged drugs using a low-level electrical current. The electrical current drives the charged drug molecules, which reside in a reservoir on a dermal patch, through the skin via an electrical potential.[66] Because lidocaine is a positively charged molecule, the electrode pad's positive charge repels the lidocaine, driving it through the skin via the sweat ducts.[67] Using iontophoresis, an area can be completely anesthetized before venipuncture within 10 minutes to a depth of 1 to 2 cm.[67] In a study by Kearns and colleagues,[68] the iontophoresis unit was shown not to deliver a significant systemic dose of lidocaine and was well tolerated in the pediatric subjects.

The future also holds promise for the development of a painless needle. A team of researchers at the University of North Carolina and a company called Laser Zentrum Hannover have recently used 2-photon polymerization to create hollow needles so fine that patients do not feel them piercing the skin. These microneedles could be clustered on a patch and deliver drugs as a standard hypodermic needle.[69] A useful and practical application of these patches would be to deliver lidocaine to a site before venipuncture. The ease of use of iontophoresis and these microneedle patches raises the possibility of a future in which medical and dental environments become significantly less threatening to patients with needle phobia.

Anxiolysis/Sedation

When anxiety becomes chronic, or when it acutely impairs normal or reasonable functioning, pharmacotherapy is indicated. Patients with needle phobia experience a high degree of situational stress that, if left unabated, may lead to syncope, hyperventilation, agitation, excitement, tachycardia, hypertension, angina, cardiac dysrhythmias, and cardiac arrest. These physiologic and behavioral changes are, at best, undesirable, and, at worst, major causes of emergent situations. Dionne and colleagues[70] and others have shown that benzodiazepines attenuate this stress response, thus paving the way for the use of benzodiazepines in procedural sedation. However, benzodiazepines and other antianxiety agents are not curative, but merely treat the symptoms of anxiety. The patient is then able to cope more effectively when stressed.

Benzodiazepines have distinct advantages compared with other oral premedicants for patients with needle phobia. They are the only drug group with specific anxiolytic properties and they have a high therapeutic index, which enhances their safety. Additionally, they cause anterograde amnesia so that patients often cannot recall the procedures performed. Oral benzodiazepines such as triazolam, diazepam, midazolam, alprazolam, or lorazepam may be indicated to provide anxiolysis before needle puncture. Larger-than-usual doses may be necessary in these cases and can be combined with nitrous oxide inhalation.

Diazepam is the prototypical benzodiazepine and is effective orally in adult doses of 2 to 20 mg and in pediatric doses of 0.15 to 0.3 mg/kg. Its onset is within 1 hour and its anxiolytic effects may last for several hours. Lorazepam is a longer-acting benzodiazepine with a clinical duration of 2 to 4 hours. It is effective orally for adults in doses of 2 to 4 mg, is well tolerated in the elderly, and is an excellent amnestic agent. Triazolam is the most commonly prescribed oral sedative for dental procedures in the United States. Its efficacy in reducing anxiety before venipuncture has been established.[71] Triazolam has a profile of rapid onset, short duration of anxiolytic and sedative action, and profound anterograde amnesia. The following day, patients have little or no recall of details associated with their appointment. If coadministered with N_2O/O_2 inhalational sedation, the sedative effects can be as profound as a combined benzodiazepine/opioid intravenous sedation.[71] It is effective in adult doses of 0.25 to 0.5 mg with a clinical duration of approximately 1 hour. Caution should be used in elderly patients because they may have an increased sensitivity to this drug. Midazolam is a popular oral sedative/anxiolytic for pediatric patients in doses of 0.25 to 1.0 mg/kg and may also be used in adults. The maximum dose should not exceed 20 mg. Its onset is within 15 to 30 minutes and it is also an excellent amnestic agent. Alprazolam 0.25 to 1.0 mg in adults may be especially effective for those whose anxiety is associated with a panic disorder.

Another useful drug class for use in patients with needle phobia is the benzodiazepinelike sedative hypnotics. The drugs in this class (zolpidem, zaleplon, and eszopiclone) are chemically unrelated to the benzodiazepines, but share a similar pharmacology. Zolpidem and zaleplon have the advantage of being rapidly absorbed after oral administration, with clinically demonstrable effects occurring in 15 to 20 minutes. Zolpidem is effective orally in doses of 5 to 10 mg, zaleplon in doses of 5 to 10 mg, and eszopiclone in doses of 2 to 3 mg.[72]

Ramelteon, a melatonin-receptor agonist in doses of 8 mg, is also effective as an anxiolytic. This drug is attractive because it is virtually without side effects. Melatonin is a naturally occurring substance secreted by the pineal gland in response to the light/dark cycle. Its action on melatonin receptors in the brain promotes sleep, thus making ramelteon useful for procedural sedation.[73] Because of the numerous pharmacologic modalities available in treating this patient population, a practitioner may want to consider consulting with a dentist anesthesiologist or other qualified practitioner trained in advanced sedation techniques.

SUMMARY

Phobias are persistent irrational and incapacitating fears of procedures or objects, and they lead to overwhelming avoidance behavior. With needle phobia, there can be profound general health, dental, societal, and legal implications that can be, at best, frustrating, and, at worst, life threatening. The prevalence is high; greater than 20% in some populations. It is a real medical condition with severe psychological, social, and physiologic consequences. There is genetic evidence for the physiologic response to needle puncture, evolving from primitive reflexes that served to improve survival from traumatic puncture wounds. There is also a significant psychological component that is familial, showing evidence of inheritance. Needle phobia is also a learned behavior.

It is important for the dental practitioner to recognize patients with needle phobia before the administration of local anesthetics to identify patients who are potentially reactive and to prevent untoward sequelae. A thorough history is necessary, including an assessment of the patient's anxiety levels and phobias. The Modified Dental Anxiety Scale is an excellent means to quantify the patient's anxiety.[74] Needle phobia is highly associated with avoidance behavior and is often responsible for missed appointments. Patients with needle phobia should be taken seriously by the dentist, and a complete description of the reaction should be obtained. The dentist must exhibit compassion, reassurance, and understanding, and show respect for the phobia and patient.

Oral premedication with benzodiazepines or other antianxiety agents must be considered for patients who are needle phobic with documented psychological and physiologic complications. Otherwise, one must be prepared to deal with bradycardia, hypotension, unconsciousness, convulsions, and possibly asystole. Management of needle phobia–induced syncope includes perioperative monitoring, oxygen administration, positioning, atropine, and vasopressors.

REFERENCES

1. Hamilton JG. Needle phobia: a neglected diagnosis. J Fam Pract 1995;41:169–75.
2. Costello CG. Fears and phobias in women. J Abnorm Psychol 1982;91:280–6.
3. Agras S, Sylvester D, Oliveau D. The epidemiology of common fears and phobias. Compr Psychiatry 1969;10:1511–56.
4. Keep PJ, Jenkins JR. From the other end of the needle. The patients experience of routine anesthesia. Anaesthesia 1978;33:830–2.
5. Cartwright PS, McLaughlin FJ, Martinez AM, et al. Teenagers' perceptions of barriers to prenatal care. South Med J 1993;86:737–41.

6. Arvidsson SB, Ekroth RH, Hansby AM, et al. Painless venipuncture. A clinical trial of iontophoresis of lidocaine for venipuncture in blood donors. Acta Anaesthesiol Scand 1984;28:209–10.
7. Oswalt RM, Napoliello M. Motivations of blood donors and nondonors. J Appl Psychol 1974;59:122–4.
8. Deacon B, Abramowitz J. Fear of needles and vasovagal reactions among phlebotomy patients. J Anxiety Disord 2006;20(7):946–60.
9. Graham DT. Prediction of fainting in blood donors. Circulation 1961;23:901–6.
10. Marks I. Blood-injury phobia: a review. Am J Psychiatry 1988;145:1207–13.
11. Callahan RC, Edelman ED, Smith MS, et al. Study of the incidence and characteristics of blood donor "reactors". Transfusion 1963;3:76–82.
12. Thyer BA, Himle J, Curtis GC. Blood-injury-illness phobia: a review. J Clin Psychol 1985;41:451–9.
13. Ost LG, Lindahl IL, Sterner U, et al. Exposure in vivo vs applied relaxation for blood phobia. Behav Res Ther 1984;22:205–16.
14. Torgersen S. The nature and origin of common phobic fears. Br J Psychiatry 1979;134:343–51.
15. Ellinwood EH, Hamilton JG. Case report of a needle phobia. J Fam Pract 1991;32: 420–3.
16. Hamilton J, Ellinwood E. Needle phobia [abstract]. South Med J 1991;84(Suppl): 2S–27.
17. Hsu LK. Novel symptom emergence after behavior therapy in a case of hypodermic injection phobia. Am J Psychiatry 1978;135:238–9.
18. Ost LG. Acquisition of blood and injection phobia and anxiety response patterns in clinical patients. Behav Res Ther 1991;29:323–32.
19. Hanson B, Tuna N, Bouchard T, et al. Genetic factors in the electrocardiogram and heart rate of twins reared apart and together. Am J Cardiol 1989;63: 606–9.
20. Losse H, Kretschmer M, Kuban G, et al. Die vegetative struktur des individuums I and II. Acta Neuroveg (Wien) 1956;13:337–99 [in German].
21. Jacobsen PB. Treating a man with needle phobia who requires daily injections of medication. Hosp Community Psychiatry 1991;42:877–8.
22. Lemasney NJ, Holland T, O'Mullane D, et al. The aetiology and treatment of needle phobia in the young patient - a review. J Ir Dent Assoc 1989;35:20–3.
23. Taggart P, Hedworth-Whitty R, Carruthers M, et al. Observations on electrocardiogram and plasma catecholamines during dental procedures: the forgotten vagus. BMJ 1976;2:787–9.
24. Marks IM. Fears phobias and rituals: panic, anxiety and their disorders. New York: Oxford University Press; 1987.
25. Gabrielsen G, Kanwisher J, Steen JB. Emotional bradycardia: a telemetry study in incubating willow grouse. Acta Physiol Scand 1977;100:255–7.
26. Lofving B. Cardiovascular adjustments induced from the rostral cingulate gyrus with special reference to sympatho-inhibitory mechanisms. Acta Physiol Scand 1961;53(Suppl 184):1–82.
27. Pool JL, Ransohoff J. Autonomic effects on stimulating rostral portion of cingulated gyrus in man. J Neurophysiol 1949;12:385–92.
28. Kremer WF. Autonomic and somatic reactions induced by stimulation of the cingular gyrus in dogs. J Neurophysiol 1947;10:371–9.
29. Engel GL. Psychological stress, vasodepressor (vasovagal) syncope, and sudden death. Ann Intern Med 1978;89:403–12.
30. Greenfield AD. An emotional faint. Lancet 1951;1:1302–3.

31. Lin JT-Y, Ziegler DK, Lai C-W, et al. Convulsive syncope in blood donors and non-donors. J Appl Psychol 1974;59:122–4.

32. Wayne HH. Syncope. Am J Med 1961;30:418–38.

33. Galena HJ. Complications occurring from diagnostic venipuncture. J Fam Pract 1992;34:582–4.

34. Caplan RA, Ward RJ, Posner K, et al. Unexpected cardiac arrest during spinal anesthesia: a closed claims analysis of predisposing factors. Anesthesiology 1988;68:5–11.

35. Schlessinger Z, Barzilay J, Stryjer D, et al. Life-threatening "vagal reaction" to emotional stimuli. Isr J Med Sci 1977;13:59–61.

36. Ziegler MG, Echon C, Wilner KD, et al. Sympathetic nervous withdrawal in the vasodepressor (vasovagal) reaction. J Auton Nerv Syst 1986;17:273–8.

37. Van Lieshout JJ, Wieling W, Karemaker JM, et al. The vasovagal response. Clin Sci 1991;81:575–86.

38. Wakita R, Ohno Y, Yamazaki S, et al. Vasovagal syncope with asystole associated with intravenous access. Oral Surg Oral Med Oral Pathol Oral Radiol Endod 2006; 102:e28–32.

39. Kinsella SM, Tucky JP. Perioperative bradycardia and asystole: relationship to vasovagal syncope and the Bezold-Jarisch reflex. Br J Anaesth 2001;86:859–68.

40. Goldstein DS, Spanarkel M, Pitterman A, et al. Circulatory control mechanisms in vasodepressor syncope. Am Heart J 1982;104:1071–5.

41. Kaufman H, Oribe E, Oliver JA. Plasma endothelin during up-right tilt: relevance for orthostatic hypotension? Lancet 1991;338:1542–5.

42. Win NN, Kohase H, Miyamoto T, et al. Decreased bispectral index as an indicator of syncope before hypotension and bradycardia in two patients with needle phobia. Br J Anaesth 2003;91(5):749–52.

43. Malamed SF. Managing medical emergencies. J Am Dent Assoc 1993;124: 40–53.

44. Hampl KF, Schneider MC. Vasovagal asystole before induction of general anaesthesia. Eur J Anaesthesiol 1994;11:131–3.

45. Mackey DC, Carpenter RL, Thompson GE, et al. Bradycardia and asystole during spinal anesthesia: a report of three cases without morbidity. Anesthesiology 1989; 70:866–8.

46. Robertson D, Hollister AS, Forman MB, et al. Reflexes unique to myocardial ischemia and infarction. J Am Coll Cardiol 1985;5:99–104.

47. Boas EP. Some immediate causes of cardiac infarction. Am Heart J 1942;23: 1–15.

48. Zukerman CM. Fatality in a blood donor; case report, with a review of the literature. Ann Intern Med 1947;26:603–8.

49. Dimsdale JE. Emotional causes of sudden death. Am J Psychiatry 1977;134:12.

50. Gustafson R, Petreman M. Myocardial necrosis in the golden-mantled squirrel. Can Med Assoc J 1963;89:900–1.

51. Selye H. Experimental cardiovascular disorders. New York: Springer-Verlag; 1970.

52. Keegan D. Psychosomatics: towards an understanding of cardiovascular disorders. Psychosomatics 1973;14:321–35.

53. Melville K. Cardiac ischemic changes induced by CNS stimulation. In: Raab W, editor. Prevention of ischemic heart disease. Springfield (IL): Charles C. Thomas; 1966. p. 31–8.

54. Wambaugh J. The blooding. New York: William Morrow; 1989. p. 210–4, 217.

55. Schmerber v California, 384 US 757, 86 SCt 1826 (1966).

56. Breithaupt v Abram, 352 US 432, 77 SCt 408 (1957).

57. South Dakota v Neville, 459 US 553, 103 SCt 916 (1983).

58. Hammer v Gross, 932 F2d 842 (USCA, 9th Cir, 1991). Cert denied 112 SCt 582 (1991).

59. Moore PA, Peskin RM, Pierce CJ. Pharmacologic desensitization for dental phobias: clinical observations. Anesth Prog 1990;37:308–11.

60. Gerschman JA. Hypnotizability and dental phobic disorders. Anesth Prog 1989; 36:131–9.

61. Gerschman JA, Burrows GD, Reade PC. Hypnosis in dentistry. In: Burrows G, Dennerstein L, editors. Handbook of hypnosis and psychosomatic medicine. Amsterdam: Elsevier/North-Holland Biomedical Press; 1980. p. 443–79.

62. Thompson KF. A rationale for suggestions in dentistry. Am J Clin Hypn 1963;5: 181–5.

63. Frankel FM. Trance capacity and the genesis of phobic behaviour. Arch Gen Phychiatry 1974;31:261–3.

64. Moore R, Brodsgaard I, Abrahamsen R. A 3-year comparison of dental anxiety treatment outcomes: hypnosis, group therapy and individual desensitization versus no specialist treatment. Eur J Oral Sci 2002;110:287–95.

65. Yamamoto LG, Boychuk RB. A blinded, randomized, paired, placebo controlled trial of 20-minute EMLA cream to reduce the pain of peripheral IV cannulation in the ED. Am J Emerg Med 1998;16:634–6.

66. Zempsky WT, Ashburn MA. Iontophoresis: noninvasive drug delivery. Am J Anesthesiol 1998;25:158–62.

67. Hamilton JG, Wrenn R, Garcia-Caro M, et al. Office management of needle fear and needle phobia by lidocaine iontophoresis. Presented at 87th Scientific Assembly, Southern Medical Association. New Orleans (LA), October 31, 1993.

68. Kearns GL, Heacock J, Daly SJ, et al. Percutaneous lidocaine administration via a new iontophoresis system in children: tolerability and absence of systemic bioavailabilty. Pediatrics 2003;112:578–82.

69. Ovsianikov A, Chichkov B, Mente P, et al. Two photon polymerization of polymer-ceramic hybrid materials for transdermal drug delivery. Int J Appl Ceram Tech 2007;4(1):22–9.

70. Dionne RA, Goldstein DS, Wirdzek PR. Effects of diazepam premedication and epinephrine-containing local anesthetic on cardiovascular and plasma catecholamine responses to oral surgery. Anesth Analg 1984;63:640–6.

71. Stopperich DS, Moore PA, Finder RL, et al. Oral triazolam pretreatment for intravenous sedation. Anesth Prog 1993;40:117–21.

72. Ganzburg SI, Dietrich T, Valeriu M, et al. Zaleplon (Sonata) oral sedation for outpatient third molar extraction surgery. Anesth Prog 2005;52:128–31.

73. Erman M, Seiden D, Zammit G, et al. An efficacy, safety, and dose-response study of ramelteon in patients with chronic primary insomnia. Sleep Med 2006; 7(1):17–24.

74. Humphris GM, Morrison T, Lindsay SJ. The Modified Dental Anxiety Scale: validation and United Kingdom norms. Community Dent Health 1995;12(3):143–50.

Needle Breakage: Incidence and Prevention

Stanley F. Malamed, DDS[a],*, Kenneth Reed, DMD[a],
Susan Poorsattar, DDS[b]

KEYWORDS

• Dental needles • Needle breakage • Incidence • Prevention

Local anesthesia forms the backbone of pain control techniques in dentistry. The injection of cocaine with epinephrine in 1885 by William Halsted enabled, for the first time, surgical procedures to be performed painlessly in a conscious human being. Before this the only option for pain-free surgery was general anesthesia, the controlled loss of consciousness, which does not prevent pain but simply prevents the patient from responding outwardly to it.

The basic local anesthetic armamentarium has, with very minor improvements, remained unchanged since Halsted's time: a syringe, needle, and a vehicle for carrying the drug, today the glass (or in some countries, plastic) dental cartridge.

Syringes have undergone change from the original Pravez glass syringe (a traditional hypodermic syringe) in 1853 to the more modern breech-loading, metallic, and cartridge-type aspirating syringe devices presently used in dentistry. New computer-controlled local anesthetic delivery systems (C-CLAD) are becoming increasingly popular.

Cook-Waite Laboratories introduced the prefilled dental cartridge into dentistry in 1920, and trademarked the now commonly used name Carpule. Before its introduction, the dentist prepared his (the use of his is correct as the profession at that time was essentially entirely male) local anesthetics daily, using a mortar and pestle to pulverize a procaine tablet. Prefilled cartridges provided the doctor with a standardized formulation of a higher quality and greater sterility. The breech-loading cartridge-type aspirating syringe was developed to accommodate the cartridge.

Needles have also undergone change since their introduction. In the early to mid-1900s needles were reusable, being cleaned, sharpened and, hopefully, sterilized between patients. Stainless steel disposable needles were introduced into dentistry in the 1960s and remain the standard today.

[a] The Herman Ostrow School of Dentistry of USC, 925 West 34th Street, Los Angeles, CA 90089-0641, USA
[b] Pediatric Dentistry, San Francisco, CA, USA
* Corresponding author.
E-mail address: malamed@usc.edu

Dent Clin N Am 54 (2010) 745–756
doi:10.1016/j.cden.2010.06.013
0011-8532/10/$ – see front matter © 2010 Elsevier Inc. All rights reserved.

dental.theclinics.com

The importance of local anesthesia to dentistry cannot be overstated. Local anesthetics represent the safest and the most effective drugs in all of medicine for the prevention and management of pain. Clinically adequate local anesthesia allows dental care to proceed safely in a pain-free environment and may represent the most important thing done for our patients to enable them to receive quality care. However it is the administration, actually the injection, of local anesthetics that represents the single most fear-inducing thing that dentists do to the patient during a typical dental visit.

Approximately 75% of medical emergencies reported in dentistry may be related to fear (stress).[1] Of 30,608 emergencies reported by Malamed,[1] 50.3% were syncope (fainting). Seeking to determine when during a dental appointment medical emergencies were most apt to occur Matsuura[2] found that 54.9% of the reported emergencies occurred during or immediately after the local anesthetic injection. Quite simply, fainting during injections is the most common medical emergency seen in dentistry.

Trypanophobia (an irrational fear of procedures involving injections) is not uncommon amongst dental patients. Dentists have all had patients state: "Doctor, do you have to give me a shot to do this?" Or "Doctor, I hate getting shots but once I am numb I'm okay." Or "Doctor, I just don't want to see the needle."

In 2004, De St Georges[3] listed the factors considered by patients when evaluating their dentist. The top 2 factors were a dentist who does not hurt, (no. 2) and one who gives a painless injection. (no. 1).

Fearful dental patients, evaluating specific dental procedures, listed seeing the needle as more fear-inducing that feeling the needle.[4] Asked specifically about which item(s) of the local anesthetic armamentarium (syringe, cartridge, needle) is most threatening, almost unanimously the response is the needle.[4]

THE LOCAL ANESTHETIC NEEDLE

The dental local anesthetic needle should permit the deposition of a local anesthetic solution in close proximity to the targeted nerve and allow for successful aspiration to prevent intravascular injection of the drug. The needle itself is composed of 1 continuous length of stainless steel metal that starts at the needle tip (**Fig. 1**) around which is placed a metal or plastic syringe adaptor and needle hub, exiting the opposite side as the portion of the needle that penetrates the diaphragm of the local anesthetic cartridge. The needle is firmly secured within its hub either by crimping of the metal hub against the needle or with glue (plastic hubbed needles). Needles have the following components in common: the bevel, the shaft (or shank), the hub, and the syringe-penetrating end (**Fig. 2**).

The bevel defines the point or tip of the needle. Manufacturers describe bevels as long, medium, and short. The greater the angle of the bevel with the long axis of the needle, the greater is the degree of deflection as the needle passes through the soft tissues of the mouth (**Fig. 3**).[5–7] As the needle bevel is eccentric, the shaft of the needle is deflected as the needle advances through soft tissue toward the target zone for anesthetic deposition. This is most obvious in injection techniques such as inferior alveolar nerve block in which more soft tissue must be penetrated (between 20 and 25 mm in the average adult patient).

The shaft or shank of the needle is 1 long piece of tubular metal running from the tip of the needle through the hub and continuing as the piece that penetrates the cartridge. Two factors to consider regarding this component of the needle are the diameter of its lumen (eg, the needle gauge) and the length of the shaft from point to hub.

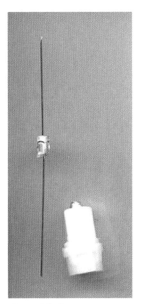

Fig. 1. Metal disposable needle, dissembled.

The hub is a plastic or metal piece through which the needle is attached to the syringe. The interior surface of the plastic and metal syringe adaptor of the needle is usually prethreaded allowing for its easy attachment to the syringe.

The syringe-penetrating end of the dental needle extends through the needle adaptor and perforates the diaphragm of the local anesthetic cartridge. Its tip lies within the cartridge.

Two factors must be considered when selecting needles for use in various injection techniques: length and gauge.

Needle Length

Needle length refers to the length of the needle shaft from the hub to the tip. Three needle lengths are used in dentistry: long, short, and extra short. Although there is some minor variation in length amongst needle manufacturers, in the United States a typical

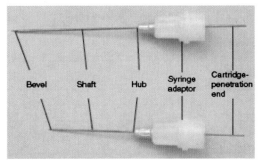

Fig. 2. Anatomy of the dental needle. (*From* Malamed SF. Handbook of local anesthesia. 5th edition. St. Louis (MO): CV Mosby; 2005. p. 99; with permission.)

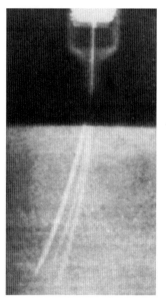

Fig. 3. Needle deflection. (*From* Robison SF, Mayhew RB, Cowan RD, et al. Comparative study of deflection characteristics and fragility of 25-, 27-, and 30-gauge short dental needles. J Am Dent Assoc 1984;109:920–4.)

long dental needle is 32 mm, a short needle is 20 mm, and an extra short needle is 10 mm (**Table 1**).

A time-honored tenet of needle usage is: "Do not insert a needle into the soft tissues to its hub, unless absolutely necessary for the success of the injection."[8–12] The significance of this statement becomes evident later.

A short needle may be used for any injection in which the penetration depth of soft tissue to the deposition site of the local anesthetic solution is less than 20 mm. Long needles are recommended for deeper penetration.

Needle Gauge

Gauge refers to the diameter of the lumen of the needle; the smaller the number, the greater the diameter of the lumen. A 30-gauge needle has a smaller internal diameter

Table 1
Industry standards for needle length

Manufacturer	25 g Long	25 g Short	27 g Long	27 g Short	30 g Long	30 g Short	30 g Extra Short
Industry Standard	32	20	32	20			
1	30		30	21	25	21	
2	32	22	32	22		21	12
3			32	21	25	21	
4	35		35	25		25	10
5	32			21		19	

All measurements obtained directly from needle manufacturers.

than a 25-gauge needle. Industry standards for needle gauge are presented in
Table 2.

There is movement amongst dentists toward the use of smaller diameter needles on
the assumption that they are less traumatic to the patient than larger diameter needles
(**Table 3**). Studies dating back to 1972 show this assumption to be unwarranted.[13–18]
Hamburg[13] reported that patients are unable to differentiate among 23-, 25-, 27-, and
30-gauge needles. Fuller and colleagues[14] reported no significant differences in
perception of pain produced by 25-, 27- and 30-gauge needles during inferior alveolar
nerve blocks in adults. Lehtinen[15] compared 27- and 30-gauge needles and found that
although insertion of the 30-gauge needle required significantly less force, the difference in pain perception was less remarkable.[17]

To avoid accidental intravascular injection, aspiration must be performed (preferably twice) before the deposition of any significant volume of local anesthetic. Trapp
and Davies[19] and Delgado-Molina and colleagues[20] reported that no significant differences existed in ability to aspirate blood through 25-, 27- and 30-gauge dental needles. However, there is increased resistance to aspiration of blood through a thinner
needle (eg, 30-gauge) compared with larger diameter needles (eg, 27- or 25-gauge).

NEEDLE BREAKAGE

Since the introduction of nonreusable, stainless steel dental local anesthetic needles,
needle breakage has become an extremely rare complication of dental local

Table 2
Industry standards for needle gauge

Specifications for Needle Gauges

Gauge	Outer Diameter (mm)	Inner Diameter (mm)
7	4.57	3.81
8	4.19	3.43
10	3.40	2.69
11	3.05	2.39
12	2.77	2.16
13	2.41	1.80
14	2.11	1.60
15	1.83	1.32
16	1.65	1.19
17	1.50	1.04
18	1.27	0.84
19	1.07	0.69
20	0.91	0.58
21	0.81	0.51
22	0.71	0.41
23	0.64	0.33
25	0.51	0.25
26	0.46	0.25
27	0.41	0.20
30	0.31	0.15

Dental needle gauge highlighted in bold type.

Table 3
Needle purchases, US dentistry, 2006

Gauge	Length	Data Provided by			
		Sullivan-Schein Inc. (2006)		Septodont Inc. (2006)	
25	Short	<1%	1%	0.6%	3%
	Long	1%		2.3%	
27	Short	10%	42%	13%	38%
	Long	32%		25%	
30	Short	50%	56%	51%	59%
	Extra short	6%		8%	

anesthetic injections. Pogrel[21] has (roughly) estimated the risk of needle breakage amongst Northern California dentists at 1 in 14 million inferior alveolar nerve blocks. In the United States 1.43 million boxes of dental needles (100 needles per box, 143,000,000 needles) were sold, by one needle manufacturer in 2004; 1.56 million boxes in 2005, and 1.43 million boxes in 2006.[22] Reports of broken dental needles in the published literature appear only infrequently, but appear they do. A MedLine search for broken dental needles from 1951 to February 2010 uncovered 26 published reports of broken dental needles, the cause, and their management.[21,23–47] Review of the 20 of these reports in which information regarding needle gauge, length, and technique of anesthesia used is available shows that 15 were inferior alveolar nerve block (IANB) and 5 were posterior superior alveolar (PSA) nerve block. All 5 PSA reports were on adult patients, whereas 9 of the 15 broken needle reports following IANB occurred in children. Needle gauge and/or length were presented in 11 papers. Ten of the 11 needles were 30-gauge short, with only 1 reported case of long needle breakage (27-gauge) with the needle remaining in the tissues.[32]

Pogrel[21] reported on 16 patients whom he evaluated following needle breakage in a 25-year period (1983–2008). Fifteen patients had received IANB and 1 a PSA. Thirteen of the 16 needles were 30-gauge short and 3 were 27-gauge short.

Independent of the cited literature, 2 of the authors have seen a total of 51 cases; 1 (SFM) has been involved in 34 cases that progressed to litigation in which broken dental needle fragments have remained within the soft tissues of the patient receiving the injection. Thirty-three of these events involved 30-gauge short needles; a 27-gauge short was involved in the other case. All but 1 involved administration of an IANB. The other case was a PSA nerve block. The second author (KR) has been involved with 17 cases, all of which were both IANB and 30-gauge short needles.

Table 4
Summary of reports of broken dental needles

	IANB	PSA	30-Gauge	27-Gauge
Refs.[23–47]	15	5	10	1
Pogrel[21]	15	1	13	3
Malamed	32	1	33	1
Reed	17	0	17	0
Manufacturer	n/a	n/a	27	0
Total	79	7	100	5

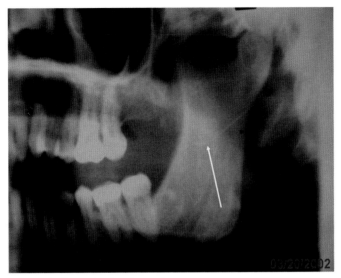

Fig. 4. Needle bent before injection (*arrow*).

A manufacturer of dental local anesthetic needles reported that in a 6-year period (1997–2002) 27 doctors contacted them reporting instances of broken dental needles. All involved 30-gauge short needles (Dentsply-MPL Technologies, Franklin Park, IL, personal communication, 2003).

There is every likelihood that long dental needles have broken during injection. However, as the long needle is unlikely to have been inserted to its full length

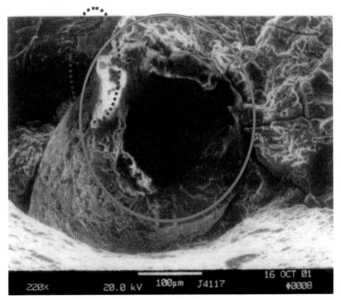

Fig. 5. Scanning electron microscopy of fractured (bent) needle. Needle lumen is outlined in blue. Bent area is indicated by red circle.

(32 mm) into soft tissue, some portion of the needle would remain visible in the patient's mouth. Retrieval of the fragment with a hemostat is easily accomplished. Litigation does not occur in such incidents.

Table 4 summarizes the accumulated findings presented here. Although it is possible that some reports may have been duplicated, the factual information clearly identifies commonalities in most cases: (1) use of 30-gauge short or extra short needles in injection techniques in which (2) the needle is inserted to its hub (hubbing the needle). All reported cases involved either the IANB or PSA nerve block. In all situations in which it is mentioned, the needle fracture occurred at the hub, never along the shaft of the needle. Additional factors include (1) intentional bending of the needle by the doctor before injection (**Figs. 4** and **5**); (2) a sudden unexpected movement by the patient while the needle is still embedded in tissue; and (3) contacting bone forcefully.

The exact cause of needle breakage is rarely discernable. In cases in which the needle has been surgically retrieved and/or forensic metallurgists have examined the hub of the needle, no evidence was found indicating manufacturing defects in the needle.

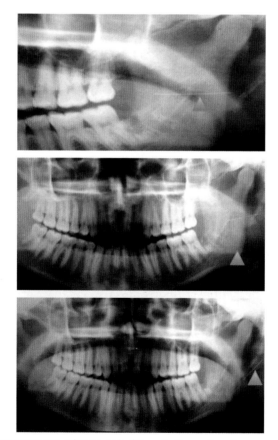

Fig. 6. Needle fragments can migrate as is shown in the series of panoramic films taken at 3-month intervals.

THE PROBLEM

Needle breakage per se is not a significant problem if the needle can be removed without surgical intervention. Ready access to a hemostat enables the doctor or assistant to grasp the visible proximal end of the needle fragment and remove it from the soft tissue.

Where the needle has been inserted to its hub and the soft tissue dimpled under pressure from the syringe, the broken fragment will not be visible when the syringe is withdrawn from the patient's mouth. The needle fragment remaining in the tissue poses a risk of serious damage being inflicted on the soft tissues for as long as the fragment remains. Although not common, needle fragments can migrate as is illustrated by the series of panoramic films taken at 3-month intervals (**Fig. 6**).

MANAGEMENT OF THE BROKEN DENTAL NEEDLE

Management of the broken dental needle involves immediate referral of the patient to an appropriate specialist (eg, oral and maxillofacial surgeon) for evaluation and possible retrieval. Conventional management involves locating the retained fragment through panoramic and computed tomographic (CT) scanning.[45] More recently three-dimensional CT scanning has been recommended to identify the location of the

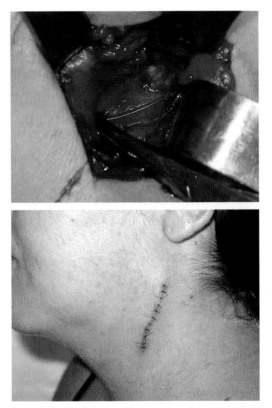

Fig. 7. Surgical excision of needle fragment (see patient from **Fig. 6**). (*Courtesy of* Dr Carlos Elias de Freitas.)

retained needle fragment.[21,48] A surgeon in the operating theater then removes the retained needle fragment while the patient is under general anesthesia (**Fig. 7**).

PREVENTION OF BROKEN DENTAL NEEDLE

Although rare, dental needle breakage can, and does, occur. Review of the literature and personal experience of the authors brings into focus several commonalities which when avoided can minimize the risk of needle breakage with the fragment being retained from occurring. These include:

- Do not use short needles for IANB in adults.
- Do not use 30-gauge needles for IANBs in adults or children.
- Do not bend needles when inserting them into soft tissue.
- Do not insert a needle into soft tissue to its hub, unless it is absolutely essential for the success of the injection.
- Observe extra caution when inserting needles in younger children or in extremely phobic adult or child patients.

REFERENCES

1. Malamed SF. Beyond the basics: emergency medicine in dentistry. J Am Dent Assoc 1997;128(7):843–54.
2. Matsuura H. Analysis of systemic complications and deaths during dental treatment in Japan. Anesth Prog 1990;36:219–28.
3. De St Georges J. How dentists are judged by patients. Dent Today 2004;23(8): 96–9.
4. Milgrom P, Weinstein P, Kleinknecht R, et al. Treating fearful dental patients: a patient management handbook. Reston (VA): Reston Publishing Co. Inc; 1985. p. 22.
5. Aldous JA. Needle deflection: a factor in the administration of local anesthetics. J Am Dent Assoc 1977;77:602–4.
6. Jeske AH, Boshart BF. Deflection of conventional versus non-deflecting dental needles in vitro. Anesth Prog 1985;32:62–4.
7. Robison SF, Mayhew RB, Cowan RD, et al. Comparative study of deflection characteristics and fragility of 25-, 27-, and 30-gauge short dental needles. J Am Dent Assoc 1984;109:920–4.
8. Monheim LM. Local anesthesia and pain control in dental practice. St Louis (MO): C.V. Mosby Co; 1957. p. 184.
9. Allen GD. Dental anesthesia and analgesia (local and general). 2nd edition. Baltimore (MD): Williams & Wilkins; 1979. p. 133.
10. Malamed SF. Needles. In: Malamed SF, editor. Handbook of local anesthesia. 5th edition. St. Louis (MO): CV Mosby; 2004. p. 103.
11. Yagiela JA, Jastack JT. Regional anesthesia of the oral cavity. St. Louis (MO): CV Mosby; 1981. p. 105.
12. Cook-Waite Laboratories Inc. Manual of local anesthesia in general dentistry. New York: Rensselaer & Springville; 1936. p. 38.
13. Hamburg HL. Preliminary study of patient reaction to needle gauge. N Y State Dent J 1972;38:425–6.
14. Fuller NP, Menke RA, Meyers WJ. Perception of pain to three different intraoral penetrations of needles. J Am Dent Assoc 1979;99(5):822–4.
15. Lehtinen R. Penetration of 27- and 30-gauge needles. Int J Oral Surg 1983;12(6): 444–5.

16. Browbill JW, Walker PO, Bourcy BD, et al. Comparison of inferior dental nerve block injections in child patients using 30-gauge and 25-gauge short needles. Anesth Prog 1987;34:215–9.

17. Lipp MD. Local anesthesia in dentistry. Chicago: Quintessence Publishing; 1993. p. 106.

18. Jeske AH, Blanton PL. Misconceptions involving dental local anesthesia. Part 2: pharmacology. Tex Dent J 2002;119(4):310–4.

19. Trapp LD, Davies RO. Aspiration as a function of hypodermic needle internal diameter in the in-vivo human upper limb. Anesth Prog 1980;27:49–51.

20. Delgado-Molina E, Tamarit-Borras M, Berini-Aytes L, et al. Evaluation and comparison of 2 needle models in terms of blood aspiration during truncal block of the inferior alveolar nerve. J Oral Maxillofac Surg 2003;61(9): 1011–5.

21. Pogrel MA. Broken local anesthetic needles: a case series of 16 patients, with recommendations. J Am Dent Assoc 2009;140:1517–22.

22. Septodont NA. Septodont reported wholesale sales. Newark (NJ): Delaware; 2006.

23. Amies AB. Broken needles. Aust Dent J 1951;55(6):403–6.

24. Muller EE, Lernoud R. Surgical extraction of needles broken during local anes-thesia of the mandibular nerve. Acta Odontol Venez 1967;5(2):229–37.

25. Dudani IC. Broken needles following mandibular injections. J Indian Dent Assoc 1971;43(1):14–7.

26. Kennett S, Curran JB, Jenkins GR. Management of a broken hypodermic needle: report of a case. J Can Dent Assoc 1972;38(11):414–6.

27. Kennett S, Curran JB, Jenkins GR. Management of a broken hypodermic needle: report of a case. Anesth Prog 1973;20(2):48–50.

28. Bump RL, Roche WC. A broken needle in the pterygomandibular space. Report of a case. Oral Surg Oral Med Oral Pathol 1973;36(5):750–2.

29. Hai HK. Retrieval of a broken hypodermic needle. A new technique of localising. Singapore Dent J 1983;8(1):27–9.

30. Orr DL 2nd. The broken needle: report of case. J Am Dent Assoc 1983;107(4): 603–4.

31. Marks RB, Carlton DM, McDonald S. Management of a broken needle in the pterygomandibular space: report of case. J Am Dent Assoc 1984;109(2): 263–4.

32. Burke RH. Management of a broken anesthetic needle. J Am Dent Assoc 1986; 112(2):209–10.

33. Fox IJ, Belfiglio EJ. Report of a broken needle. Gen Dent 1986;34(2):102–6.

34. Pietruszka JF, Hoffman D, McGivern BE Jr. A broken dental needle and its surgical removal: a case report. N Y State Dent J 1986;52(7):28–31.

35. Chaikin L. Broken needles. N Y State Dent J 1987;53(1):8.

36. Burgess JO. The broken dental needle–a hazard. Spec Care Dentist 1986;8(2): 71–3.

37. Ho KH. A simple technique for localizing a broken dental needle in the pterygo-mandibular region. Aust Dent J 1988;33(4):308–9.

38. Mima T, Shirasuna K, Morioka S, et al. A broken needle in the pterygomandibular space. Osaka Daigaku Shigaku Zasshi 1989;34(2):418–22.

39. McDonogh T. An unusual case of trismus and dysphagia. Br Dent J 1996;180(12): 465–6.

40. Bhatia S, Bounds G. A broken needle in the pterygomandibular space: report of a case and review of the literature. Dent Update 1998;25(1):35–7.

41. Bedrock RD, Skigen A, Dolwick MF. Retrieval of a broken needle in the pterygo-mandibular space. J Am Dent Assoc 1999;130(5):685–7.
42. Faura-Sole M, Sanchez-Garces MA, Berini-Aytes L, et al. Broken anesthetic injection needles: report of 5 cases. Quintessence Int 1999;30(7):461–5.
43. Dhanrayani PJ, Jonaidel O. A forgotten entity: 'broken needle while inferior dental block'. Dent Update 2000;27(2):101.
44. Murray M. A forgotten entity: 'broken needle while administering inferior dental block'. Dent Update 2000;27(6):306.
45. Zeltser R, Cohen C, Casap N. The implications of a broken needle in the pterygomandibular space: clinical guidelines for prevention and retrieval. Pediatr Dent 2002;24(2):153–6.
46. Thompson M, Wright S, Cheng LH, et al. Locating broken dental needles. Int J Oral Maxillofac Surg 2003;32(6):642–4.
47. Baart JA, van Amerongen WE, de Jong KJ, et al. Needle breakage during mandibular block anaesthesia: prevention and retrieval. Ned Tijdschr Tandheelkd 2006;113(12):520–3.
48. Ethunandan M, Tran AL, Anand R, et al. Needle-breakage following inferior alveolar nerve block: implications and management. Br Dent J 2007;202(7):395–7.

Advanced Techniques and Armamentarium for Dental Local Anesthesia

Taylor M. Clark, DDS[a], John A. Yagiela, DDS, PhD[a,b,*]

KEYWORDS

- Dental anesthesia • Local anesthesia • Intraosseous anesthesia

Effective local anesthesia is arguably the single most important pillar upon which modern dentistry stands.[1,2] Paradoxically, the injection of local anesthetic is also perhaps the greatest source of patient fear,[3,4] and inability to obtain adequate pain control with minimal discomfort remains a significant concern of dental practitioners.[5,6] Although the traditional aspirating syringe is the most common method by which local anesthetics are administered, newer technologies have been developed that can assist the dentist in providing enhanced pain relief with reduced injection pain and fewer adverse effects. This discussion will focus on the clinical uses of computer-controlled local anesthesia delivery (C-CLAD) devices and intraosseous (IO) systems for local anesthetic injection.

C-CLAD SYSTEMS
Available Devices

Milestone Scientific (Piscataway, NJ, USA) introduced the first C-CLAD system in the United States in 1997. Originally known as the Wand, subsequent versions were sequentially renamed the Wand Plus and then CompuDent, the current designation. In 2001, the Comfort Control Syringe (Dentsply International, York, PA, USA) was marketed as an alternative to the Wand. Examples of similar products originating and available outside of the United States include the QuickSleeper and SleeperOne devices (Dental Hi Tec, Cholet, France) and the Anaeject (Nippon Shika Yakuhin, Shimonoseki, Japan) and Ora Star (Showa Uyakuhin Kako, Tokyo, Japan) syringes.

[a] Dental Anesthesiology Residency Program, School of Dentistry, University of California, Los Angeles, 10833 Le Conte Avenue, Los Angeles, CA 90095-1668, USA
[b] Division of Diagnostic and Surgical Sciences, School of Dentistry, University of California, Los Angeles, 10833 Le Conte Avenue, Los Angeles, CA 90095-1668, USA
* Corresponding author. Dental Anesthesiology Residency Program, School of Dentistry, University of California, Los Angeles, 10833 Le Conte Avenue, Los Angeles, CA 90095-1668.
E-mail address: jyagiela@dentistry.ucla.edu

Dent Clin N Am 54 (2010) 757–768
doi:10.1016/j.cden.2010.06.017
0011-8532/10/$ – see front matter © 2010 Elsevier Inc. All rights reserved.

Milestone Scientific Products

The CompuDent system has three components: a base unit, a foot pedal, and a disposable handpiece assembly. The base unit contains a microprocessor and connects to both the foot pedal and the end of the handpiece assembly that accepts the local anesthetic cartridge. The microprocessor controls a piston that expresses local anesthetic by pushing the local anesthetic plunger up into the cartridge. The anesthetic solution is then forced through the microbore tubing, Wand handpiece, and attached needle into the tissue. Pressing lightly on the foot pedal activates a slow injection rate (0.005 mL/s) appropriate for needle insertion, periodontal ligament (PDL) injection, and palatal administration. Heavier pressure on the pedal increases injection speed to deliver the entire content of the cartridge in 1 minute (ie, 0.03 mL/s), which is normally used for buccal infiltrations and nerve blocks. In 2005, a third, higher rate (0.06 mL/s) was added in response to practitioner requests. Release of the foot pedal stops injection, and if the aspiration feature is enabled, causes an aspiration cycle in which the piston retracts, drawing blood into the tubing if the needle tip is located intravascularly. The CompuDent system costs approximately $1500; each disposable Wand assembly is $2 to $3 per set.

In 2007, Milestone Scientific added the STA (Single Tooth Anesthesia) system to its product line (**Fig. 1**). The STA unit adds dynamic pressure sensing (DPS) technology, which provides continuous feedback to the user about pressure at the needle tip to help identify ideal needle placement for PDL injections. In this STA mode there is a single, slow rate of injection. Selecting the normal mode emulates the original CompuDent device. A third mode, called turbo, adds the third, faster rate of injection (0.06 mL/s). The cost for the STA system is approximately $2000.

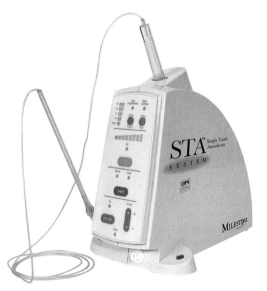

Fig. 1. The STA single tooth anesthesia system. Shown are the base unit and the STA Wand handpiece assembly. (*Courtesy of* Milestone Scientific, Livingston, NJ; with permission.)

Comfort Control Syringe

The Comfort Control Syringe differs from the Milestone products in that there is no foot pedal. It has two main components: a base unit and a syringe. Several functions of the unit—most importantly injection and aspiration—can be controlled directly from the syringe, possibly making its use easier to master for practitioners accustomed to the traditional manual syringe.

The Comfort Control Syringe ($1200, $1 per cartridge sleeve) has five different basic injection rate settings designed for specific injections: block, infiltration, PDL, IO, and palatal. Each rate is selected by the push of a button. The unit uses a two-stage delivery rate for every injection. It initially expresses the anesthetic solution at an extremely low rate. After 10 seconds, the rate slowly increases to the pre-programmed value for the selected injection. The basic speed of each injection also can be doubled by pushing a button on the syringe or the base unit. Although use of the Comfort Control Syringe may be more intuitive than that of the Milestone devices in the sense that the injection is controlled by hand, the syringe is bulky and more cumbersome to use than the Wand handpiece. A comparison between the traditional dental syringe and the Comfort Control Syringe revealed no meaningful differences in ease of administration, injection pain and efficacy, and acceptance by patients.[6]

Potential advantages

Several potential advantages have been ascribed to C-CLAD systems in general and to the Milestone products in particular. These include more accurate needle insertion for deeper nerve blocks, less pain on injection, and less fear of injection.

Because the Wand handpiece is approximately the same size as a ballpoint pen, it is easily held in a pen grasp, which facilitates fine motor control and often allows the fingers to be significantly closer to the needle tip than is the case with the traditional dental syringe.[7] The net result is a more controlled insertion of the needle. Furthermore, the ability to rotate the handpiece back and forth during needle insertion may reduce the needle deflection that occurs in response to the straight insertion of a dental needle whose needle tip is not coincident with the central axis of the shaft.[8] At this time, there is no compelling evidence that these potential advantages in needle placement actually foster increased anesthetic efficacy.

Three features of C-CLAD support the assertion that there may be less pain on injection. First, the ability to administer small amounts of local anesthetic continuously during needle insertion helps to anesthetize tissues immediately ahead of the advancing needle. Second, the steady infusion of anesthetic solution once the needle has reached its target may reduce discomfort associated with less controlled injections. Third, the reduced force required for needle insertion using the bidirectional rotation Wand technique[9] may translate into improved comfort. Various investigators[10-12] have reported no difference in injection pain, whereas others[13-18] have found significantly reduced pain with the Milestone products. Numerous differences in study design and the inherent inability to perform double-blind comparisons complicate interpretation of these results. The authors nevertheless conclude the following

With the important exception of palatal injections, C-CLAD does not materially reduce the discomfort of needle insertion

Most reductions in injection pain can be attributed to the significantly reduced rates of local anesthetic infusion used in studies reporting beneficial effects of C-CLAD on injection pain.

In support of the latter inference is the study by Kudo,[19] which documented a direct relationship between initial injection pressure and subsequent patient reports of pain and anxiety.

Reduced fear of injection would be an expected outcome of decreased pain. The relatively unthreatening appearance of the Wand handpiece also may help alleviate anxiety. Experimental support for lower apprehension with C-CLAD is limited, however. Although Krochak and Friedman[20] noted decreased anxiety in subjects given Wand injections compared with traditional methods, Versloot and colleagues[21] found that this potential benefit of C-CLAD was lost in highly anxious children, perhaps because their fear of treatment overwhelmed any technique-sensitive differences in nociception.

Alternative injections

The ability of C-CLAD devices to administer local anesthetics at a slow, controlled rate has been used to advantage with respect to three injections: the anterior middle superior alveolar (AMSA), the palatal approach to the anterior superior alveolar (P-ASA), and the PDL.

The AMSA injection, described in 1998 by Friedman and Hochman,[22] is intended to provide pulpal anesthesia of the ipsilateral incisor, canine, and premolar teeth and their associated palatal soft tissues. Using a C-CLAD device, a 30-gauge ultrashort needle is placed along the line bisecting the premolar teeth at the point halfway between the midpalatine suture and the free gingival margin. With the assistance of pressure anesthesia from a cotton-tipped applicator, the bevel of the needle is placed against the palatal tissue, and the slow flow of anesthetic is started. After approximately 8 seconds, the needle is slipped beneath the palatal mucosa with a gentle twisting motion and then advanced laterally and superiorly very slowly (0.25 mm/s) until bone is gently contacted. Generally, and after a negative aspiration, the entire contents of the local anesthetic cartridge are administered over a 4-minute period.

The P-ASA injection (**Fig. 2**), also described by Friedman and Hochman,[23] was designed to anesthetize the six maxillary anterior maxillary teeth with a single injection. Anesthetized soft tissues include those overlying the anterior palate (nasopalatine nerve distribution) and, to a lesser extent, the labial gingiva. The technique of needle penetration is similar to that described for the AMSA injection except that the needle is placed initially just lateral to the incisive papilla. Once the needle has penetrated the mucosa, 5 to 6 seconds should elapse before the needle is reoriented more vertically

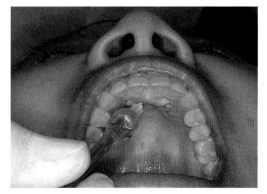

Fig. 2. The P-ASA injection.

to enter the nasopalatine canal. After a very slow (0.25 mm/s) insertion of 0.5 to 1 cm—at which point the bony wall of the canal should be felt and a negative aspiration obtained—the rest of the cartridge is deposited in about 4 minutes.

The PDL injection using a C-CLAD device is similar in technique to that using a traditional syringe or dedicated periodontal ligament syringe. The infusion of anesthetic, however, is quite different. Much larger volumes (up to 0.9 mL for a single-rooted tooth or 1.8 mL for a multirooted tooth) are injected much more slowly (eg, 0.005 mL/s). The STA device by Milestone, with its ability to monitor fluid pressure at the needle tip, helps to ensure that both leakage of anesthetic and overpressure are avoided during the PDL injection.

These three injections using C-CLAD share certain attributes. They all tend to limit anesthesia of the cheek and lip and preserve motor control, an important criterion for cosmetic dentistry. They also provide useful alternative injection techniques when primary methods (eg, maxillary supraperiosteal injection and inferior alveolar nerve block) are contraindicated or ineffective. Whether they should be used routinely as primary techniques is less clear.

At least in adults, these injections can produce moderate levels of pain during needle insertion (AMSA, P-ASA)[16,24,25] or after the procedure (PDL).[26] To minimize local tissue irritation, a rate of injection comparable with the lowest rate of the CompuDent device should be used. Presumably because of anecdotal reports, Milestone Scientific recommends that reduced volumes of anesthetic be administered if 4% anesthetic solutions are used and that formulation alternatives with higher concentrations of epinephrine (ie, 2% lidocaine with 1:50,000 epinephrine or 4% articaine with 1:100,000 epinephrine) be avoided.[27] Perhaps the biggest concern regarding the routine reliance on the AMSA and P-ASA injections is the potential for incomplete anesthesia. Electric pulp testing studies have shown that the extent of anesthesia is often less than was originally proposed for the techniques, and sometimes the depth of anesthesia is less than that produced with supraperiosteal injections.[24,28,29] Interestingly, recent studies[30,31] also have shown that the extent of anesthesia achieved with traditional maxillary and infraorbital nerve blocks is also significantly less than previously thought.

One use in which the palatal injections shine is in periodontal therapy of the maxilla. A single AMSA injection, for example, may produce sufficient pain control to treat the entire hemimaxilla.[15,32] This approach avoids the need for multiple injections and can result in significantly less local anesthetic being administered. Likewise, PDL injections using C-CLAD devices, especially the STA system, are highly effective for short-duration single-tooth anesthesia and compare favorably with alternative PDL methods.[33,34]

Pediatric use

Special mention should be made regarding the use of C-CLAD devices in pediatric dentistry. Although several studies[10,11] found no benefit when the Wand was used essentially to replace the traditional syringe, Palm and colleagues[17] recorded a reduction in pain with the inferior alveolar nerve block. Possible differences in injection rates used for the C-CLAD and traditional syringe may have contributed to this finding. Of greater significance are the investigations that have focused on the use of palatal injections for pulpal anesthesia. Most,[35–38] but not all,[21] of these studies have found that the AMSA and P-ASA injections administered by C-CLAD devices may be better tolerated or produce less disruptive behavior than supraperiosteal injections delivered with traditional syringes, especially when supplemental palatal infiltrations have to be performed. There is also general agreement that the palatal C-CLAD injections produce comparable efficacy to traditional alternatives, even for pulpotomies and extractions.[37–39] Finally, two reports[40,41] comparing PDL injections with the Wand to conventional anesthesia (buccal infiltration and inferior alveolar nerve block with a standard aspirating syringe) found the PDL injection to be accepted more positively. Although anesthetic efficacy was the same in young children (2 to 4 years) receiving dental treatment in the upper anterior maxilla,[40] the PDL injection was less effective than mandibular blockade in relieving pain during treatment for children aged 6 to 10 years.[41] Nevertheless, patients still preferred the Wand by a 2 to 1 margin.

IO LOCAL ANESTHESIA

Although IO-induced local anesthesia has been used in clinical dentistry for over a century, the original technique was too invasive for widespread adoption, requiring a gingival flap to be raised to gain access to the buccal cortical bone for perforation with a small round bur. IO anesthesia became even less important with the discovery and marketing of lidocaine in the 1940s. Nevertheless, in 1975 Lilienthal[42] described a technique in which a handpiece-driven root canal reamer was used to perforate the cortical plate. This use of a motor-driven perforator to penetrate the buccal gingiva and bone may be considered the first modern technique of IO anesthesia and the foundation upon which all current methods are based.

Available Devices

Several systems have been developed to achieve IO anesthesia. Although significant differences exist among them, they all aim to inject local anesthetic solution into the cancellous bone adjacent to the apex of the tooth. Three systems are available in the United States: Stabident (Fairfax Dental, Miami, Florida), X-tip (X-tip Technologies, Lakewood, NJ, USA), and IntraFlow (Pro-Dex Incorporated, Santa Ana, CA, USA).

Stabident

The Stabident system for IO anesthesia includes a solid 27-gauge perforator needle with a simple beveled tip and a plastic base designed to fit in a latch-type slow-speed contra-angle hand piece (**Fig. 3**). The operator uses the perforator to create a small tunnel through the attached gingiva, periosteum, and alveolar bone. The typical insertion point is on the attached gingiva, 2 mm below the facial gingival margin, and midway between the tooth of interest and an immediately adjacent (preferably distal) tooth. Local anesthesia should be administered to anesthetize the local gingival tissue if it is not already numb from a previous injection. The angle of perforation is not critical

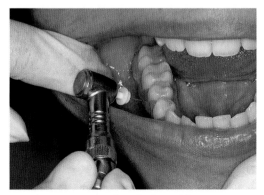

Fig. 3. The Stabident perforator penetrating the buccal bone.

but is usually adjusted in the mandibular incisor region (where the mesiodistal width is quite narrow) so that perforator travels in an apical direction. A more perpendicular angle is advantageous in the mandibular molar region to help avoid bending the perforator against the dense cortical bone. Penetration is made using short bursts with light pressure. A 27-gauge ultrashort (8 mm) needle is then inserted through the hole to deposit anesthetic solution into the cancellous bone. Up to an entire cartridge can be administered; a slow initial rate of injection is critical to patient comfort. The component cost per injection is about $1.

X-tip

The X-tip Anesthesia Delivery System was designed to solve the primary technical difficulty encountered with the Stabident system—finding the hole and inserting the needle. The X-tip system comprises three parts ($3 per set): the drill (perforator), a 25-gauge guide sleeve that fits over the 27-gauge drill, and an ultrashort needle of the same diameter. The drill leads the guide sleeve through the cortical plate into the cancellous bone. The drill portion is then removed, leaving the guide sleeve in place. The guide sleeve is then used to direct the needle into the cancellous bone to deposit the anesthetic solution (**Fig. 4**). The primary differences in using the X-tip device are

> The penetration need not be performed through the attached gingiva
> The guide sleeve must be carefully removed with a hemostat after the injection is performed.

IntraFlow

The IntraFlow HTP Anesthesia Delivery System is designed as an all-in-one system that allows the user to perforate bone and deposit anesthetic solution in a single intraoral step. The IntraFlow device is essentially a dental handpiece equipped with an injection system built into the body (**Fig. 5**). A 24-gauge hollow perforator is used to penetrate the bone and infuse the local anesthetic solution. Anesthetic from the dental cartridge is routed to the perforator by a disposable transfuser that also serves to cover the switch used to select between perforator rotation and anesthetic infusion modes. In contrast to the Stabident and X-tip techniques, penetration with this low-speed, high-torque device is effected by a single, steady insertion using direct pressure (**Fig. 6**). The insertion point and penetrator angulation are similar to that described for the X-tip. The interested reader is referred to the Pro-Dex Web site[43] for detailed

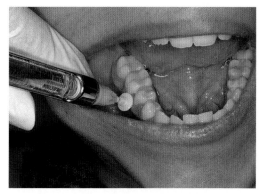

Fig. 4. Intraosseous injection using the X-tip system.

Transfuser

Cartridge (not included)

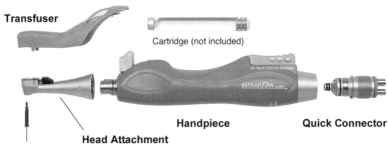

Handpiece **Quick Connector**

Head Attachment

Perforator

Fig. 5. Expanded view of the IntraFlow system. (*Courtesy of* Pro-Dex Medical Devices, Irvine, CA; with permission.)

instructions regarding use of the device. The initial cost is approximately $1300 for the handpiece, with disposable costs (penetrator and transfuser) of about $3 per patient.

Clinical uses

Although multiple IO injections can provide anesthesia for quadrant dentistry, the most common application of IO systems is for anesthesia of single teeth. The IO approach may be used as the primary method of pain control or as a supplementary technique when a different primary technique proves inadequate.

Assessments of IO anesthesia used alone demonstrate effectiveness at least comparable to those of more conventional approaches to local anesthesia. Coggins and colleagues[44] showed, for instance, that 2% lidocaine with 1:100,000 epinephrine achieved anesthesia success in 75% of mandibular first molars and 93% of maxillary first molars. Replogle and colleagues[45] reported that 2% lidocaine with 1:100,000 was successful 74% of the time in providing anesthesia of the mandibular first molar, compared with a success rate of only 45% with 3% mepivacaine. Although the lidocaine formulation would be acceptable for short procedures (<30 minutes), the weak and evanescent action of plain mepivacaine argues against its use. Subsequent studies,[46,47] collectively using all three IO devices, found that lidocaine with epinephrine had even higher success rates (87% to 95%) for mandibular anesthesia.

Most dentists who use IO systems on an occasional basis do so to achieve profound anesthesia when conventional techniques (eg, inferior alveolar nerve blocks) fail. One common instance where this occurs is in mandibular molars diagnosed with

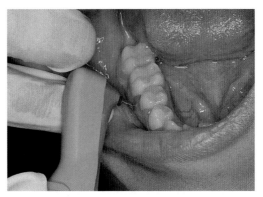

Fig. 6. Intraosseous penetration using the IntraFlow system.

irreversible pulpitis. Several groups[48–50] have studied patients requiring endodontic treatment in whom conventional local anesthetic injections failed to provide adequate pain relief for accessing the pulp. A supplemental IO injection of 2% lidocaine with 1:100,000 provided complete anesthesia in 82% to 89% of these subjects. Four percent articaine with 1:100,000 epinephrine[51] and even 3% mepivacaine plain[52] elicited similar successes. IO anesthesia is unsurpassed for this application.

IO anesthesia also may be helpful in treating children and adolescents. The quick onset, limited duration, and minimal collateral anesthesia with the IO approach can be especially beneficial in this population. One study[53] reported an overall success rate of 91% when IO anesthesia was used as the primary technique for various procedures in subjects 4 to 16 years of age.

Side effects and complications

The most common side effect of IO anesthesia is tachycardia from the injected vasoconstrictor. As noted by Lilienthal and Reynolds,[54] the heart rate accelerates within seconds after injection and remains elevated for several minutes thereafter. More recent evaluations have revealed that up to 90% of patients will subjectively report tachycardia.[55–57] Objective heart rate increases in response to a single cartridge of 2% lidocaine, with 1:100,000 clustering around 30 beats/min, although increases above 50 beats/min occasionally occur. Warning patients that they will likely experience transient cardiac stimulation is essential to avoid acute anxiety. IO injection of solutions containing epinephrine or levonordefrin should be limited or avoided in patients with significant cardiac disease.

Separation of the perforator drill/needle from its plastic holder may happen, especially when perforation is difficult and the drill heats up from overuse. Almost always, the perforator shaft is embedded in the bone and easily removed with a hemostat. Care, including the placement of a gauze barrier, is indicated when removing the shaft or an X-tip guide sleeve to avoid the possibility of ingestion or aspiration of the foreign body.

Although the incidence of adverse reactions is low with IO injections, local tissue damage becomes more likely when difficulties are encountered by inexperienced clinicians attempting to penetrate tough cortical bone as found in the mandibular molar region of large adult males. Overheating the bone and macerating the overlying soft tissue may cause pain, swelling with or without an inflammatory exudate at the injection site, and localized infection. Postinjection hyperocclusion is relatively common. Moderate postinjection pain also may develop in 0% to 15% of patients, and severe pain may develop in 0% to 2% of patients. In one study,[58] a 5% incidence of postoperative swelling at the injection site and soreness to chewing was noted after use of the Stabident device. Significantly higher incidences of postoperative swelling (20%) and chewing soreness (15%) developed in subjects treated with the X-tip system. This disparity may have been related to the more apical location of the X-tip perforation in alveolar mucosa. Finally, dentinal tooth damage and osteonecrosis of bone may rarely occur after an IO injection.[59]

REFERENCES

1. Davis MJ, Vogel LD. Local anesthetic safety in pediatric patients. N Y State Dent J 1996;62(2):32–5.
2. Feck AS, Goodchild JH. The use of anxiolytic medications to supplement local anesthesia in the anxious patient. Compend Contin Educ Dent 2005;26(3):183–6, 188, 190.
3. Milgrom P, Weinstein P, Getz T. Treating fearful dental patients. A patient management handbook. 2nd edition. Seattle (WA): Continuing Dental Education, University of Washington; 1995.

4. Al-Omari WM, Al-Omiri MK. Dental anxiety among university students and its correlation with their field of study. J Appl Oral Sci 2009;17(3):199–203.
5. Kaufman E, Weinstein P, Milgrom P. Difficulties in achieving local anesthesia. J Am Dent Assoc 1984;108(2):205–8.
6. Grace EG, Barnes DM, Reid BC, et al. Computerized local dental anesthetic systems: patient and dentist satisfaction. J Dent 2003;31(1):9–12.
7. Friedman MJ, Hochman MN. A 21st century computerized injection system for local pain control. Compend Contin Educ Dent 1997;18(10):995–1000.
8. Hochman MN, Friedman MJ. In vitro study of needle deflection: a linear insertion technique versus a bidirectional rotation insertion technique. Quintessence Int 2000;31(1):33–9.
9. Hochman MN, Friedman MJ. An in vitro study of needle force penetration comparing a standard linear insertion to the new bidirectional rotation insertion technique. Quintessence Int 2001;32(10):789–96.
10. Asarch T, Allen K, Petersen B, et al. Efficacy of a computerized local anesthesia device in pediatric dentistry. Pediatr Dent 1999;21(7):421–4.
11. Ram D, Peretz B. The assessment of pain sensation during local anesthesia using a computerized local anesthesia (Wand) and a conventional syringe. J Dent Child 2003;70(2):130–3.
12. Versloot J, Veerkamp JS, Hoogstraten J. Pain behaviour and distress in children during two sequential dental visits: comparing a computerised anaesthesia delivery system and a traditional syringe. Br Dent J 2008;205(1):E2.
13. Hochman M, Chiarello D, Hochman CB, et al. Computerized local anesthetic delivery vs. traditional syringe technique. NY State Dent J 1997;63(7):24–9.
14. Saloum FS, Baumgartner JC, Marshall G, et al. A clinical comparison of pain perception to the Wand and a traditional syringe. Oral Surg Oral Med Oral Pathol Oral Radiol Endod 2000;89(6):691–5.
15. Loomer PM, Perry DA. Computer-controlled delivery versus syringe delivery of local anesthetic injections for therapeutic scaling and root planing. J Am Dent Assoc 2004;135(3):358–65.
16. Nusstein J, Lee S, Reader A, et al. Injection pain and postinjection pain of the anterior middle superior alveolar injection administered with the Wand or conventional syringe. Oral Surg Oral Med Oral Pathol Oral Radiol Endod 2004;98(1):124–31.
17. Palm AM, Kirkegaard U, Poulsen S. The Wand versus traditional injection for mandibular nerve block in children and adolescents: perceived pain and time of onset. Pediatr Dent 2004;26(6):481–4.
18. Yenisey M. Comparison of the pain level of computer-controlled and conventional anesthesia techniques in prosthodontic treatment. J Appl Oral Sci 2009;17(5):414–20.
19. Kudo M. Initial injection pressure for dental local anesthesia: effects on pain and anxiety. Anesth Prog 2005;52(3):95–101.
20. Krochak M, Friedman N. Using a precision-metered injection system to minimize dental injection anxiety. Compend Contin Educ Dent 1998;19(2):137–40, 142, 143, 146.
21. Versloot J, Veerkamp JS, Hoogstraten J. Computerized anesthesia delivery system vs. traditional syringe: comparing pain and pain-related behavior in children. Eur J Oral Sci 2005;113(6):488–93.
22. Friedman MJ, Hochman MN. The AMSA injection: a new concept for local anesthesia of maxillary teeth using a computer-controlled injection system. Quintessence Int 1998;29(5):297–303.
23. Friedman MJ, Hochman MN. P-ASA block injection: a new palatal technique to anesthetize maxillary anterior teeth. J Esthet Dent 1999;11(2):63–71.

24. Fukayama H, Yoshikawa F, Kohase H, et al. Efficacy of anterior and middle superior alveolar (AMSA) anesthesia using a new injection system: the Wand. Quintessence Int 2003;34(7):537–41.

25. Nusstein J, Burns Y, Reader A, et al. Injection pain and postinjection pain of the palatal-anterior superior alveolar injection, administered with the Wand Plus system, comparing 2% lidocaine with 1:100,000 epinephrine to 3% mepivacaine. Oral Surg Oral Med Oral Pathol Oral Radiol Endod 2004;97(2):164–72.

26. Nusstein J, Berlin J, Reader A, et al. Comparison of injection pain, heart rate increase, and postinjection pain of articaine and lidocaine in a primary intraligamentary injection administered with a computer-controlled local anesthetic delivery system. Anesth Prog 2004;51(4):126–33.

27. STA. Single tooth anesthesia system operating manual. Livingston (NJ): Milestone Scientific; 2008.

28. Lee S, Reader A, Nusstein J, et al. Anesthetic efficacy of the anterior middle superior alveolar (AMSA) injection. Anesth Prog 2004;51(3):80–9.

29. Burns Y, Reader A, Nusstein J, et al. Anesthetic efficacy of the palatal–anterior superior alveolar injection. J Am Dent Assoc 2004;135(9):1269–76.

30. Broering R, Reader A, Drum M, et al. A prospective randomized comparison of the anesthetic efficacy of the greater palatine and high tuberosity second division nerve blocks. J Endod 2009;35(10):1337–42.

31. Karkut B, Reader A, Drum M, et al. A comparison of the local anesthetic efficacy of the extraoral versus the intraoral infraorbital nerve block. J Am Dent Assoc 2010;141(2):185–92.

32. Acharya AB, Banakar C, Rodrigues SV, et al. The AMSA (anterior middle superior alveolar) injection is effective in providing anesthesia extending to the last molar in maxillary periodontal surgery. J Periodontol 2010. [Epub ahead of print].

33. Berlin J, Nusstein J, Reader A, et al. Efficacy of articaine and lidocaine in a primary intraligamentary injection administered with a computer-controlled local anesthetic delivery system. Oral Surg Oral Med Oral Pathol Oral Radiol Endod 2005;99(3):361–6.

34. Ferrari M, Cagidiaco MC, Vichi A, et al. Efficacy of the computer-controlled injection system STA, the Ligmaject, and the dental syringe for intraligamentary anesthesia in restorative patients. Int Dent SA 2009;11(1):4–12.

35. Gibson RS, Allen K, Hutfless S, et al. The Wand vs. traditional injection: a comparison of pain related behaviors. Pediatr Dent 2000;22(6):458–62.

36. Allen KD, Kotil D, Larzelere RE, et al. Comparison of a computerized anesthesia device with a traditional syringe in preschool children. Pediatr Dent 2002;24(4):315–20.

37. Klein U, Hunzeker C, Hutfless S, et al. Quality of anesthesia for the maxillary primary anterior segment in pediatric patients: comparison of the P-ASA nerve block using CompuMed delivery system vs traditional supraperiosteal injections. J Dent Child (Chic) 2005;72(3):119–25.

38. Ram D, Kassirer J. Assessment of a palatal approach-anterior superior alveolar (P-ASA) nerve block with the Wand in paediatric dental patients. Int J Paediatr Dent 2006;16(5):348–51.

39. Amoudi NA, Feda M, Sharaf A, et al. Assessment of the anesthetic effectiveness of anterior and middle superior alveolar injection using a computerized device versus traditional technique in children. J Clin Pediatr Dent 2008;33(2):97–102.

40. Ran D, Peretz B. Assessing the pain reaction of children receiving periodontal ligament anesthesia using a computerized device (Wand). J Clin Pediatr Dent 2003;27(3):247–50.

41. Öztaş N, Ulusu T, Bodur H, et al. The Wand in pulp therapy: an alternative to inferior alveolar nerve block. Quintessence Int 2005;36(7–8):559–64.

42. Lilienthal B. A clinical appraisal of intraosseous dental anesthesia. Oral Surg Oral Med Oral Pathol 1975;39(5):692–7.

43. IntraFlow operating manual. Available at: http://www.pro-dex.com/media/Intraflow_Manual_English.pdf. Accessed June 1, 2010.

44. Coggins R, Reader A, Nist R, et al. Anesthetic efficacy of the intraosseous injection in maxillary and mandibular teeth. Oral Surg Oral Med Oral Pathol Oral Radiol Endod 1996;81(6):634–41.

45. Replogle K, Reader A, Nist R, et al. Anesthetic efficacy of the intraosseous injection of 2% lidocaine (1:100,000 epinephrine) and 3% mepivacaine in mandibular first molars. Oral Surg Oral Med Oral Pathol Endod 1997;83(1):30–7.

46. Gallatin J, Reader A, Nusstein J, et al. A comparison of two intraosseous anesthetic techniques in mandibular posterior teeth. J Am Dent Assoc 2003;134(11):1476–84.

47. Remmers T, Glickman G, Spears R, et al. The efficacy of IntraFlow intraosseous injection as a primary anesthesia technique. J Endod 2007;34(3):280–3.

48. Nusstein J, Reader A, Nist R, et al. Anesthetic efficacy of the supplemental intraosseous injection of 2% lidocaine with 1:100,000 epinephrine in irreversible pulpitis. J Endod 1998;24(7):487–91.

49. Parente SA, Anderson RW, Herman WW, et al. Anesthetic efficacy of the supplemental intraosseous injection for teeth with irreversible pulpitis. J Endod 1998;24(12):826–8.

50. Nusstein J, Kennedy S, Reader A, et al. Anesthetic efficacy of the supplemental X-tip intraosseous injection in patients with irreversible pulpitis. J Endod 2003;29(11):724–8.

51. Bigby J, Reader A, Nusstein J, et al. Articaine for supplemental intraosseous anesthesia in patients with irreversible pulpitis. J Endod 2006;32(11):1044–7.

52. Reisman D, Reader A, Nist R, et al. Anesthetic efficacy of the supplemental intraosseous injection of 3% mepivacaine in irreversible pulpitis. Oral Surg Oral Med Oral Pathol Oral Radiol Endod 1997;84(6):676–81.

53. Sixou JL, Barbosa-Rogier ME. Efficacy of intraosseous injections of anesthetic in children and adolescents. Oral Surg Oral Med Oral Pathol Oral Radiol Endod 2008;106(2):173–8.

54. Lilienthal B, Reynolds AK. Cardiovascular responses to intraosseous injections containing catecholamines. Oral Surg Oral Med Oral Pathol 1975;40(5):574–83.

55. Replogle K, Reader A, Nist R, et al. Cardiovascular effects of intraosseous injections of 2 percent lidocaine with 1:100,000 epinephrine and 3 percent mepivacaine. J Am Dent Assoc 1999;130(5):649–57.

56. Stabile P, Reader A, Gallatin E, et al. Anesthetic efficacy and heart rate effects of the intraosseous injection of 1.5% etidocaine (1:200,000 epinephrine) after an inferior alveolar nerve block. Oral Surg Oral Med Oral Pathol Oral Radiol Endod 2000;89(4):407–11.

57. Susi L, Reader A, Nusstein J, et al. Heart rate effects of intraosseous injections using slow and fast rates of anesthetic solution deposition. Anesth Prog 2008;55(1):9–15.

58. Gallatin J, Nusstein J, Reader A, et al. A comparison of injection pain and postoperative pain of two intraosseous anesthetic techniques. Anesth Prog 2003;50(3):111–20.

59. Woodmansey KF, White RK, He J. Osteonecrosis related to intraosseous anesthesia: report of a case. J Endod 2009;35(2):288–91.

Local Anesthesia Administration by Dental Hygienists

Sean G. Boynes, DMD, MS[a],*, Jayme Zovko, RDH, BS[b],
Robert M. Peskin, DDS[c]

KEYWORDS

- Anesthesia • Dental hygienists

Within the last 30 years, many states have expanded the scope of practice for dental hygienists to include the administration of local anesthesia.[1,2] Several studies have been performed to assess practice characteristics and effectiveness of these changes in state licensure regulations. Findings indicate an acceptance of this expansion in dental hygiene practice, with prominent rates of employer delegation of local anesthesia administration to dental hygienists, successful injection administration, and positive benefits to dental practice.[3] Although these various outcomes support the use of this modality by dental hygienists, the delegation of these pain control procedures remains controversial.[1,4,5] To address this controversy, the authors have reviewed of current literature to assess the practice of local anesthesia administration by dental hygienists.

SCOPE OF PRACTICE

Regulations permitting the administration of local anesthesia by dental hygienist have been slowly implemented into the scope of dental hygiene practice since Washington approved regulations in 1971. As of the writing of this article, 42 US dental boards allow dental hygienists to deliver local anesthetic injections, and two additional states (Indiana and Maryland) have regulations pending for the implementation of this modality.[6] New York and South Carolina are the only states in which dental hygienists are limited to local infiltration injections (Maryland's proposed regulations will also limit use to infiltration injections).[7] Texas, Mississippi, Alabama, Georgia, North Carolina,

[a] Department of Anesthesiology, University of Pittsburgh School of Dental Medicine, 622 Salk Hall, 3501 Terrace Street, Pittsburgh, PA 15261, USA
[b] Department of Anesthesiology, University of Pittsburgh School of Dental Medicine, G-87 Salk Hall, 3501 Terrace Street, Pittsburgh, PA 15261, USA
[c] Department of Hospital Dentistry and Dental Anesthesiology, School of Dental Medicine, Stony Brook University, East Loop Road, Stony Brook, NY 11794, USA
* Corresponding author.
E-mail address: sebst54@pitt.edu

Dent Clin N Am 54 (2010) 769–778
doi:10.1016/j.cden.2010.06.014
0011-8532/10/$ – see front matter © 2010 Published by Elsevier Inc.

and Florida have not included a provision for the administration of local anesthesia injections within the scope of practice of dental hygienists.

As shown in **Fig. 1**, most state dental boards require dental hygienists to administer local anesthesia under the direct supervision of a dentist. Under direct supervision, the dentist responsible for the procedure must be present in the dental office or facility, personally diagnose the condition to be treated, personally authorize the procedure and, before dismissal of the patient, personally examine the condition after treatment is completed. It does not require the dentist to be physically present in the operatory as the injection is being administered.

It should be noted, however, that within the jurisdictions of 6 dental boards (Alaska, Colorado, Idaho, Minnesota, Nevada, and Oregon), the dental hygienist is permitted to administer local anesthetics under general supervision. General supervision means that the dentist has authorized the procedures to be performed for a patient but does not require that a dentist is physically present within the office or facility when the procedures are performed.

In the 2007 Survey of Dental Hygienists in the United States, dental hygienists were asked not only to describe the clinical services provided at their worksites, but also to indicate the amount of time spent weekly providing each service and the level of required supervision for each task.[8] An analysis of required supervision for specific dental hygiene clinical services revealed that there were differences across states in the supervision required for many of the tasks. Mean supervision scores were computed based on a scale in which direct supervision for a task was scored as 4, indirect supervision was scored as 3, general supervision was scored as 2, and no supervision was scored as 1. According to the survey, the mean national supervision scores for administration of local anesthesia (3.06) were among the highest for any dental hygiene service. The range in mean supervision scores for local anesthesia (2.0 to 4.0) was greater than for prophylaxis.

EDUCATION AND TRAINING REQUIREMENTS

In the United States, professional licensure regulations establishing the policies of oral health personnel are the responsibility of individual state governments. Each state's governing body operates with a specific board or committee that oversees dental professionals and the statutes that govern the dental profession. Of the 42 states that allow dental hygienists to administer local anesthesia, most require the successful completion of a state board-approved continuing education course or competency training via a Commission on Dental Accreditation (CODA)-recognized dental hygiene program.[7] However, a significant variation exists between the individual state dental boards on specific education requirements and the prerequisite of examination before certification.

As is true with dental sedation/anesthesia guidelines, the largest variation with dental hygienists wishing to achieve local anesthesia permit status relates to the amount and type of instructional hours needed.[9] Depending on which state is being referenced, the legal requirements for instruction hours for dental hygiene local anesthesia courses are usually described in one of three categories: the general total course hours needed, specific course hours established by a set amount of didactic and clinical hours, or no specific hourly requirement.

Twenty-eight states have general hourly requirements on local anesthesia instruction; 18 of those states specifically describe the amount of coursework to be dedicated didactically (mean = 15.4 hours) and clinically (mean = 11.5 hours). Currently, 14 states do not provide general instructional hour requirements in their regulation

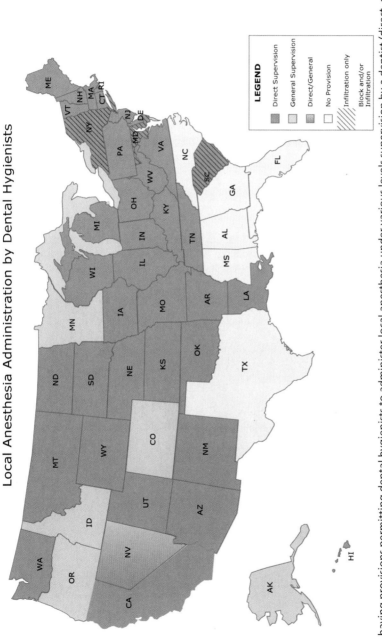

Local Anesthesia Administration by Dental Hygienists

LEGEND
Direct Supervision
General Supervision
Direct/General
No Provision
Infiltration only
Block and/or Infiltration

Fig. 1. States having provisions permitting dental hygienists to administer local anesthesia under various levels supervision by a dentist (direct, general, or both). Two states (*hash fill*) limit local anesthesia administration to infiltration anesthesia. Six states (*no fill*) have not passed laws expanding dental hygienists' scope of practice to include the administration of local anesthesia.

guidelines. However, all of these states require that the courses receive state board approval before granting permit status to students. As demonstrated in **Fig. 2**, additional evaluation of the 28 states that have general instructional hour requirements reveals a mean of 32.7 total hours of instruction needed for permit status with the minimum number of hours of 12 (Kansas) and the maximum number of hours of 72 (Louisiana).

Twenty-seven of the 42 dental boards (63.4%) also require the successful completion of clinical or written examinations for certification. The type of examination varies between the individual dental boards. Fifteen dental boards require a board-approved examination given through the training course or accredited program; five dental boards only certify applicants through regional board examination (North East Regional Board [NERB] - 3 and Western Regional Examination Board [WREB] – 2). Two dental boards require both a regional board and state-approved examination, and four dental boards accept either regional board or state-approved examinations.

PRACTICE ACTIVITY

In a randomized survey completed as part of the University of Pittsburgh Dental Hygiene Local Anesthesia Initiative (UPDHLI), 429 dental hygienists located throughout the United States completed a questionnaire submitted to obtain data on practice characteristics and training. The demographics of this sample demonstrated representation of 296 dental hygiene training programs and included practice sites of equal distribution within 51 United States' dental boards.

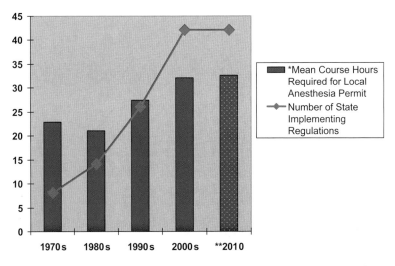

* The mean course hours were calculated by decade and only represent the dental boards passing regulation during that time period. The numbers used for the data set were the general course hours given when the regulations were first passed. Therefore, each decade has a unique set of numbers used and the information is not cumulative.

** The data set for" 2010" uses cumulative numbers. Therefore, the information relayed in the" 2010" area of the chart is a representation of current mean number of hours and total number of dental boards with regulations allocating local anesthesia administration to dental hygiene practitioners.

Fig. 2. Decadal analysis of mean course hours required for a local anesthesia permit and number of dental boards implementing regulation for local anesthesia administration by dental hygienists.

The survey found that 59.5% (257 respondents) of United States' dental hygienists currently administer local anesthesia in their hygiene practice, while 40.5%(175 respondents) do not. It was also revealed that 58.4% of the respondents who reported administering injections (n = 257), administered local anesthesia for the procedures in which the dentist was to perform total care. Additional regional analysis demonstrated that a higher percentage of hygienists administered injections for the dentist in practice locations where the date of hygiene-related local anesthesia regulation implementation was the oldest.

As demonstrated in **Table 1**, the UPDHLI survey also determined the type of local anesthetic injections used by the respondents administering local anesthesia (n = 257). The questions were grouped into four categories: infiltration/supraperiosteal injections, nerve block injections, field block injections, and topical anesthetic application without injection. The results demonstrated that nerve block injections (two to three times per week) and infiltration/supraperiosteal injections (two to three times per week) were the most commonly administered injection techniques while field block injections (one to two times per week) were administered by the respondents with lesser frequency. It should be noted that the survey also determined that topical anesthetic (ie, Oraqix) application without injection was the most common form of local anesthesia to be employed by those administering injections. Higher frequency of topical anesthesia use is likely related to the fact that topical anesthetics may sometimes be used as a substitute to injectable anesthesia (ie, long buccal and palatal injections), which can be distressing for the patient but necessary for quadrant management.

Previous studies also demonstrated that use of local anesthesia by dental hygienists varies by practice type, with the highest frequency of usage occurring in periodontal practices. In a survey of Minnesota dental hygienists, Anderson found that 47.6% of dental hygienists working in periodontal offices reported administering local anesthesia for three to six patients each week, while 63% of hygienists working in general practice administered local anesthesia for one or two patients each week.[3] In this

Table 1
University of Pittsburgh Dental Hygiene Local Anesthesia Initiative Survey: mean distribution of local anesthetic injection type used according to the dental hygiene respondents main practice activity[a]

Local Anesthesia Modality	Total Response (n = 257)	Periodontal Setting	Public Health Setting	Academic/ University Setting	General Dentistry Setting	Pediatric Setting
Infiltration injection	2.02	2.87	2.33	1.62	1.64	0.75
Nerve block injection	2.12	2.38	1.64	2.25	1.72	0.67
Field block injection	1.52	2.06	1.64	2.25	1.15	0.67
Topical anesthesia without injection	2.38	2.65	2.17	2.62	2.09	1.75

[a] The respondent was asked to select a single numeric answer for the amount of each local anesthesia modality performed from the choices: 0, never (0); 1, rarely (1–2 times per week); 2, occasionally (2–3 times per week); 3, often (4-5 times per week); 4, most often (more than 5 times per week).

same report, Anderson also revealed that, overall, hygienists were most frequently (92%) using local anesthesia for periodontal root planing and debridement.

SAFETY AND EFFICACY

Of prime importance in the delegation of local anesthesia administration to dental hygienists is safety and efficacy. Numerous studies have been completed, which assess these significant concerns. Methods employed by investigators interested in evaluating the safety of local anesthesia administration by dental hygienists have included surveys to ascertain aspiration rates before injection, complication rates, and surveys to quantify disciplinary actions against dental hygienists associated with local anesthesia administration.

The safety of local anesthesia administration by dental hygienists has been assessed indirectly through determining whether dental hygienists consistently employ recommended safety techniques, such as aspiration before injection, to reduce the risk of adverse reactions. In a survey of Minnesota dental hygienists, Anderson found that 86% of respondents reported the use of consistent aspiration before injecting; 7% reported the use of aspiration most of the time, and 3% reported infrequently aspirating before injection.[3] In comparison, Malamed[10] found that, of dentists he surveyed, 23% routinely administered local anesthesia with a nonaspirating syringe, making it impossible to assure the location of the needle tip before injection.

In spite of this apparent lapse of adherence to ideal protocol by dentists, there are approximately 300 million local anesthetic administrations provided per year in the United States with few significant adverse drug reactions reported.[10,11] Presumably, higher rates of aspiration before injection, as reported by the Minnesota dental hygienists, would contribute to an equally respectable record of safety.

Further insight into the safety of local anesthesia administration by dental hygienists has been obtained through the investigation of complication rates. Although information is limited in this area, both Anderson[3] and Lobene[12] reported minimal rates of complications resulting from the administration of local anesthesia by dental hygienists. Approximately 30 years ago, Lobene addressed this important concern for an experimental program designed to train dental hygienists in expanded functions. Lobene[12] reported that out of 19,849 anesthetizations by dental hygienists, only three cases of temporary paresthesia were identified. In the more recent study, Anderson's survey reported that 88% of dental hygienists reported no complications when administering local anesthesia.[3]

The safety of local anesthesia administration by dental hygienists also has been substantiated through the lack of reported disciplinary actions. No formal complaints associated with local anesthesia administration against dental hygienists were known to state dental boards or American Dental Hygienists' Association constituent presidents based on surveys reported in 1990 and again in 2005.[11,13] It should be noted that 28% of the dental boards responding to the 2005 survey reported that this information was unavailable, most likely due to dental practice act limitations in certain states.

Along with the prime concern of patient safety, when assessing the wisdom of the delegation of local anesthesia administration to dental hygienists, consideration must be given to the ability of dental hygienists to provide effective injections. During the experimental training program conducted by Lobene[12] in the 1970s, it was determined that dental hygienists could be trained to provide local anesthesia with a high rate of success. Out of 19,849 injections performed by dental hygienists, Lobene reported a success rate of 96.7% with infiltrations and an 85.7% success rate with blocks.

Success of local anesthesia administration by dental hygienists also has been examined through dental hygienists' self report, faculty ratings of dental hygiene students, and surveys to determine employer satisfaction. Anderson found that within 4 to 12 months of completing a Minnesota continuing education course, 76% of the dental hygienists surveyed reported successful anesthetization 90% to 100% of the time, and 16% reported success 75% to 89% of the time.[3] Sisty-LePeau and colleagues[13] analyzed data from an experimental program designed to train dental hygienists in expanded functions. Through evaluations completed by restorative dentistry and periodontics faculty, it was determined that out of 3926 injections administered by dental hygiene students, adequate anesthesia was achieved 95% of the time.[14] Indirect evaluation of the success of local anesthesia administration by dental hygienists has been accomplished through determining employer satisfaction hygienists' ability to provide this service. In a survey of Arkansas dental hygienists, DeAngelis and Goral[15] found that 92% of dentist employers were satisfied with their dental hygienists' ability in administering local anesthesia.

Considering another aspect of successful injections, Malamed[10] comments on the ability of dental hygienists to provide comfortable injections, noting that patients are aware of the difference between injections administered by dental hygienists and those administered by dentists. Whether due to slower administration rates, attention to detail, or greater empathy, patient satisfaction with a dental hygienist providing local anesthesia is generally positive.

PRACTICE IMPLICATIONS

Another significant consideration in assessing the advisability of local anesthesia administration by dental hygienists is the impact this provision has on the individual dental practice. Numerous studies have examined this issue through surveys of dentists and dental hygienists that incorporate questions on general value to practice, improvement to schedules, patient satisfaction, patient comfort, and improved hygienist productivity. Anderson[3] reported that besides administering anesthesia for their own patients, dental hygienists are administering local anesthesia for patients whose care is to be provided by the dentist. In providing pain control for the dentist's patients as well as their own, hygienists are able to contribute to improved workflow and time savings for the practice.

Anderson[3] also reported that 58% of responding dentists revealed that their ability to administer local anesthesia was very valuable to their practice, with 64.4% reporting that their practice ran more smoothly, and 53.1% reporting that they were more thorough in their treatment. In addition, 76.9% of responding dental hygienists indicated that they provide more comfortable treatment as a result of their ability to provide local anesthesia for their patients. In similar findings, Cross-Poline and colleagues[16] reported that most dentists identified a benefit to both their practices and their patients as a result of the administration of local anesthesia by their dental hygienist. Additionally, DeAngelis and Goral[15] reported that most dentists indicated that local anesthesia administration by dental hygienists produced positive effects on their practice in the form of smoother schedules, patient satisfaction and comfort, and improved hygienist productivity. Benefit to patients and improvement in patient comfort are not insignificant findings when correlated with the findings by Sisty-LePeau and colleagues,[5] who reported 69.5% of practicing hygienists not currently administering local anesthesia injections indicated they treat a median of two to three patients per month who need but do not receive anesthesia. Reasons selected for why pain control was not provided ranged from lack of time to interruption

Table 2
Synopsis of local anesthesia administration safety and efficacy studies with dental hygienists

	Category	Subject	Findings
Anderson[3]	Safety	Aspiration safety protocol	86% of responding hygienists reported the use of consistent aspiration before injection; 7% reported the use of aspiration most of the time, and 3% reported infrequently aspirating before injection
Anderson[3]	Safety	Complication rates	87.8% of dental hygienists signified no complications when administering local anesthesia injections
Anderson[3]	Efficacy	Self-reporting of success	76% of surveyed dental hygienists reported successful anesthetization 90%–100% of the time, and 16% reported success 75%–89% of the time
Cross-Poline et al[16]	Efficacy	Employer/dentist observer ratings	Dentists (n = 57) identified a benefit to both their practices and their patients as a result of the administration of local anesthesia by their dental hygiene employees; the mean percentage of agreement with this statement was reported at 80.4%
DeAngelis and Goral[15]	Efficacy	Employer/dentist observer ratings	92% of dentist employers were satisfied with their dental hygienists' ability in administering local anesthesia injections
Lobene[12]	Safety	Complication rates	Out of 19,849 anesthetizations by dental hygienists, only three cases of temporary paresthesia were identified
Lobene[12]	Efficacy	Success rates	Out of 19,849 injections performed by dental hygienists, a success rate of 96.7% with infiltrations and an 85.7% success rate with nerve block techniques were found with dental hygienists
Rich and Smorang[17]	Safety/efficacy	Continued delegation of anesthesia administration to hygienists	100% of periodontists and 86% of general dentists delegated the administration of local anesthesia to dental hygienists based on this survey of California dental hygiene graduates
Scofield et al[11]	Safety	Disciplinary reports	No formal complaints associated with local anesthesia administration against dental hygienists were known to state dental boards or American Dental Hygienists' Association constituent presidents based on surveys reported in 1990 and again in 2005
Sisty-LePeau et al[14]	Efficacy	Adequacy of anesthesia with dental hygiene students	Through evaluations completed by restorative dentistry and periodontics faculty, it was determined that out of 3926 injections administered by dental hygiene students, adequate anesthesia was achieved 95% of the time

of the dentist's schedule. Delegation of local anesthesia to dental hygienists will help prevent these unfortunate occasions where a patient needlessly endures a painful procedure because his or her hygienist is not legally allowed to administer local anesthesia.

SUMMARY

This literature review confirms patient and dentist satisfaction with dental hygienists providing local anesthesia. With the preponderance of dental hygienists reporting a need for this modality, this practice appears to be a substantial addition to total dental care.

Taking into account the consistent record of safety and success with local anesthesia administration by dental hygienists documented in the reviewed studies and the existing evidence of overall benefit to dental practices through increased patient comfort and improved practice workflow, continued support for the delegation of local anesthesia administration to dental hygienists appears to be warranted **(Table 2)**.

REFERENCES

1. Minervini R, Harrington M, Stindt D. Assessing expanded functions performed by hygienists in Missouri. Dent Hyg (Chic) 1981;55(5):36–41.
2. McCloskey FS. Survey of nontraditional functions performed by hygienists. J Dent Educ 1977;41:693–4.
3. Anderson JM. Use of local anesthesia by dental hygienists who completed a Minnesota CE course. J Dent Hyg 2002;76(1):35–46.
4. Powell WO, Sinkford JC, Henry JL, et al. Comparison of clinical performance of dental therapist trainees and dental sudents. J Dent Educ 1974;38:268–72.
5. Sisty-LePeau N, Nielson-Thompson N, Lutjen D. Use, need and desire for pain control by Iowa hygienists. J Dent Hyg 1992;66:137–46.
6. American Dental Hygiene Association. States where dental hygienists may administer local anesthesia: reference map. Available at: http://www.adha.org/governmental_affairs/downloads/localanesthesiamap.pdf. Accessed June 12, 2009.
7. American Dental Hygiene Association. Local anesthesia administration by dental hygienists: state chart. Available at: http://www.adha.org/governmental_affairs/downloads/localanesthesia.pdf. Accessed June 12, 2009.
8. American Dental Hygiene Association. Survey of dental hygienists in the united states, 2007: executive survey. 2009. Available at: http://www.adha.org/downloads/DH_pratitioner_Survey_Exec_Summary.pdf. Accessed February 27, 2009.
9. Boynes SG. Dental anesthesiology: a guide to the rules and regulations of the United States of America. 2008–2009 edition. Pittsburgh (PA): Slavia Printing Company, Incorporated; 2008.
10. Malamed SF. Handbook of local anesthesia. 5th edition. St. Louis (MO): Mosby; 2004.
11. Scofield JC, Gutmann ME, DeQald JP, et al. Disciplinary actions associated with the administration of local anesthetics against dentists and dental hygienists. J Dent Hyg 2005;79(1):8. Available at: http://www.ingentaconnect.com. Accessed September 9, 2009.
12. Lobene RR. The Forsyth experiment. Boston (MA): Harvard University Press; 1979.

13. Sisty-LePeau N, Boyer EM, Lutjen D. Dental hygiene licensure specifications on pain control procedures. J Dent Hyg 1990;64(4):179–85.

14. Sisty NL, Henderson WG, Martin JF. The administration of local anesthesia by dental hygiene students. Dent Hyg 1986;60:28–32.

15. DeAngelis S, Goral V. Utilization of local anesthesia by Arkansas dental hygienists, and dentists' delegation/satisfaction relative to this function. J Dent Hyg 2000;74:196–204.

16. Cross-Poline GN, Passon JC, Tillis TS, et al. Effectiveness of a continuing education course in local anesthesia for dental hygienists. J Dent Hyg 1992;66:130–6.

17. Rich SK, Smorang J. Survey of 1980 California dental hygiene graduates to determine expanded-function utilization. J Pub Health Dent 1984;44:22–7.

Index

Note: Page numbers of article titles are in **boldface** type.

A

Allergic reactions, and adverse effects of local anesthetics, differentiated, 656
    to formulations of local anesthetics, **655–664**
    to local anesthetic preservatives, 660–662
Allergy testing procedures, 656–658
Amide local anesthetics, 603–604
    allergic reactions to, 658
    cross-reactivity procedures and, 660
Anesthesia, infiltration. See *Infiltration anesthesia*.
    local, administration by dental hygienists, **769–778**
        practice activity, 772–774
        practice implications of, 775–777
        safety and efficacy of, 774–775, 776
        scope of practice, 769–770
      dental, advanced techniques and armamentarium for, **757–768**
      intraosseous, 762–765
        clinical uses of, 764–765
        devices available for, 762–764
        IntraFlow system, 763–784
        side effects and complications of, 765
        Stabident system, 762–763
        X-tip system, 763
    neuraxial, 606–608
      epidural technique for, 607–608
      spinal technique for, 606–607
    primary surgical, 604
    regional, 601
    soft tissue, lingering, quality-of-life issues and, 632
Anesthesia prefilled dental cartilage, 745
Anesthetic delivery systems, 745
Anesthetics, injectable, local anesthetics and, 668–669
    local, administration to children, 594
      adverse effects of, and allergic reactions to, differentiated, 656
      allergic reactions to, 658–660
        treatment of, 661–662
      amide, 603–604
        allergic reactions to, 658
        cross-reactivity procedures and, 660
      and coagulation, 705
      and general anesthesia, combined, 608
      and ocular complications. See *Ocular complications*.
      clinical pharmacology of, 587–592

Dent Clin N Am 54 (2010) 779–785
doi:10.1016/S0011-8532(10)00096-0
0011-8532/10/$ – see front matter © 2010 Elsevier Inc. All rights reserved.

dental.theclinics.com

United States Postal Service

Statement of Ownership, Management, and Circulation
(All Periodicals Publications Except Requestor Publications)

1. Publication Title	2. Publication Number									3. Filing Date
Dental Clinics of North America	5	6	6	-	4	8	0			9/15/10

4. Issue Frequency	5. Number of Issues Published Annually	6. Annual Subscription Price
Jan, Apr, Jul, Oct	4	$224.00

7. Complete Mailing Address of Known Office of Publication (*Not printer*) (*Street, city, county, state, and ZIP+4®*)

Elsevier Inc.
360 Park Avenue South
New York, NY 10010-1710

Contact Person
Stephen Bushing

Telephone (*Include area code*)
215-239-3688

8. Complete Mailing Address of Headquarters or General Business Office of Publisher (*Not printer*)

Elsevier Inc., 360 Park Avenue South, New York, NY 10010-1710

9. Full Names and Complete Mailing Addresses of Publisher, Editor, and Managing Editor (*Do not leave blank*)

Publisher (*Name and complete mailing address*)

Kim Murphy, Elsevier, Inc., 1600 John F. Kennedy Blvd. Suite 1800, Philadelphia, PA 19103-2899

Editor (*Name and complete mailing address*)

John Vassallo, Elsevier, Inc., 1600 John F. Kennedy Blvd. Suite 1800, Philadelphia, PA 19103-2899

Managing Editor (*Name and complete mailing address*)

Catherine Bewick, Elsevier, Inc., 1600 John F. Kennedy Blvd. Suite 1800, Philadelphia, PA 19103-2899

10. Owner (*Do not leave blank. If the publication is owned by a corporation, give the name and address of the corporation immediately followed by the names and addresses of all stockholders owning or holding 1 percent or more of the total amount of stock. If not owned by a corporation, give the names and addresses of the individual owners. If owned by a partnership or other unincorporated firm, give its name and address as well as those of each individual owner. If the publication is published by a nonprofit organization, give its name and address.*)

Full Name	Complete Mailing Address
Wholly owned subsidiary of	4520 East-West Highway
Reed/Elsevier, US holdings	Bethesda, MD 20814

11. Known Bondholders, Mortgagees, and Other Security Holders Owning or Holding 1 Percent or More of Total Amount of Bonds, Mortgages, or Other Securities. If none, check box □ None

Full Name	Complete Mailing Address
N/A	

12. Tax Status (*For completion by nonprofit organizations authorized to mail at nonprofit rates*) (*Check one*)
The purpose, function, and nonprofit status of this organization and the exempt status for federal income tax purposes:
□ Has Not Changed During Preceding 12 Months
□ Has Changed During Preceding 12 Months (*Publisher must submit explanation of change with this statement*)

PS Form **3526**, September 2007 (Page 1 of 3 (Instructions Page 3)) PSN 7530-01-000-9931 PRIVACY NOTICE: See our Privacy policy in www.usps.com

---

13. Publication Title		14. Issue Date for Circulation Data Below
Dental Clinics of North America		July 2010

15. Extent and Nature of Circulation			Average No. Copies Each Issue During Preceding 12 Months	No. Copies of Single Issue Published Nearest to Filing Date
a. Total Number of Copies (*Net press run*)			1835	1750
b. Paid Circulation (By Mail and Outside the Mail)	(1)	Mailed Outside-County Paid Subscriptions Stated on PS Form 3541. (*Include paid distribution above nominal rate, advertiser's proof copies, and exchange copies*)	671	656
	(2)	Mailed In-County Paid Subscriptions Stated on PS Form 3541 (*Include paid distribution above nominal rate, advertiser's proof copies, and exchange copies*)		
	(3)	Paid Distribution Outside the Mails Including Sales Through Dealers and Carriers, Street Vendors, Counter Sales, and Other Paid Distribution Outside USPS®	405	363
	(4)	Paid Distribution by Other Classes Mailed Through the USPS (e.g. First-Class Mail®)		
c. Total Paid Distribution (*Sum of 15b (1), (2), (3), and (4)*)		▲	1076	1019
d. Free or Nominal Rate Distribution (By Mail and Outside the Mail)	(1)	Free or Nominal Rate Outside-County Copies Included on PS Form 3541	74	57
	(2)	Free or Nominal Rate In-County Copies Included on PS Form 3541		
	(3)	Free or Nominal Rate Copies Mailed at Other Classes Through the USPS (e.g. First-Class Mail)		
	(4)	Free or Nominal Rate Distribution Outside the Mail (Carriers or other means)		
e. Total Free or Nominal Rate Distribution (*Sum of 15d (1), (2), (3) and (4)*)		▲	74	57
f. Total Distribution (*Sum of 15c and 15e*)		▲	1150	1076
g. Copies not Distributed (*See instructions to publishers #4 (page #3)*)		▲	685	674
h. Total (*Sum of 15f and g*)		▲	1835	1750
i. Percent Paid (15c divided by 15f times 100)			93.57%	94.70%

16. Publication of Statement of Ownership

□ If the publication is a general publication, publication of this statement is required. Will be printed in the **October 2010** issue of this publication. □ Publication not required

17. Signature and Title of Editor, Publisher, Business Manager, or Owner	Date
Stephen R. Bushing	September 15, 2010
Stephen R. Bushing – Fulfillment/Inventory Specialist	

I certify that all information furnished on this form is true and complete. I understand that anyone who furnishes false or misleading information on this form or who omits material or information requested on the form may be subject to criminal sanctions (including fines and imprisonment) and/or civil sanctions (including civil penalties).

PS Form **3526**, September 2007 (Page 2 of 3)

Moving?

Make sure your subscription moves with you!

To notify us of your new address, find your **Clinics Account Number** (located on your mailing label above your name), and contact customer service at:

Email: journalscustomerservice-usa@elsevier.com

800-654-2452 (subscribers in the U.S. & Canada)
314-447-8871 (subscribers outside of the U.S. & Canada)

Fax number: 314-447-8029

Elsevier Health Sciences Division
Subscription Customer Service
3251 Riverport Lane
Maryland Heights, MO 63043

*To ensure uninterrupted delivery of your subscription, please notify us at least 4 weeks in advance of move.

ELSEVIER

Portland Community College